Clinical Microbiology for the General Dentist

Editors

ARVIND BABU RAJENDRA SANTOSH
ORRETT E. OGLE

DENTAL CLINICS OF NORTH AMERICA

www.dental.theclinics.com

April 2017 • Volume 61 • Number 2

ELSEVIER

1600 John F. Kennedy Boulevard • Suite 1800 • Philadelphia, Pennsylvania, 19103-2899

http://www.dental.theclinics.com

DENTAL CLINICS OF NORTH AMERICA Volume 61, Number 2
April 2017 ISSN 0011-8532, ISBN: 978-0-323-52402-5

Editor: John Vassallo; j.vassallo@elsevier.com
Developmental Editor: Kristen Helm

Dental Clinics of North America (ISSN 0011-8532) is published quarterly by Elsevier Inc., 360 Park Avenue South, New York, NY 10010-1710. Months of issue are January, April, July, and October. Business and Editorial Offices: 1600 John F. Kennedy Boulevard, Suite 1800, Philadelphia, PA 19103-2899. Periodicals postage paid at New York, NY and additional mailing offices. Subscription prices are $288.00 per year (domestic individuals), $569.00 per year (domestic institutions), $100.00 per year (domestic students/residents), $350.00 per year (Canadian individuals), $737.00 per year (Canadian institutions), $422.00 per year (international individuals), $737.00 per year (international institutions), and $200.00 per year (international and Canadian students/residents). International air speed delivery is included in all *Clinics* subscription prices. All prices are subject to change without notice. **POSTMASTER:** Send address changes to *Dental Clinics of North America*, Elsevier Health Sciences Division, Subscription Customer Service, 3251 Riverport Lane, Maryland Heights, MO 63043. **Customer Service (orders, claims, online, change of address): Elsevier Health Sciences Division, Subscription Customer Service, 3251 Riverport Lane, Maryland Heights, MO 63043. Tel: 1-800-654-2452 (U.S. and Canada). Fax: 314-447-8029. E-mail: journalscustomer service-usa@elsevier.com (for print support); journalsonlinesupport-usa@elsevier.com (for online support).**

Reprints. For copies of 100 or more, of articles in this publication, please contact the Commercial Reprints Department, Elsevier Inc., 360 Park Avenue South, New York, NY 10010-1710. Tel.: 212-633-3874; Fax: 212-633-3820; E-mail: reprints@elsevier.com.

The Dental Clinics of North America is covered in *MEDLINE/PubMed (Index Medicus), Current Contents/Clinical Medicine, ISI/BIOMED* and *Clinahl.*

Contributors

EDITORS

ARVIND BABU RAJENDRA SANTOSH, BDS, MDS
Lecturer and Research Coordinator, Dentistry Program, Faculty of Medical Sciences, The University of the West Indies, Mona, Kingston, Jamaica, West Indies

ORRETT E. OGLE, DDS
Oral and Maxillofacial Surgeon, Atlanta, Georgia; Former Chief and Director of Residency Training Program, Oral and Maxillofacial Surgery, Woodhull Hospital, Brooklyn, New York; Visiting Lecturer, Dental Program, The University of the West Indies, Kingston, Jamaica, West Indies; Douglasville, Georgia

AUTHORS

SAIF ABDULATEEF, DMD
Chief Resident, Department of Oral and Maxillofacial Surgery, Woodhull Medical Center, Brooklyn, New York

CARL M. ALLEN, DDS, MS
Professor, Division of Oral and Maxillofacial Pathology and Radiology, College of Dentistry, The Ohio State University, Columbus, Ohio

IMANI H. ASHER, DDS
Chief Resident, Department of Oral and Maxillofacial Surgery, University Health Oral and Maxillofacial Surgery Clinic, Kansas City, Missouri

SCOTT BARBER, DDS
Attending Physician, Department of Oral and Maxillofacial Surgery, University Health Oral and Maxillofacial Surgery Clinic, Kansas City, Missouri

EARL CLARKSON, DDS
Program Director, Department of Oral and Maxillofacial Surgery, Woodhull Medical Center, NYU Langone, Brooklyn, New York

HARRY DYM, DDS
Program Director and Chair, Department of Dentistry and Oral Maxillofacial Surgery, The Brooklyn Hospital Center, Brooklyn, New York

BRETT L. FERGUSON, DDS
Chairman of Oral and Maxillofacial Surgery Residency Program, University of Missouri-Kansas City, Oral and Maxillofacial Surgery, Head and Neck Clinic, University Health, Chairman of Hospital Dentistry, Truman Medical Center, Vice President, American Association of Oral and Maxillofacial Surgery, Kansas City, Missouri

LESLIE R. HALPERN, DDS, MD, PhD, MPH
Associate Professor, Program Director, Residency Program, Oral and Maxillofacial Surgery, Meharry Medical College, Nashville, Tennessee

JOHN D. HARVEY, DDS, MS
Department of Anatomy, Howard University, Washington, DC; Formerly, Assistant Professor and Chairman, Department of Periodontics, Meharry Medical College, Nashville, Tennessee

NIRAJ KARKI, MD
Infectious Diseases, Internal Medicine, Clinical Assistant Professor, University of New England College of Osteopathic Medicine, Biddeford, Maine; Infectious Diseases, The Aroostook Medical Center, Presque Isle, Maine

TARUN KIRPALANI, DDS
Resident, Department of Oral and Maxillofacial Surgery, The Brooklyn Hospital Center, Brooklyn, New York

SUSAN MAHABADY, MS
PhD Candidate, Division of Periodontology, Diagnostic Sciences and Dental Hygiene, USC Center for Biofilms, Ostrow School of Dentistry, University of Southern California, Los Angeles, Los Angeles, California

MICHAEL W. MARSHALL, DDS, FICD, FACD
Oral & Maxillofacial Surgery, Private Practice: Huntington Beach Oral & Maxillofacial Surgery, Huntington Beach, California; Long Beach Memorial Medical Center, Long Beach, California; Oral & Maxillofacial Surgery, Assistant Clinical Professor, Division of Otolaryngology, University of California, Irvine School of Medicine, Orange, California

FATIMA MASHKOOR, DDS
Chief Resident, Department of Oral and Maxillofacial Surgery, Woodhull Medical Center, Brooklyn, New York

VICTOR H. MATSUBARA, PhD, DDS, MSc
School of Dentistry, University of São Paulo, São Paulo, Brazil

CHARLES MOUTON, MD, MS
Professor, Department of Family and Community Medicine, Meharry Medical College, School of Medicine, Nashville, Tennessee

ALISON NICHOLSON, MBBS, DM (Medical Microbiology)
Consultant Medical Microbiologist, Director, Department of Microbiology, The University of the West Indies, Mona, Kingston, Jamaica, West Indies

ORRETT E. OGLE, DDS
Oral and Maxillofacial Surgeon, Atlanta, Georgia; Former Chief and Director of Residency Training Program, Oral and Maxillofacial Surgery, Woodhull Hospital, Brooklyn, New York; Visiting Lecturer, Dental Program, The University of the West Indies, Kingston, Jamaica, West Indies; Douglasville, Georgia

ARVIND BABU RAJENDRA SANTOSH, BDS, MDS
Lecturer and Research Coordinator, Dentistry Program, Faculty of Medical Sciences, The University of the West Indies, Mona, Kingston, Jamaica, West Indies

THOMAS E. RAMS, DDS, MHS, PhD
Professor, Department of Periodontology and Oral Implantology; Director, Oral
Microbiology Testing Service Laboratory, Temple University School of Dentistry,
Department of Microbiology and Immunology, Temple University School of Medicine,
Philadelphia, Pennsylvania

BADDAM VENKAT RAMANA REDDY, MDS
Professor and Head, Department of Oral and Maxillofacial Pathology, SIBAR Institute of
Dental Sciences, Guntur, Andhra Pradesh, India

**GLENDEE REYNOLDS-CAMPBELL, BSc(Hons), BMedSc, MBBS, DM
(Medical Microbiology)**
Consultant Medical Microbiologist, Department of Microbiology, The University of the
West Indies, Mona, Kingston, Jamaica, West Indies

MIRIAM R. ROBBINS, DDS, MS
Chair, Department of Dental Medicine, Winthrop University Hospital, Mineola, New York;
Clinical Associate Professor, Department of Oral and Maxillofacial Pathology, Radiology
and Medicine, New York University College of Dentistry, New York, New York

LAKSHMAN SAMARANAYAKE, DSc, DDS, FRCPath, FDSRCS, FDSRCPS, FRACDS
Professor Emeritus, Faculty of Dentistry, University of Hong Kong, Hong Kong, China;
Honorary Professor, University of Queensland, Brisbane, Australia; Professor of
Bioclinical Sciences, Kuwait University, Kuwait

FRANCESCO R. SEBASTIANI, DMD
Resident, Department of Oral and Maxillofacial Surgery, The Brooklyn Hospital Center,
Brooklyn, New York

PARISH P. SEDGHIZADEH, DDS, MS
Assistant Professor, Director, USC Center for Biofilms, Division of Periodontology,
Diagnostic Sciences and Dental Hygiene, Ostrow School of Dentistry, University of
Southern California, Los Angeles, Los Angeles, California

DAVID R. TELLES, DDS
Assistant Clinical Professor, Oral & Maxillofacial Surgery, Herman Ostrow USC School
of Dentistry, Los Angeles, California; Oral & Maxillofacial Surgery, Private Practice:
Huntington Beach Oral & Maxillofacial Surgery, Huntington Beach, California; Long Beach
Memorial Medical Center, Long Beach, California; Fountain Valley, California; Orange
Coast Memorial Medical Center, Orange County Global Medical Center, Santa Ana,
California

CAMILLE-ANN THOMS-RODRIGUEZ, BMedSc, MBBS, DM (Medical Microbiology)
Consultant Medical Microbiologist, Department of Microbiology, The University of the
West Indies, Mona, Kingston, Jamaica, West Indies

ARIE J. VAN WINKELHOFF, PhD
Professor, Center for Dentistry and Oral Hygiene; Department of Medical Microbiology,
University Medical Center Groningen, Faculty of Medical Sciences, University of
Groningen, Groningen, The Netherlands

DWIGHT WILLIAMS, DDS
Attending Surgeon, Oral and Maxillofacial Surgery, Woodhull Hospital, Brooklyn,
New York

CHALMERS R. WOOD, DDS
Chief Resident, Department of Oral and Maxillofacial Surgery, University Health Oral and Maxillofacial Surgery Clinic, Kansas City, Missouri

EDWARD F. WOODBINE, DDS
Department of Dentistry/Oral and Maxillofacial Surgery, Woodhull Medical Center, Brooklyn, New York

JOSEPH ZEIDAN, DMD
Resident, Department of Oral and Maxillofacial Surgery, The Brooklyn Hospital Center, Brooklyn, New York

Contents

Clinical oral microbiology may help dental professionals identify infecting pathogenic species and evaluate their in vitro antimicrobial susceptibility. Saliva, dental plaque biofilms, mucosal smears, abscess aspirates, and soft tissue biopsies are sources of microorganisms for laboratory testing. Microbial-based treatment end points may help clinicians better identify patients in need of additional or altered dental therapies before the onset of clinical treatment failure, and help improve patient oral health outcomes. Microbiological testing appears particularly helpful in periodontal disease treatment planning. Further research and technological advances are likely to increase the availability and clinical utility of microbiological analysis in modern dental practice.

The oral ecosystem comprises the oral flora, so-called oral microbiome, the different anatomic microniches of the oral cavity, and its bathing fluid, saliva. The oral microbiome comprises a group of organisms and includes bacteria, archaea, fungi, protozoa, and viruses. The oral microbiome exists suspended in saliva as planktonic phase organisms or attached to oral surfaces as a plaque biofilm. Homeostasis of the plaque biofilm and its symbiotic relationship with the host is critical for oral health. Disequilibrium or dysbiosis within the plaque biofilms is the initiating event that leads to major oral diseases, such as caries and periodontal disease.

Dental caries and periodontal disease are the most common dental infections and are constantly increasing worldwide. Distribution, occurrence of dental caries, gingivitis, periodontitis, odontogenic infections, antibiotic resistance, oral mucosal infections, and microbe-related oral cancer are important to understand the public impact and methods of controlling such disease. Distribution of human papilloma virus and human immunodeficiency virus -related oral cancers in the US population is presented.

The pathogenesis of odontogenic infection is polymicrobial, consisting of various facultative and strict anaerobes. The dominant isolates are strictly anaerobic gram-negative rods and gram-positive cocci. The periapical infection is the most common form of odontogenic infection. Although odontogenic infections are usually confined to the alveolar ridge vicinity, they can spread into deep fascial spaces. Cavernous sinus thrombosis, brain abscess, airway obstruction, and mediastinitis are possible complications of dental infections. The most important element in treating odontogenic infections is elimination of the primary source of the infection with antibiotics as adjunctive therapy.

This article provides a review of current information about periodontal bacteria, their activities within dental plaque biofilm, their interactions with the host immune system, and the infections with which they are associated. Periodontal disease, plaque formation, and the host immune response are also discussed, as are antimicrobial measures used to control the bacteria and the disease.

Osteomyelitis is an inflammation of bone marrow with a tendency for progression, involving the cortical plates and often periosteal tissues, with most cases occurring after trauma to bone or bone surgery or secondary to vascular insufficiency. Antimicrobial therapy and surgical débridement are the primary modalities of osteomyelitis treatment, although often it is associated with a prolonged course, requiring a large commitment between patient and clinician as well as sizable health care costs. Despite surgical and chemotherapeutic advancements, osteomyelitis remains difficult to treat, and no universally accepted protocol for treatment exists.

Oral mucosal infections appear as localized or generalized lesions. Symptoms range from almost unnoticeable lesions to severe pain. Systemic disease, age, immunocompromised condition, and medication use are common causes. Local causes include dentures, poor oral hygiene, traumatized epithelium, ulcerations, dentures, implants, oral piercing, and reduced salivary secretion. Oral mucosal infections are underdiagnosed and microbiological diagnosis should be more frequently used. Candidiasis is most frequently diagnosed. Clinical appearances are not always clear and are varied, creating a diagnostic challenge. Thorough understanding of clinical appearance and updated information on diagnostic and therapeutic management are essential for successful patient outcome.

The human oral cavity contains more than 500 different bacterial species. These organisms belong to several phyla including Bacteroidetes,

Firmicutes, Tenericutes, Actinobacteria, Proteobacteria, Euryarchaeota, Chlamydiae, and Spirochaetes. Many of these have the ability to colonize the gingival crevices and the outer surface of the tooth forming biofilms often leading to dental plaque formation. These bacteria produce acid that erode teeth causing cavities or infections. The diagnosis of these infections is often clinical and antibiotics are used empirically to treat some infections or as prophylaxis. The characterization, definitive diagnosis, and susceptibility testing of oral bacterial infections are valuable in guiding appropriate therapy and in prevention of disease.

Oral and maxillofacial fungal infections can appear in high-risk patients, including those immunocompromised. This article explores common oral manifestations of fungal infections in the oral cavity as primary lesions or as a result of disseminated disease. By far the most common oral fungal infection experienced in dentistry is oral candidiasis, which is reviewed in depth from simple oral infections to invasive candidiasis. The review aids the dental practitioner in understanding the full scope of *Candida* infections and other fungal infections. In addition to candidiasis, various other fungal infections are reviewed, including mucormycosis, aspergillosis, blastomycosis, histoplasmosis, cryptococcosis, and coccidioidomycosis.

This article focuses on common viral infections in the oral cavity with associated systemic manifestations. Discussed are the clinical features, histopathology, diagnosis, treatment, and prevention of viral infections in oral cavity. This will be a useful aid for general practitioners and other dental personnel wanting to expand their pathologic knowledge. This article discusses herpes simplex, varicella zoster, mononucleosis, cytomegalovirus, enteroviruses, rubeola, rubella, mumps, and human papillomavirus. After reviewing this topic, the dentist or hygienist will minimally be competent to diagnose the appropriate oral cavity viral infectious diseases and help patients get the appropriate care they need.

Human immunodeficiency virus (HIV) infection has become a chronic condition. HIV is not a valid reason to deny, delay, or withhold dental treatment. There are no absolute contraindications and few complications associated with comprehensive oral health care treatment delivered in an outpatient setting for asymptomatic HIV-infected patients and clinically stable patients with AIDS. Consultation with the patient's medical provider and modifications in the delivery of dental treatment may be necessary when treating patients with advanced HIV disease or other comorbid conditions. Oral health care is an integral and important part of comprehensive health care for all patients with HIV/AIDS.

An opportunistic infection (OI) is a disease of microbial cause or pathogenesis generally thought to occur in hosts with weakened immunity. Oral OIs are associated with many risk factors and pathogens. Causative organisms for oral OIs have unique modes of transmission. The clinical presentation of oral OIs is heterogeneous and diagnosis can be challenging. Therefore, laboratory identification of causative pathogens is useful for definitive diagnosis and targeted therapeutics, and can be achieved by biological, serologic, histologic, and/or molecular methods. Clinical risk assessment and history with review of systems, and accurate diagnosis, treatment, and follow-up, are essential.

Oral health care professionals are at risk for the transmission of bacterial and viral microorganisms. Providers need to be knowledgeable about the exposure/transmission of life-threatening infections and options for prevention. This article is designed to increase the oral health care provider's awareness of the latest assessment of vaccine-preventable diseases that pose a high risk in the dental health care setting. Specific dosing strategies are suggested for the prevention of infections based on available evidence and epidemiologic changes. This information will provide a clear understanding for prevention of vaccine-preventable diseases that pose a public health consequence.

The role of bacterial and viral carcinogenesis in the oral cavity is increasingly of interest, as a means to provide more methods of cancer prevention. There may be relationships between bacteria and multiple strains of viruses in the progression of malignancy. Cancer cause is closely related to the type of carcinogen, as well as the synergistic or additive actions of combined risk factors, the susceptibility of the host, and duration of interaction between host and exposure to risk factor. Much research is underway to further define the role of microbial and bacterial agents in the progression of malignancy.

The goal of an infection control program is to provide a safe working environment for dental health care personnel and their patients. Practitioners can achieve this by adopting measures that reduce health care–associated infections among patients and occupational exposures among dental health care personnel. It is crucial for all dental practitioners to be up to date on current Centers for Disease Control and Prevention guidelines, equipment, and techniques for proper infection control. Continuous evaluation of infection control practices is important. Patients and dental providers should be confident that oral health care can be delivered and received in a safe manner.

DENTAL CLINICS OF NORTH AMERICA

FORTHCOMING ISSUES

July 2017
Evidence-based Pediatric Dentistry
Donald L. Chi, *Editor*

October 2017
Dental Biomaterials
Jack Ferracane, Luiz E. Bertassoni, and
Carmem S. Pfeifer, *Editors*

January 2018
Dental Public Health
Michelle Henshaw and Astha Singhal,
Editors

RECENT ISSUES

January 2017
Endodontics: Clinical and Scientific Updates
Mo K. Kang, *Editor*

October 2016
**Impact of Oral Health on Interprofessional
Collaborative Practice**
Linda M. Kaste and Leslie R. Halpern,
Editors

July 2016
Special Care Dentistry
Burton S. Wasserman, *Editor*

ISSUE OF RELATED INTEREST

Oral and Maxillofacial Surgery Clinics of North America
February 2017 (Vol. 29, No. 1)
Emerging Biomaterials and Techniques in Tissue Regeneration
Alan S. Herford, *Editor*
Available at: www.oralmaxsurgery.theclinics.com

THE CLINICS ARE AVAILABLE ONLINE!
Access your subscription at:
www.theclinics.com

Erratum

In the April 2016 issue (Volume 60, number 2), in the article, "Updates of Topical and Local Anesthesia Agents," co-authored by Ricardo A. Boyce, Tarun Kirpalani, and Naveen Mohan, the following corrections should be noted:

In Table 2 on page 452, in the "Lidocaine" section under the "Vasoconstrictor" column, the MRD in the first row should be 4.5 mg/kg, instead of 4.4 kg. Also the MRD value for both "Epi (1:100,000)" should be 7.0 mg/kg. The section of the revised table:

Drug	LA (%)	Vasoconstrictor	Duration	MRD
1. Lidocaine	2	None *short acting*	Pulpal = 5–10 min Soft Tissue = 1–2 h	4.5 mg/kg 2.0/lb Max = 300
		Epi (1:50,000) for *hemostasis*	Pulpal = 1.0–1.5 h Soft tissue = 3–5 h	7.0 mg/kg 2.0/lb Max = 300
		Epi (1:100,000)	Pulpal = 1.0–1.5 h Soft tissue = 3–5 h	7.0 mg/kg 2.0/lb Max = 300

2. In Table 3 on page 453, under the "Facts" column in the "Lidocaine" section, please note:
   - pH (with epi) = 3.5
   - pKa = 7.9
   - Onset = 3–5 min
3. In Table 3 on page 453, under the "Facts" column in the "Mepivacaine" section, please note:
   - pH (plain solution) = 6.0–6.5
   - Onset = 3–5 min
4. In Table 3 on page 454, under the "Facts" column in the "Articaine" section, please note:
   - pH (with epi) = 3.5–4.0

Preface

Clinical Microbiology for the General Dentist

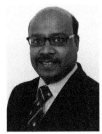
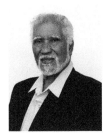

Arvind Babu Rajendra Santosh, BDS, MDS   Orrett E. Ogle, DDS

Editors

As early as 5000 BC, the Sumerians described a "tooth worm" as the cause of dental caries, and this belief lasted for over 6000 years until the mid-1700s. During the 1800s, it was clearly established that dental caries and periodontal disease, the two major dental diseases, were both due to microorganisms. Today, modern research has correlated the oral microbiota from poor oral health with the ability of this oral microbiota to invade the body and affect other organ systems, most significantly, cardiac health. It is evident, therefore, that oral microbiology is the foundation for modern dentistry, and in fact, dentistry, more than any other health care profession, exists primarily because of the effects of microbes.

With the excitement over new composites, ceramics, other nanomaterials, cosmetic dentistry, cosmetic oral surgical procedures, and dental implants, we may have forgotten the genesis of our profession. However, it is very important to be reminded that microorganisms still play a big role in multiple oral diseases.

Clinical microbiology is defined as a branch of science dealing with the interrelation of macroorganisms and microorganisms with their host under normal and pathological conditions along with the dynamics of the infectious process with the aim of arriving at a complete cure through the appropriate use of various antibiotics to inhibit or kill the isolated microorganisms.

Evidently, the above-said definition indicates that the duties of clinical microbiologists are to assist the physician and dentist in diagnosing pathological conditions and guiding in the treatment of microbial diseases. To further advance these goals, these professionals conduct research on the pathogenesis, mechanism of action of antibiotics, and other immunological preparations (such as vaccine) and culture methods to diagnose the pathogenic organism involved in disease process. Advancements in the field of microbiology allow these professionals to render state-of-the-art

Dent Clin N Am 61 (2017) xv–xvii
http://dx.doi.org/10.1016/j.cden.2017.01.001
dental.theclinics.com

blood culture methods and rapid development in diagnostic methods that help them to support the clinician in rapid and appropriate antibiotic de-escalation.

Considering the scope of clinical microbiology and advancements in diagnostic methods, this issue was proposed and developed to emphasize the clinical microbiology aspects in dentistry. General dentists need to have a good understanding of microbial involvement in dental and/or oral infections and their susceptibility and/or resistance to antimicrobial agents.

We believe that this issue of the *Dental Clinics of North America* should serve as a useful reference on oral microbiology. The topics cover the full gamut of oral infections, along with some basic laboratory microbiology.

We are very thankful to all the authors who took the time to contribute to this issue of *Dental Clinics of North America*. We cannot express our gratitude to each of the esteemed authors in enough words here as to how pleased we are with their submissions to this issue that should now serve as an effective reference on the clinical microbiology aspects for all dentists, without whose contribution it is doubtful that readers of *Dental Clinics of North America* would now be holding this issue in their hand. We are also extremely thankful and honored from the support received from the editorial staff of the *Dental Clinics of North America*. We are extremely pleased for the opportunity and support from Mr John Vassallo, Editor, and Ms Kristen Helm, Developmental Editor, at Elsevier from the beginning of this project to the successful publishing of this issue.

ACKNOWLEDGMENTS

From Dr Santosh: I am deeply grateful to the following individuals who motivated, supported, and guided me in my life and professional path:

Prof Naresh Lingaraju, past Head of Oral Medicine and Radiology, Farooqia Dental College and Hospital, Mysuru, Karnataka, India. Prof Kumaraswamy KL, Oral and Maxillofacial Pathology, Farooqia Dental College and Hospital, Mysuru, Karnataka, India. Prof Ramana Reddy BV, Head of Oral and Maxillofacial Pathology, SIBAR Institute of Dental Sciences, Andhra Pradesh, India. Prof Ratheesh Kumar Nandan, Head of Oral and Maxillofacial Pathology, Kamineni Institute of Dental Sciences, Telangana, India.

I am very appreciative of the ongoing support of the coeditor, Dr Orrett Ogle, immediate past Chief of Oral and Maxillofacial Surgery, Woodhull Medical Center, Brooklyn, NY, without whose guidance from the initiation of this project along every single step to reach the final stage of bringing out this issue would have been challenging. My sincere thanks and respect for his dedication and deserved grateful recognition for his indispensable help.

My sincere thanks to the following officials of my current institution, The University of the West Indies, Jamaica, for their unflinching support and for allowing me to take valuable time in editing this issue: Prof Archibald McDonald, Principal, The University of the West Indies, Jamaica; Prof Horace Fletcher, Dean; Prof John Lindo, Deputy Dean, Research, Faculty of Medical Sciences; Prof Russell Pierre, MBBS Programme Director; Dr Thaon Jones, Dentistry Programme Director; and Dr Christine Cummings, Faculty of Social Sciences, The University of the West Indies, Jamaica.

Finally, I owe a huge debt to my parents, sister, wife, Ramyaa, and my son, Ryaan, for their patience and support during this project.

From Dr Ogle: As coeditor, it was my pleasure working on this issue of *Dental Clinics of North America*. Thanks to my wife, children, and grandchildren, from whom I took valuable time. Also, thanks to my patients, residents, and students from whom I have learned and gained invaluable experience over the last 40-plus years.

Arvind Babu Rajendra Santosh, BDS, MDS
Dentistry Program
Faculty of Medical Sciences
The University of the West Indies
Mona, Kingston-7
Jamaica, West Indies

Orrett E. Ogle, DDS
Atlanta, GA, USA

Residency Training Program
Oral and Maxillofacial Surgery
Woodhull Hospital
Brooklyn, NY 11206, USA

Dental Program
The University of the West Indies
Kingston, Jamaica, West Indies

4974 Golf Valley Court
Douglasville, GA 30135, USA

E-mail addresses:
arvindbabu2001@gmail.com (A.B. R. Santosh)
oeogle@aol.com (O.E. Ogle)

Introduction to Clinical Microbiology for the General Dentist

Thomas E. Rams, DDS, MHS, PhD[a,b],*, Arie J. van Winkelhoff, PhD[c,d]

KEYWORDS

- Oral microbiology • Clinical microbiology technology
- Antimicrobial susceptibility testing • Microbial risk assessment
- Microbiological testing

KEY POINTS

- Many oral diseases have a microbial cause that can be characterized and monitored by microbiological testing.
- Clinical oral microbiology helps identify infecting pathogenic agents in oral infections and evaluate their in vitro antimicrobial susceptibility.
- Microbiological analysis supplementing conventional diagnostic procedures may aid dental professionals in clinical decision making and selection of the most appropriate treatment of individual dental patients.
- Microbial-based dental care end points may help reduce clinical treatment failures and improve patient oral health outcomes.
- Recent technological advances in clinical oral microbiology are increasing its utility and value to dental professionals.

Disclosures: T.E. Rams has nothing to disclose. A.J. van Winkelhoff is a co-owner of LabOral Diagnostics, LabOral International, and BlueClinics, which provide clinical microbiology services for dental professionals.
[a] Department of Periodontology and Oral Implantology, Oral Microbiology Testing Service Laboratory, Temple University School of Dentistry, 3223 North Broad Street, Philadelphia, PA 19140, USA; [b] Department of Microbiology and Immunology, Temple University School of Medicine, 3500 North Broad Street, Philadelphia, PA 19140, USA; [c] Center for Dentistry and Oral Hygiene, University Medical Center Groningen, Faculty of Medical Sciences, University of Groningen, Antonius Deusinglaan 1, Groningen 9713 AV, The Netherlands; [d] Department of Medical Microbiology, University Medical Center Groningen, Faculty of Medical Sciences, University of Groningen, Hanzeplein 1, Groningen GZ 9713, The Netherlands
* Corresponding author. Department of Periodontology and Oral Implantology, Temple University School of Dentistry, 3223 North Broad Street, Philadelphia, PA 19140.
E-mail address: trams@temple.edu

Dent Clin N Am 61 (2017) 179–197
http://dx.doi.org/10.1016/j.cden.2016.11.001
0011-8532/17/© 2016 Elsevier Inc. All rights reserved.

dental.theclinics.com

INTRODUCTION

Major diseases that dental professionals treat daily in clinical practice are primarily of microbial cause and include dental caries, periodontitis, and odontogenic infections. However, in contrast with management of infectious diseases in medicine, there seems to be at present little use of clinical microbiology laboratory testing in the diagnostic assessment and care of dental patients. Treatment of most dental diseases remains largely focused on provision of mechanical-surgical debridement and/or drainage of lesions, with adjunctive local and/or systemic broad-spectrum antimicrobial drug therapy potentially used and empirically selected by the treating clinician without microbiological testing. Although effective in many patients, this mechanical-surgical treatment model may be inadequate in addressing certain types of oral infections, resulting in clinical therapeutic failures. This article provides an overview of the present status of clinical microbiology in dentistry, and how it may be used by dental professionals to better optimize selection of therapy and potentially improve patient oral health care outcomes, with emphasis on management of chronic periodontitis.

ORAL DISEASES OF INFECTIOUS ORIGIN

A wide range of disorders may occur in the human oral cavity from the effects of microbial infections, developmental defects, adverse host immunologic-autoimmune reactions, and growth of different types of benign tumors and cancer. Details on bacterial, viral, and fungal infections in the oral cavity are provided in other articles of this issue, but are summarized for the following oral diseases (**Table 1**).

Dental caries is a multifactorial process driven by acidogenic and acid-tolerant bacterial species fermenting dietary carbohydrates, particularly sucrose, which leads to lowered dental plaque biofilm pH levels and demineralization/cavitation of susceptible tooth surfaces.[1] In United States population-based surveys conducted in 2011 to 2012, 91% of adults aged 20 to 64 years showed evidence of dental caries in permanent teeth, with 27% yielding untreated carious lesions.[2] Among those greater than or equal to 65 years of age, 19% were fully edentulous,[2] mainly as a result of untreated and progressive dental caries.[3] Similar or greater levels of dental caries are found worldwide in various countries and population groups.[4]

High levels of streptococci (in particular *Streptococcus mutans* and *Streptococcus sobrinus*), lactobacilli, Bifidobacteriaceae species, *Scardovia wiggsiae*, and other organic acid-producing bacteria in dental plaque biofilms confer an increased risk for coronal dental caries on smooth tooth surfaces and in occlusal pit and fissures.[5] A similar array of species plus proteolytic/amino acid–degrading bacteria contribute to the development of root surface caries.[6]

Chronic periodontitis is another prevalent oral disease in the United States. Nearly 50% of dentate adults aged 30 years or older, representing 64.7 million people, were estimated to have periodontitis in United States 2009 to 2012 national surveys, with 8.9% revealing severe chronic periodontitis,[7] which is in a similar range to other countries and population groups throughout the world.[8] Risk factors known to modulate expression of chronic periodontitis include subgingival colonization by microbial pathogens; male gender; African American (black) and Hispanic racial identification; smoking; obesity; poor coping with psychosocial stress; certain genetic polymorphisms; poorly controlled diabetes mellitus; and nutritional deficiencies in calcium, vitamin D, and vitamin C.[9]

Several anaerobic bacterial species are frequently increased in the subgingival microbiome of untreated chronic periodontitis, including *Porphyromonas gingivalis*,

Table 1
Microorganisms associated with selected oral diseases

Oral Disease	Gram-Positive Aerobic or Facultative Bacteria	Gram-Positive Anaerobic Bacteria	Gram-Negative Aerobic or Facultative Bacteria	Gram-Negative Anaerobic Bacteria	Herpesvirus	Yeasts
Dental caries	++	—	—	—	—	—
Chronic periodontitis	+	++	+	++	+	—
Aggressive periodontitis (localized)	—	+	++	+	+	—
Aggressive periodontitis (generalized)	+	++	++	++	+	—
Refractory periodontitis	+	++	++	++	+	+
Periimplantitis	+	++	+	++	+	—
Endodontic infection (primary)	++	+	++	++	+	—
Endodontic infection (refractory)	++	+	+	+	—	+
Infective stomatitis	++	+	++	+	++	++
Halitosis	—	+	+	++	—	—

Symbols: ++, usually prominent; +, may be prominent; —, absent or uncommonly prominent.

Tannerella forsythia, Treponema denticola, Prevotella intermedia, Parvimonas micra, Fusobacterium nucleatum, Selenomonas noxia, Selenomonas sputigena, Eubacterium nodatum, Campylobacter rectus, Filifactor alocis, Fretibacterium fastidiosum, and *Dialister pneumosintes.*[5,10] Several uncultivated bacterial phylotypes identified only by their 16S ribosomal RNA (rRNA) gene sequences[10]; certain herpesviruses, including Epstein-Barr virus and cytomegalovirus[11]; and the nonbacterial Archaea species *Methanobrevibacter oralis*[12] have also been associated with chronic periodontitis lesions. Longitudinal studies have shown the clinical onset and early progression of chronic periodontitis to be related to subgingival colonization by spirochetes, *P gingivalis, T forsythia, T denticola, S noxia, C rectus,* and the gram-negative capnophilic coccobacillus *Aggregatibacter actinomycetemcomitans.*[13–18] In contrast, these species are in only low abundance or not detected in the core subgingival microbiome of periodontally healthy sites, which is instead dominated by various *Actinomyces, Rothia, Streptococcus,* and *Burkholderia* species.[19]

Localized aggressive periodontitis, with its characteristic molar-incisor interproximal pattern of periodontal attachment loss and crestal alveolar bone resorption, is found less frequently than chronic periodontitis. It is uncommon in the United States, with an estimated prevalence of 0.53% in teenagers 14 to 17 years old,[20] but is more prevalent in Africa and populations of African descent.[21]

A actinomycetemcomitans, particularly strains belonging to the highly leukotoxic JP2 clone, has been strongly associated since the mid-1970s with the onset and progression of localized aggressive periodontitis.[22] A prospective study found that oral carriage of the *A actinomycetemcomitans* JP2 clone in periodontally healthy adolescents of West African or North African descent rendered an 18 times greater risk of onset of localized aggressive periodontitis over a 2-year period.[23] More recently, *F alocis*[24] and selected herpesviruses[11] have additionally been implicated in the pathogenesis of localized aggressive periodontitis.

Generalized aggressive periodontitis, which is estimated to occur in 0.13% of United States teenagers 14 to 17 years old,[20] is associated with subgingival *A actinomycetemcomitans* plus many high-abundance putative bacterial pathogens found in patients with moderate to severe chronic periodontitis.[25]

Refractory periodontitis occurs in a subset of treated patients with periodontitis who have marked progressive periodontal attachment loss during posttreatment time periods despite institution of meticulous patient home plaque control, thorough subgingival root debridement (with or without access flap surgery), periodontal maintenance care at regular short intervals, and administration of local and/or systemic antimicrobial chemotherapy. Microbiological analysis of patients with chronic periodontitis with widespread progressive periodontal attachment loss following modified Widman flap surgery and systemic amoxicillin-metronidazole drug therapy revealed subgingival persistence of increased numbers of *P gingivalis, T forsythia, F alocis, P micra, Prevotella* species, *Eubacterium* species, *Dialister* species, *Selenomonas* species, *Catonella morbi,* and *Streptococcus intermedius/Streptococcus constellatus,* as well as several uncultivated/unrecognized bacterial phylotypes.[26] Rams and colleagues[27] reported a 2.5 relative risk for recurrent periodontal breakdown within 12 months in patients with treated chronic periodontitis yielding at posttreatment increased subgingival proportions of 1 or more species among *P gingivalis, P intermedia, P micra, C rectus,* and/ or *A actinomycetemcomitans.* Patients with refractory periodontitis may also develop subgingival colonization by opportunistic medical pathogens not commonly associated with periodontitis lesions, including *Escherichia coli; Pseudomonas aeruginosa;* other Enterobacteriaceae, Pseudomonadaceae, and *Acinetobacter* species; *Staphylococcus aureus;* and various *Candida* species.[28–30]

Periimplantitis is an inflammatory lesion around dental implants that induces progressive destruction of periimplant soft tissues and supporting alveolar bone, resulting in increased periimplant probing depths, loss of crestal alveolar bone height, and ultimately loss of the dental implant from the oral cavity.[31] The cause of human periimplantitis is controversial and not well understood at present, but increased submucosal numbers of 5 bacterial species recognized as periodontal pathogens on natural teeth (*P gingivalis*, *T forsythia*, *T denticola*, *P intermedia*, and *C rectus*) have been linked to periimplant breakdown,[32] which supports the concept of a bacterial contribution to periimplantitis.

Untreated infected root canals, with or without symptomatic periradicular lesions, generally yield *Porphyromonas endodontalis*, *Pseudoramibacter alactolyticus*, and many of the major suspected bacterial pathogens associated with chronic periodontitis.[33] In contrast, *Enterococcus faecalis* is most frequently recovered from treated root canals with persistent endodontic lesions,[33] possibly because of the lack of antimicrobial activity against *E faecalis* by the calcium hydroxide pastes used in endodontic therapy to disinfect dentinal tubules,[34] and/or introduction via mastication of viable food-borne *E faecalis* (such as in certain aged cheese products) into root canal spaces by oral fluid leakage adjacent to temporary restorations.[35]

Oral mucosal lesions of infective origin, also known as infective stomatitis, can potentially yield a wide range of infectious agents, including viruses (eg, human papillomavirus, coxsackievirus, various herpesviruses, measles morbillivirus, and mumps paramyxovirus); bacterial pathogens such as various *Actinomyces* species in actinomycosis and bisphosphonate-related osteonecrosis of the jaw, *Neisseria gonorrhoeae*, *Mycobacterium* species, fungi (such as *Candida* in candidiasis), and various parasites.[36–38]

Halitosis, also known as oral malodor, is characterized by an unpleasant, foul, offensive odor of expired air originating from the oral cavity.[39] The dorsoposterior region of the tongue is the main origin of intraoral, physiologic, halitosis. Anaerobic bacteria within dorsum tongue coatings, as part of their metabolic activities, release malodorous volatile sulfur compounds (hydrogen sulfide, methylmercaptan), short-chain fatty acids (butyric acid, propionic acid, valeric acid), and cadaverine into expired air.[40]

Organisms most associated with halitosis include *Solobacterium moorei*, *Fusobacterium periodonticum*, *Eubacterium sulci*, and *Atopobium parvulum*, whereas *Streptococcus salivarius* is most predominant on the tongue of patients without halitosis, and is typically absent from persons with halitosis.[40]

DENTAL CLINIC INFECTION CONTROL

The dental clinic can be a source of infectious risk to patients and dental professionals. In particular, the microbiological quality of water passing through dental unit waterlines has been an ongoing source of concern. High numbers of aerobic heterotrophic microorganisms have been recovered from water originating from dental unit tubing.[41] The inner surface of narrow-diameter waterline tubing in dental units provides a specialized ecologic niche that permits microorganisms normally present in low numbers in municipal tap water to form adherent, growing, multispecies bacterial biofilms, particularly when the water is warmed for patient comfort or allowed to stagnate during overnight and weekend periods of nonuse. These biofilms localize on the inner lumen of narrow waterline tubing, and release bursts of planktonic cells into water expended into the mouth of patients undergoing dental care, and into the dental office operatory environmental atmosphere. Without frequent disinfection, narrow waterline tubing in dental units may rapidly develop internal biofilm growth of bacterial species that are potentially pathogenic in immunocompromised patients, such as *Sphingomonas paucimobilis*, *Acinetobacter calcoaceticus*, *Methylobacterium mesophilicum*, and *P aeruginosa*, within 5 days after installation.[42]

Legionella species, including *Legionella pneumophila*, the causal agent of legionnaires' disease and Pontiac fever, may also be isolated from dental unit water.[43] In one study, 62% of 47 dental operatory waterline samples in Maryland and California tested positive for *Legionella* species before the introduction of daily disinfection procedures.[44] Only limited evidence to date links dental waterline *Legionella* colonization to an increased risk of human disease, most likely because of a general lack of epidemiologic surveillance systems and resources available to track individual *Legionella* infections back to specific dental clinic appointments and waterline sources. However, Ricci and colleagues[45] reported a fatal case of legionnaires' disease likely acquired from dental unit water by an 82-year-old woman during routine dental care, which led to fulminant and irreversible septic shock. Droplet inhalation of aerosolized water from the dental clinic's high-speed turbine instruments was the most likely source and route of the patient's infection. *L pneumophila* serogroup 1 isolates with genetically identical patterns, as detected in amplified fragment length polymorphism typing, were recovered in high numbers from dental unit water serving the high-speed turbine instruments, and from the patient's bronchial aspirates, but not from any of the patient's home water sources.

In addition to this case, occupational workplace exposure to *Legionella* species was suspected in the death of a California dentist from legionnaires' disease in the 1990s, in which the infecting organisms were isolated from the dentist's own dental unit water.[46] Increased serum antibody titers to *Legionella* species have been detected in dental office personnel[47] and dental clinic patient populations[48] compared with general population-based control groups.

For prevention, biannual testing should be performed to examine for *Legionella* species in dental unit water. In addition, only water meeting the United States Environmental Protection Agency regulatory standard threshold for drinking water of less than 500 colony-forming units per milliliter of heterotrophic bacteria should be used in routine dental care procedures.[49]

Proper cleaning and sterilization of dental instruments is also critical to dental professionals and patients in attaining effective infection control in dental practice settings. The American Dental Association recommends that steam autoclaves attain a temperature of 121°C to 124°C at a pressure of 1.1 to 1.25 bar for a minimum of 15 minutes, or reach 134°C to 137°C at 2.1 to 2.3 bar for a minimum of 3 minutes.[50]

Testing of dental office autoclave sterilization efficacy with spore-based biological indicators must be performed on either a weekly or monthly basis in the United States, depending on individual state dental board regulations. A recent survey of dental offices in a region of Mexico found that 17% of 230 autoclaves still yielded positive bacterial growth after testing with biological indicators,[51] which underscores the importance of properly operating autoclaves and frequently testing their efficacy in obtaining sterilization of contaminated dental instruments.

CLINICAL ORAL MICROBIOLOGY IN DENTAL PRACTICE

Oral microorganisms may be sampled and removed from diseased sites or lesions in the oral cavity in specimens of saliva, dental plaque, mucosal smears, and soft tissue biopsies. Methods commercially available to analyze oral microbial samples include microbial culture, various nucleic acid hybridization and amplification procedures, and even direct microscopic examination. How these may be applied in the management of oral infectious diseases is addressed as follows.

DENTAL CARIES

For a microbiologically based assessment of dental caries risk, saliva samples may be readily and noninvasively obtained that contain bacteria originating from a wide array of intraoral soft tissue surfaces and tooth sites. An in-office commercial caries risk assay (Dentocult-SM Strip Mutans; Orion Diagnostica Oy, Finland[52]) uses saliva for detection and quantitation of selected cariogenic species in dental patients. After a patient chews on paraffin wax to shed adherent bacteria from tooth surfaces, saliva is acquired from the dorsum of the patient's tongue with a plastic test strip possessing a rough surface to enhance adherence and growth of mutans streptococci. The plastic test strips can also be inoculated with dental plaque removed from interproximal tooth sites with dental floss.[53] The inoculated plastic strip is immersed in a capped vial containing a selective broth medium for mutans streptococci (MSB [mitis salivarius-bacitracin] medium modified with 30% sucrose), and incubated aerobically at 37°C for 48 hours. Mutans streptococci growing on the rough surface of the plastic strip appear as light to dark blue, raised-surface colonies. The density of microbial growth on the strip is visually compared with a reference chart to semiquantitatively determine the mutans streptococci counts per milliliter of saliva.[52] A level of greater than or equal to 1 million mutans streptococci per milliliter of saliva indicates a high caries risk, compared with levels of 1000/mL to 10,000/mL for a low caries risk.[53]

Salivary mutans streptococci levels of greater than or equal to 1,000,000/mL in a recent systematic review provided a pooled positive likelihood ratio of 3.98 (from 3 clinical studies) for future dental caries in children aged 2 to 7 years with primary teeth at baseline.[53] However, only low sensitivity, but high specificity, was found for salivary mutans streptococci as a predictor of future dental caries when all studies were considered,[53] which limits their overall clinical prognostic utility in dental practice. However, periodic testing of salivary mutans streptococci levels has value as an aid in motivating dental patients to alter dietary intake patterns and reduce high fermentable carbohydrate/sucrose consumption.

ORAL MUCOSAL AND ODONTOGENIC INFECTIONS

Swab smears of oral mucosal lesions, and aspirates from odontogenic abscesses, can be subjected to anaerobic and aerobic microbial culture to identify likely bacterial and/or fungal pathogens, and provide in vitro susceptibility of isolated organisms to various antibiotics or antifungal agents. A recent systematic review found the Levine swab technique to be superior to a Z-swab for obtaining microbial specimens from infected wounds.[54] Ultrasonography can be used to direct needle aspiration of microbial specimens from deep-seated orofacial infections, as was described for a lateral masticator space infection.[55] Such specimens need to be collected with a minimum of contamination from adjacent tissues, preferably before antibiotic administration, and transported to the microbiology laboratory as quickly as possible using holding or transport media (ie, Stuart or Aimes transport media) recommended by the laboratory to maintain microbial viability.[56] Microbiological insight derived from the samples may be particularly valuable with regard to management of recalcitrant cases that are poorly responsive to standard empirically selected therapies.

For suspected oral yeast infections, stained smears of mucosal lesion scrapings or soft tissue biopsies may be examined with light microscopy to detect the presence of virulent and invasive hyphae-forming yeasts.[57]

HALITOSIS

In patients with halitosis, hydrogen sulfide (H_2S) and methylmercaptan (CH_3SH) concentrations may be measured in expired mouth air with a portable volatile sulfide monitor (Halimeter, Interscan Corp., Simi Valley, CA; or OralChroma, Abimedical Corp., Osaka, Japan). These volatile sulfur gases may be considered as surrogate markers for colonizing microbial species like *P gingivalis*, *T forsythia*, *T denticola*, *P micra*, *P endodontalis*, *Fusobacterium* species, *Eubacterium* species, *Selenomonas* species, *Prevotella* species, *Peptostreptococcus* species, *Streptococcus anginosus*, and *Centipeda periodontii*, which are the most active hydrogen sulfide and/or methylmercaptan producers among oral species.[58–60] However, other malodorous compounds potentially contributing to halitosis, such as cadaverine, putrescine, urea, and indole, are not detected by the instrument, but rarely occur in the absence of volatile sulfur gases, and do not produce halitosis by themselves.

Another microbiologically based test for halitosis estimates dorsum tongue levels of proteolytic bacteria in a colorimetric assay detecting trypsinlike proteolytic enzyme production via degradation on a test strip of benzoyl-DL-arginine-a-naphthylamide (BANA), a synthetic trypsin substrate (BANA-Zyme, OraTec Corp., Manassas, VA). Although BANA test scores correlate significantly with organoleptic measurements of halitosis,[61] they do not identify specific bacterial species in tested tongue specimens.[62]

PERIODONTITIS

The most frequent use of clinical microbiology in dentistry is currently in periodontal disease diagnosis and treatment. Starting in the late 1970s, analysis of subgingival microbial morphotypes with either phase-contrast or darkfield microscopy was proposed for periodontal risk assessment.[63–65] Microbial morphotypes in direct wet-mount preparations of subgingival biofilm specimens were microscopically characterized by their cell shape and motility. In clinical studies in which bacterial cell morphotypes alone were monitored in subgingival biofilms, increased baseline proportions of spirochetes and motile rods were significantly associated with chronic periodontitis progression in treated patients when periodontal maintenance care was discontinued for a year,[66] or administered after extended customized time intervals.[67] In comparison, no significant microscopic morphotype relationships with progressive disease were found when a periodontal prophylaxis was performed on patients at regular 3-month intervals.[67] As a result of these latter findings, and the increased availability of more sophisticated microbiological testing of subgingival biofilms with culture and molecular biology methods, use of phase-contrast and darkfield microscopy in clinical dental practice has waned, with few practitioners now using the technology in patient assessments.

However, in a recent secondary analysis of a previously completed clinical study,[68] phase-contrast microscopic morphotype analysis of posttreatment subgingival spirochete and crevicular leukocyte levels, as simplified biomarkers of subgingival biofilm pathogenicity and host-derived inflammatory responses in periodontal pockets, respectively, were shown to provide added diagnostic value compared with the use of conventional periodontal parameters in posttreatment risk assessment of patients with chronic periodontitis.[69] A posttreatment joint occurrence of high spirochete and high crevicular leukocyte counts, as seen with phase-contrast microscopic examination of subgingival biofilms during periodontal maintenance evaluations, showed a strong statistically significant association (odds ratio, 10.1; $P = .004$) with clinical progression of chronic periodontitis in patients over a mean 4.5-year posttreatment period, in contrast with the absence of any statistically significant relationships between various clinical and radiographic parameters and chronic periodontitis progression.[69] In addition, the 100% negative predictive value found with phase-contrast microscopic evaluations suggests that, if no or only low spirochete and crevicular leukocyte counts are attained and maintained in subgingival biofilms by periodontal treatment procedures, then the risk of chronic periodontitis disease progression posttreatment seems to be minimal.[69]

An advantage of phase-contrast microscopy analysis is that it can be performed rapidly at chairside in dental practice, unlike the need to send microbial specimens to an outside microbiology laboratory when seeking culture and/or molecular testing. An added value is the potential to better educate and motivate patients in their performance of home oral hygiene procedures, and to attain enhanced reductions in supragingival plaque levels,[70] when patients view phase-contrast microscopic video projections of motile microorganisms in their own subgingival biofilm samples.[63] Among the limitations of periodontal phase-contrast microscopy is an inability to provide identification of specific bacterial species in biofilm samples, an inability to distinguish nonmotile periodontal pathogens from nonmotile health-associated species, an inability to determine in vitro antibiotic susceptibility of observed biofilm species, and uncertainty about therapeutic steps to take when high-risk bacterial and/or crevicular leukocyte levels are detected in subgingival biofilm specimens.

Microbial culture was for many years the gold standard in clinical periodontal microbiology. The first commercial periodontal microbiology testing laboratory was established by Benjamin F. Hammond and D. Walter Cohen at the University of Pennsylvania School of Dental Medicine in 1982 with culture of major putative bacterial pathogens (the laboratory is presently located at Temple University School of Dentistry). Other commercial periodontal microbiology testing laboratories offering microbial culture were subsequently established and operate in the United States[71] and Europe.[72]

Microbial culture has the advantages of enabling recovery and identification to a genus and species level of a wide range of cultivable oral microorganisms, determining their proportional representation among total cultivable counts in subgingival biofilm samples, and facilitating in vitro susceptibility testing of isolates to various antimicrobial agents of potential therapeutic interest.

Periodontal microbial culture services require timely delivery of viable organisms from dental practice sites to be successful. Effective microbial transport media, such as viability medium göteborg anaerobically prepared and sterilized (VMGA) III and reduced transport fluid,[73] are essential for maintaining viability of microorganisms, particularly anaerobic bacteria, during a 24-hour to 48-hour maximum time period of transit to the microbiology testing laboratory after curette or paper-point sampling of plaque biofilms from periodontal pockets (**Fig. 1**). Other limitations with periodontal microbial culture are a need for specialized laboratory personnel expertise and experience in cultivation of periodontal bacteria (conventional hospital medical microbiology laboratories cannot be used), an inability to successfully cultivate all known putative periodontal bacterial pathogens, and an inability to easily differentiate between highly virulent versus less virulent strains of periodontal pathogens. In some laboratories, the lack of standard operating procedures and adequate quality control measures hamper their reliability in evaluating subgingival microbial specimens.[72] Periodontal microbial culture and identification is also costly (not usually covered by

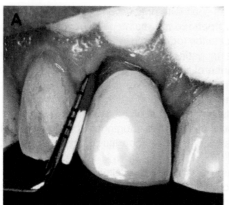
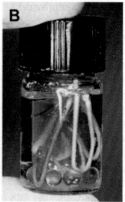

Fig. 1. (*A*) Paper-point sampling of subgingival biofilm (periodontal probe used to aid apical advancement of paper-point into periodontal pocket). (*B*) Multiple paper-point subgingival biofilm specimens pooled into VMGA III transport medium for shipment to microbiology laboratory.

dental insurance in the United States) and time consuming to perform, with results not available to clinicians for 7 to 14 days to permit adequate growth of slow-growing anaerobic species.

Fig. 2 outlines an example of a specimen processing protocol used for periodontal microbiology culture analysis by the Oral Microbiology Testing Service Laboratory at Temple University School of Dentistry, which is subject to the same Pennsylvania Health Department licensing, inspections, and quality control/proficiency testing standards applied to high-complexity clinical medical microbiology laboratories in hospitals.[74] Dilutions of subgingival biofilm samples are plated onto nonselective enriched *Brucella* blood agar (EBBA), and onto Hammond's selective medium for *Campylobacter* species (WOL), with anaerobic incubation for 7 days and 3 days, respectively,

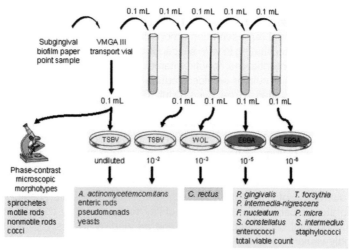

Fig. 2. Example of laboratory processing protocol for periodontal microbiology culture analysis. EBBA, enriched *Brucella* blood agar; TSBV, tryptic soy serum bacitracin vancomycin agar; WOL, hammond's selective medium for Campylobacter species.

for recovery of various anaerobic and facultative putative periodontal pathogens. Other laboratories use blood agar plates (Oxoid no. 2, Basingstoke, United Kingdom), supplemented with sheep blood, hemin, and menadione as nonselective medium.[75] Another selective medium, tryptic soy serum bacitracin vancomycin agar (TSBV), is incubated in air plus 5% CO_2 for 3 days for potential recovery of *A actinomycetemcomitans*, gram-negative facultative enteric rods and pseudomonads, and yeasts. Modified Dentaid-1 medium is a low-cost, effective alternative to TSBV medium used by some other periodontal microbiology testing laboratories.[76] A quasiuniversal culture medium with high levels of ascorbic acid added as an antioxidant has the potential to provide reliable recovery of both aerobic and anaerobic bacteria on a single culture medium,[77] but needs further validation of its efficacy specific to mixed subgingival biofilm populations. Microbial culture uniquely enables antibiotic susceptibility testing of cultivable subgingival biofilm isolates with either agar or broth dilution assays, or antibiotic gradient strips (Etest, bioMérieux, Durham, NC), to determine minimal inhibitory and/or minimal bactericidal drug concentrations.

A direct plating method may also be used to identify microorganism resistance to critical antibiotic threshold concentrations.[74] With the direct plating method, subgingival biofilm specimens are plated simultaneously on EBBA culture medium with and without test antibiotic drugs at concentrations internationally recognized as nonsusceptible/resistant breakpoint levels for anaerobic bacteria, such as those recommended by the United States Clinical and Laboratory Standards Institute (CLSI) or the European Committee on Antimicrobial Susceptibility Testing (EUCAST). In vitro resistance of a bacterial species to a specific antibiotic breakpoint is detected when the organism is found to grow both on EBBA medium prepared without any antibiotics and also on EBBA culture plates supplemented with the antibiotic threshold concentration.[74] This simplified rapid screening method shows nearly perfect correlation ($r^2 = 0.99$) with more labor-intensive and time-consuming CLSI-approved agar dilution susceptibility assays that require subculturing of primary isolation plates to identify antibiotic-resistant periodontal microorganisms.[78]

An important limitation of conventional in vitro susceptibility testing of periodontal bacterial pathogens is that it likely overestimates the potential in vivo activity of antimicrobial agents. Bacterial species form biofilms within periodontal pockets, which are many times more resistant to antimicrobial agents than when the organisms are disaggregated into planktonic cell suspensions for in vitro antibiotic susceptibility testing.[79] Thus, it may be more important to identify antibiotic resistance than susceptibility with in vitro testing, because a drug that is ineffective in vitro against periodontal bacterial pathogens under ideal laboratory testing conditions with planktonic cells can be confidently ruled out as unlikely to be of therapeutic benefit for in vivo administration.

An important development in microbial culture analysis is the enhanced genus and species identification of cultivable isolates offered by matrix-assisted laser desorption/ionization time-of-flight (MALDI-TOF) mass spectrometry. MALDI-TOF mass spectrometry uses proteomic spectral fingerprinting of microbial ribosomal proteins to definitively identify cultivable bacteria by matching mass spectra from clinical specimens to unique mass spectra of known microorganisms in its large reference library of bacterial protein profiles.[80]

Overall, microbial culture, when properly performed on viable biofilm samples,[81] has the ability to provide dental professionals with reasonably reproducible data on the subgingival occurrence, levels, and antimicrobial susceptibility of most major periodontal bacterial pathogens, and shows close agreement with findings of real-time polymerase chain reaction (PCR) for detection of subgingival *P gingivalis*, *T forsythia*, *P intermedia*, *P micra*, *F nucleatum*, and *A actinomycetemcomitans*.[82,83]

The past 2 decades have witnessed revolutionary advances in molecular DNA-based analysis of subgingival biofilms. Nucleic acid hybridization and amplification procedures have the advantages of being culture independent, not requiring viable microorganisms, and testing for a wider range of microbial species than culture. Some molecular methodologies may be used to detect uncultivated/unrecognized phylotypes. However, most molecular testing methods are not at present commercially available for diagnostic purposes to dental professionals, and none have the capability to assess the in vitro antibiotic susceptibility of subgingival biofilm species. Molecular methods applied at a research level for evaluation of oral microbial specimens include end point and real-time PCR[82,83]; loop-mediated isothermal amplication[84]; and, as recently reviewed,[85] denaturing and temperature gradient gel electrophoresis, restriction fragment length polymorphism, DNA-DNA checkerboard hybridization, DNA microarrays with reverse-capture 16S ribosomal DNA (rDNA) taxa-specific oligonucleotide probes, 16S rRNA gene sequencing with 454 pyrosequencing and other next-generation sequencing platforms, 16S rDNA profiling, whole-genome shotgun metagenome sequencing, and microbial metatranscriptomic sequencing.

Commercial laboratory testing services in the United States (MyPerioPath; OralDNA Labs, Eden Prairie, MN) and Europe[86] offer PCR or DNA-DNA hybridization–based analysis of subgingival biofilms. However, most of the laboratories have limited disclosure, publication, or outside evaluation of their quality control outcomes. In this regard, the agreement and reproducibility of 3 European periodontal testing laboratories regarding detection of *P gingivalis*, *T forsythia*, *T denticola*, and *A actinomycetemcomitans* was recently investigated by sending each laboratory portions of subgingival biofilm samples taken from 20 patients with severe chronic or aggressive periodontitis.[86] The results found only poor intertest agreement between the laboratories, and only 1 laboratory attained 100% intratest reproducibility.[86] Another study using only mock subgingival specimens made from mixtures of 12 reference strains of various oral microorganisms found better identification and agreement between the 3 laboratories.[87] Diagnostic testing services may become more available in the future for laboratories using next-generation sequencing technology supplemented with in silico 16S rDNA probe analysis (HOMI*N*GS, The Forsyth Institute, Cambridge, MA),[88] which presently is for research purposes only.

MICROBIAL TESTING IN CHRONIC PERIODONTITIS TREATMENT PLANNING

An urgent need exists for improved diagnostic risk assessment for patients with chronic periodontitis, because conventional clinical and radiographic parameters show little predictive utility in identifying future destructive periodontal disease activity.[89] Microbiological analysis of subgingival biofilms has the potential to enhance clinical decision making in periodontics by aiding in identification of patients at increased risk of progressive periodontitis. For example, Mombelli and colleagues[90] found that 59% of 17 chronic periodontitis patients remained subgingival *P gingivalis* culture positive after extensive periodontal root scaling therapy, with a statistically significant relationship noted between *P gingivalis* subgingival persistence and the number of 5 mm or greater posttreatment probing depths. Persistence of subgingival *P gingivalis* after nonsurgical root instrumentation was also associated with an increased risk of subsequent progressive alveolar bone loss (odds ratio, 31.9; positive predictive value, 84%), with radiographic alveolar bone gains found only when subgingival *P gingivalis* was absent posttreatment.[91] The occurrence of increased posttreatment numbers of subgingival *P gingivalis* and *T denticola* showed a 62% and 130% excess risk, respectively, for clinical periodontal break-down occurring 3 months later in patients with treated chronic periodontitis on maintenance care.[92] Charalampakis and colleagues[93] reported that increased post-treatment levels of 1 or more of the 3 red complex species (*P gingivalis*, *T forsythia*, *T denticola*), or at least 2 A-complex species (*F alocis*, *P endodontalis*, *Prevotella tannerae*), or at least 2 B-complex species (*P intermedia*, *F nucleatum*, *C rectus*) showed statistically significant odds ratio relationships of 39.3, 28.5, and 61.9, respectively, with subsequent clinical periodontal breakdown ($\geq$2-mm loss of clin-ical periodontal attachment together with $\geq$2-mm increase in probing depth) occur-ring over a 2-year period in patients with treated chronic periodontitis. These studies suggest that microbial-based treatment end points may markedly help cli-nicians better identify patients in need of additional or altered periodontal therapies before the onset of clinical treatment failure, and contribute to improved patient oral health outcomes.

More recently, Bizzarro and colleagues[94] found the subgingival microbiome compo-sition in patients with chronic periodontitis at pre-treatment to be predictive of 12-month posttreatment clinical responses to periodontal debridement therapy used with or without a systemic metronidazole plus amoxicillin drug regimen. Patients at pretreatment with a highly diverse subgingival microbiome composed mainly of oral taxa traditionally associated with periodontitis were more likely to have a good treat-ment outcome with mechanical periodontal debridement therapy alone, unless there was a posttreatment persistence of *Filifactor*, Synergistaceae, *Treponema*, and *Palu-dibacter* species, for which systemic metronidazole plus amoxicillin therapy was found to be beneficial.[94] In contrast, patients at pretreatment with low microbial diversity, and higher proportions of Pseudomonadaceae, such as *P aeruginosa*, responded less favorably to nonsurgical periodontal therapy regardless of their use of systemic metronidazole plus amoxicillin.[94]

For patients with chronic periodontitis, similar to those discussed earlier, who pre-sent with subgingival gram-negative enteric rods and/or pseudomonads, such as *P aeruginosa*, adjunctive systemic ciprofloxacin alone, or in combination with metroni-dazole if additional metronidazole-susceptible periodontal pathogens are present, may be more appropriately considered for administration[95] because mechanical peri-odontal debridement alone does not reliably suppress large subgingival populations of gram-negative enteric rods and pseudomonads,[29] and the species are usually resis-tant to therapeutic concentrations of both metronidazole and amoxicillin.[74] It is in clin-ical situations such as these that clinical oral microbiology testing encompassing in vitro antibiotic susceptibility analysis is most helpful to dental professionals in their selection of periodontal treatment modalities, and reduces the risk of therapeutic fail-ures attributable to subgingival persistence of antibiotic-resistant periodontal pathogens.

Perhaps the best example of this was described more than 20 years ago by Daniel H. Fine[96] in several patient case reports. For patients with refractory periodon-titis, who had had repeated clinical treatment failures and harbored periodontal bacterial pathogens resistant to antibiotics conventionally used in periodontal prac-tice, more appropriate systemic antibiotic therapies were identified and administered based on microbiological testing and in vitro antibiotic susceptibility testing.[96] This approach resulted in suppression of persistent pathogenic bacterial species, and sus-tained clinical resolution and stabilization of destructive periodontal disease in each of the patients.

Further guidance on the role of clinical oral microbiology in periodontal treatment planning may be found in previously published reviews and position papers.[95,97,98]

SUMMARY

- Many oral diseases have well-characterized infectious causes, including dental caries, various forms of periodontitis, endodontic lesions, halitosis, and odontogenic infections.
- Saliva, dental plaque, mucosal smears, abscess aspirates, and soft tissue biopsies may all serve as sources for obtaining microorganisms for clinical oral microbiology laboratory testing.
- Methods commercially available to analyze oral microbial samples include direct microscopic examination, microbial culture, various PCR and DNA-DNA hybridization–based molecular biology technologies, and next-generation sequencing platforms.
- Microbiological testing may be particularly helpful for patients with chronic periodontitis in selection of antimicrobial therapy and performing posttreatment periodontal risk assessments.
- Further research and technological advances are likely to increase the availability and clinical utility of microbiological analysis in modern dental practice.

REFERENCES

1. Selwitz RH, Ismail AI, Pitts NB. Dental caries. Lancet 2007;369:51–9.
2. Dye B, Thornton-Evans G, Li X, et al. Dental caries and tooth loss in adults in the United States, 2011-2012. NCHS Data Brief 2015;197:1–7.
3. Saunders RH Jr, Meyerowitz C. Dental caries in older adults. Dent Clin North Am 2005;49:293–308.
4. Jin LJ, Lamster IB, Greenspan JS, et al. Global burden of oral diseases: emerging concepts, management and interplay with systemic health. Oral Dis 2015;22:609–19.
5. Tanner AC. Anaerobic culture to detect periodontal and caries pathogens. J Oral Biosci 2015;57:18–26.
6. Takahashi N, Nyvad B. Ecological hypothesis of dentin and root caries. Caries Res 2016;50:422–31.
7. Eke PI, Dye BA, Wei L, et al. Update on prevalence of periodontitis in adults in the United States: NHANES 2009 to 2012. J Periodontol 2015;86:611–22.
8. Petersen PE, Ogawa H. The global burden of periodontal disease: towards integration with chronic disease prevention and control. Periodontol 2000 2012;60: 15–39.
9. Genco RJ, Borgnakke WS. Risk factors for periodontal disease. Periodontol 2000 2013;62:59–94.
10. Pérez-Chaparro PJ, Gonçalves C, Figueiredo LC, et al. Newly identified pathogens associated with periodontitis: a systematic review. J Dent Res 2014;93: 846–58.
11. Slots J. Periodontal herpesviruses: prevalence, pathogenicity, systemic risk. Periodontol 2000 2015;69:28–45.
12. Nguyen-Hieu T, Khelaifia S, Aboudharam G, et al. Methanogenic archaea in subgingival sites: a review. APMIS 2013;121:467–77.
13. Riviere GR, DeRouen TA, Kay SL, et al. Association of oral spirochetes from sites of periodontal health with development of periodontitis. J Periodontol 1997;68: 1210–4.
14. Tanner A, Maiden MF, Macuch PJ, et al. Microbiota of health, gingivitis, and initial periodontitis. J Clin Periodontol 1998;25:85–98.

15. Tran SD, Rudney JD, Sparks BS, et al. Persistent presence of *Bacteroides forsythus* as a risk factor for attachment loss in a population with low prevalence and severity of adult periodontitis. J Periodontol 2001;72:1–10.
16. Van der Velden U, Abbas F, Armand S, et al. Java project on periodontal diseases. The natural development of periodontitis: risk factors, risk predictors and risk determinants. J Clin Periodontol 2006;33:540–8.
17. Tanner AC, Paster BJ, Lu SC, et al. Subgingival and tongue microbiota during early periodontitis. J Dent Res 2006;85:318–23.
18. Tanner AC, Kent R Jr, Kanasi E, et al. Clinical characteristics and microbiota of progressing slight chronic periodontitis in adults. J Clin Periodontol 2007;34:917–30.
19. Abusleme L, Dupuy AK, Dutzan N, et al. The subgingival microbiome in health and periodontitis and its relationship with community biomass and inflammation. ISME J 2013;7:1016–25.
20. Löe H, Brown LJ. Early onset periodontitis in the United States of America. J Periodontol 1991;62:608–16.
21. Susin C, Haas AN, Albandar JM. Epidemiology and demographics of aggressive periodontitis. Periodontol 2000 2014;65:27–45.
22. Könönen E, Müller HP. Microbiology of aggressive periodontitis. Periodontol 2000 2014;65:46–78.
23. Haubek D, Ennibi OK, Poulsen K, et al. Risk of aggressive periodontitis in adolescent carriers of the JP2 clone of *Aggregatibacter* (*Actinobacillus*) *actinomycetemcomitans* in Morocco: a prospective longitudinal cohort study. Lancet 2008;371(9608):237–42.
24. Fine DH, Markowitz K, Fairlie K, et al. A consortium of *Aggregatibacter actinomycetemcomitans*, *Streptococcus parasanguinis*, and *Filifactor alocis* is present in sites prior to bone loss in a longitudinal study of localized aggressive periodontitis. J Clin Microbiol 2013;51:2850–61.
25. Ximenez-Fyvie LA, Almaguer-Flores A, Jacobo-Soto V, et al. Subgingival microbiota of periodontally untreated Mexican subjects with generalized aggressive periodontitis. J Clin Periodontol 2006;33:869–77.
26. Colombo AP, Bennet S, Cotton SL, et al. Impact of periodontal therapy on the subgingival microbiota of severe periodontitis: comparison between good responders and individuals with refractory periodontitis using the human oral microbe identification microarray. J Periodontol 2012;83:1279–87.
27. Rams TE, Listgarten MA, Slots J. Utility of 5 major putative periodontal pathogens and selected clinical parameters to predict periodontal breakdown in patients on maintenance care. J Clin Periodontol 1996;23:346–54.
28. Slots J, Rams TE, Listgarten MA. Yeasts, enteric rods and pseudomonads in the subgingival flora of severe adult periodontitis. Oral Microbiol Immunol 1988;3:47–52.
29. Slots J, Feik D, Rams TE. Prevalence and antimicrobial susceptibility of Enterobacteriaceae, Pseudomonadaceae and *Acinetobacter* in human periodontitis. Oral Microbiol Immunol 1990;5:149–54.
30. Colombo AP, Boches SK, Cotton SL, et al. Comparisons of subgingival microbial profiles of refractory periodontitis, severe periodontitis, and periodontal health using the human oral microbe identification microarray. J Periodontol 2009;80:1421–32.
31. Rams TE, Degener JE, van Winkelhoff AJ. Antibiotic resistance in human peri-implantitis microbiota. Clin Oral Implants Res 2014;25:82–90.

32. Pérez-Chaparro PJ, Duarte PM, Shibli JA, et al. The current weight of evidence of the microbiological profile associated with peri-implantitis: a systematic review. J Periodontol 2016;15:1–16.

33. Siqueira JF Jr, Rocas IN. Diversity of endodontic microbiota revisited. J Dent Res 2009;88:969–81.

34. Stevens RH, Grossman LI. Evaluation of the antimicrobial potential of calcium hydroxide as an intracanal medicament. J Endod 1983;9:372–4.

35. Kampfer J, Göhring TN, Attin T, et al. Leakage of food-borne *Enterococcus faecalis* through temporary fillings in a simulated oral environment. Int Endod J 2007;40:471–7.

36. Rivera-Hidalgo F, Stanford TW. Oral mucosal lesions caused by infective microorganisms. I. Viruses and bacteria. Periodontol 2000 1999;21:106–24.

37. Stanford TW, Rivera-Hidalgo F. Oral mucosal lesions caused by infective microorganisms. II. Fungi and parasites. Periodontol 2000 1999;21:125–44.

38. De Ceulaer J, Tacconelli E, Vandecasteele SJ. *Actinomyces* osteomyelitis in bisphosphonate-related osteonecrosis of the jaw (BRONJ): the missing link? Eur J Clin Microbiol Infect Dis 2014;33:1873–80.

39. Kapoor U, Sharma G, Juneja M, et al. Halitosis: current concepts on etiology, diagnosis and management. Eur J Dent 2016;10:292–300.

40. Kazor CE, Mitchell PM, Lee AM, et al. Diversity of bacterial populations on the tongue dorsa of patients with halitosis and healthy patients. J Clin Microbiol 2003;41:558–63.

41. O'Donnell MJ, Boyle MA, Russell RJ, et al. Management of dental unit waterline biofilms in the 21st century. Future Microbiol 2011;6:1209–26.

42. Barbeau J, Tanguay R, Faucher E, et al. Multiparametric analysis of waterline contamination in dental units. Appl Environ Microbiol 1996;62:3954–9.

43. Szymanska J. Risk of exposure to *Legionella* in dental practice. Ann Agric Environ Med 2004;11:9–12.

44. Williams HN, Paszko-Kolva C, Shahamat M, et al. Molecular techniques reveal high prevalence of *Legionella* in dental units. J Am Dent Assoc 1996;127:1188–93.

45. Ricci ML, Fontana S, Pinci F, et al. Pneumonia associated with a dental unit waterline. Lancet 2012;379(9816):684.

46. Atlas RM, Williams JF, Huntington MK. *Legionella* contamination of dental-unit waters. Appl Environ Microbiol 1995;61:1208–13.

47. Reinthaler FF, Mascher F, Stunzner D. Serological examinations for antibodies against *Legionella* species in dental personnel. J Dent Res 1988;67:942–3.

48. Fotos PG, Westfall HN, Snyder IS, et al. Prevalence of *Legionella*-specific IgG and IgM antibody in a dental clinic population. J Dent Res 1985;64:1382–5.

49. Kohn WG, Harte JA, Malvitz DM, et al. Guidelines for infection control in dental health care settings–2003. J Am Dent Assoc 2004;135:33–47.

50. American Dental Association. Guidelines for infection control in the dental office and the commercial dental laboratory. J Am Dent Assoc 1996;127:672–80.

51. Patiño-Marín N, Martínez-Castañón GA, Zavala-Alonso NV, et al. Biologic monitoring and causes of failure in cycles of sterilization in dental care offices in Mexico. Am J Infect Control 2015;43:1092–5.

52. Jensen B, Bratthall D. A new method for the estimation of mutans streptococci in human saliva. J Dent Res 1989;68:468–71.

53. Senneby A, Mejàre I, Sahlin NE, et al. Diagnostic accuracy of different caries risk assessment methods. A systematic review. J Dent 2015;43:1385–93.

54. Copeland-Halperin LR, Kaminsky AJ, Bluefeld N, et al. Sample procurement for cultures of infected wounds: a systematic review. J Wound Care 2016;25:S4–6, S8–10.
55. Sivarajasingam V, Sharma V, Crean SJ, et al. Ultrasound-guided needle aspiration of lateral masticator space abscess. Oral Surg Oral Med Oral Pathol Oral Radiol Endod 1999;88:616–9.
56. Winn WC, Allen SD, Janda WM, et al. Koneman's color atlas and textbook of diagnostic microbiology. 6th edition. Baltimore (MD): Lippincott Williams & Wilkins; 2006.
57. Mayer FL, Wilson D, Hube B. *Candida albicans* pathogenicity mechanisms. Virulence 2013;4:119–28.
58. Persson S, Edlund MB, Claesson R, et al. The formation of hydrogen sulfide and methyl mercaptan by oral bacteria. Oral Microbiol Immunol 1990;5:195–201.
59. Yoshida A, Yoshimura M, Ohara N, et al. Hydrogen sulfide production from cysteine and homocysteine by periodontal and oral bacteria. J Periodontol 2009;80:1845–51.
60. Basic A, Blomqvist S, Carlén A, et al. Estimation of bacterial hydrogen sulfide production in vitro. J Oral Microbiol 2015;7:28166.
61. Kozlovsky A, Gordon D, Gelernter I, et al. Correlation between the BANA test and oral malodor parameters. J Dent Res 1994;73:1036–42.
62. van den Broek AM, Feenstra L, de Baat C. A review of the current literature on aetiology and measurement methods of halitosis. J Dent 2007;35:627–35.
63. Keyes PH, Wright WE, Howard SA. The use of phase-contrast microscopy and chemotherapy in the diagnosis and treatment of periodontal lesions–an initial report (I). Quintessence Int Dent Dig 1978;9:51–6.
64. Listgarten MA, Helldén L. Relative distribution of bacteria at clinically healthy and periodontally diseased sites in humans. J Clin Periodontol 1978;5:115–32.
65. Keyes PH, Rams TE. A rationale for management of periodontal diseases: rapid identification of microbial 'therapeutic targets' with phase-contrast microscopy. J Am Dent Assoc 1983;106:803–12.
66. Listgarten MA, Levin S. Positive correlation between the proportions of subgingival spirochetes and motile bacteria and susceptibility of human subjects to periodontal deterioration. J Clin Periodontol 1981;8:122–38.
67. Listgarten MA, Schifter CC, Sullivan P, et al. Failure of a microbial assay to reliably predict disease recurrence in a treated periodontitis population receiving regularly scheduled prophylaxes. J Clin Periodontol 1986;13:768–73.
68. Rams TE, Keyes PH, Wright WE, et al. Long-term effects of microbiologically modulated periodontal therapy on advanced adult periodontitis. J Am Dent Assoc 1985;111:429–41.
69. Keyes PH, Rams TE. Subgingival microbial and inflammatory cell morphotypes associated with chronic periodontitis progression in treated adults. J Int Acad Periodontol 2015;17:49–57.
70. Acharya S, Goyal A, Utreja AK, et al. Effect of three different motivational techniques on oral hygiene and gingival health of patients undergoing multibracketed orthodontics. Angle Orthod 2011;81:884–8.
71. Rams TE. Availability of laboratory testing services for identification of periodontal pathogens in dental plaque. Clin Prev Dent 1989;11(4):18–21.
72. Rautemaa-Richardson R, van der Reijden WA, Dahlén G, et al. Quality control for diagnostic oral microbiology laboratories in European countries. J Oral Microbiol 2011;3. http://dx.doi.org/10.3402/jom.v3i0.8395.

73. Dahlén G, Pipattanagovit P, Rosling B, et al. A comparison of two transport media for saliva and subgingival samples. Oral Microbiol Immunol 1993;8:375–82.

74. Rams TE, Degener JE, van Winkelhoff AJ. Antibiotic resistance in human chronic periodontitis microbiota. J Periodontol 2014;85:160–9.

75. van Winkelhoff AJ, Rurenga P, Wekema-Mulder GJ, et al. Non-oral gram-negative facultative rods in chronic periodontitis microbiota. Microb Pathog 2016;94: 117–22.

76. Rurenga P, Raangs E, Singadji Z, et al. Evaluation of three selective media for isolation of *Aggregatibacter actinomycetemcomitans*. J Periodontal Res 2013; 48:549–52.

77. Dione N, Khelaifia S, La Scola B, et al. A quasi-universal medium to break the aerobic/anaerobic bacterial culture dichotomy in clinical microbiology. Clin Microbiol Infect 2016;22:53–8.

78. Feres M, Haffajee AD, Goncalves C, et al. Systemic doxycycline administration in the treatment of periodontal infections (II). Effect on antibiotic resistance of subgingival species. J Clin Periodontol 1999;26:784–92.

79. Olsen I. Biofilm-specific antibiotic tolerance and resistance. Eur J Clin Microbiol Infect Dis 2015;34:877–86.

80. Rams TE, Sautter JD, Getreu A, et al. Phenotypic identification of *Porphyromonas gingivalis* validated with matrix-assisted laser desorption/ionization time-of-flight mass spectrometry. Microb Pathog 2016;94:112–6.

81. Cohen L, Rams T, Slots J, et al. Independent analysis of microbiological samples by three oral testing laboratories. J Dent Res 2001;80(Special Issue):219 [abstract: 1465].

82. Boutaga K, van Winkelhoff AJ, Vandenbroucke-Grauls CM, et al. Comparison of real-time PCR and culture for detection of *Porphyromonas gingivalis* in subgingival plaque samples. J Clin Microbiol 2003;41:4950–4.

83. Boutaga K, van Winkelhoff AJ, Vandenbroucke-Grauls CM, et al. Periodontal pathogens: a quantitative comparison of anaerobic culture and real-time PCR. FEMS Immunol Med Microbiol 2005;45:191–9.

84. Miyagawa J, Maeda H, Murauchi T, et al. Rapid and simple detection of eight major periodontal pathogens by the loop-mediated isothermal amplification method. FEMS Immunol Med Microbiol 2008;53:314–21.

85. Krishnan K, Chen T, Paster BJ. A practical guide to the oral microbiome and its relation to health and disease. Oral Dis 2016. http://dx.doi.org/10.1111/odi. 12509.

86. Untch M, Schlagenhauf U. Inter- and intra-test agreement of three commercially available molecular diagnostic tests for the identification of periodontal pathogens. Clin Oral Investig 2015;19:2045–52.

87. Santigli E, Leitner E, Wimmer G, et al. Accuracy of commercial kits and published primer pairs for the detection of periodontopathogens. Clin Oral Investig 2016; 20(9):2515–28.

88. Mougeot JL, Stevens CB, Cotton SL, et al. Concordance of HOMIM and HOMINGS technologies in the microbiome analysis of clinical samples. J Oral Microbiol 2016;8:30379.

89. Armitage GC. Learned and unlearned concepts in periodontal diagnostics: a 50-year perspective. Periodontol 2000 2013;62:20–36.

90. Mombelli A, Schmid B, Rutar A, et al. Persistence patterns of *Porphyromonas gingivalis*, *Prevotella intermedia/nigrescens*, and *Actinobacillus actinomyetemcomitans* after mechanical therapy of periodontal disease. J Periodontol 2000;71: 14–21.

91. Chaves ES, Jeffcoat MK, Ryerson CC, et al. Persistent bacterial colonization of *Porphyromonas gingivalis*, *Prevotella intermedia*, and *Actinobacillus actinomycetemcomitans* in periodontitis and its association with alveolar bone loss after 6 months of therapy. J Clin Periodontol 2000;27:897–903.
92. Byrne SJ, Dashper SG, Darby IB, et al. Progression of chronic periodontitis can be predicted by the levels of *Porphyromonas gingivalis* and *Treponema denticola* in subgingival plaque. Oral Microbiol Immunol 2009;24:469–77.
93. Charalampakis G, Dahlén G, Carlén A, et al. Bacterial markers vs. clinical markers to predict progression of chronic periodontitis: a 2-yr prospective observational study. Eur J Oral Sci 2013;121:394–402.
94. Bizzarro S, Laine ML, Buijs MJ, et al. Microbial profiles at baseline and not the use of antibiotics determine the clinical outcome of the treatment of chronic periodontitis. Sci Rep 2016;6:20205.
95. Slots J, Research, Science and Therapy Committee. Systemic antibiotics in periodontics. J Periodontol 2004;75:1553–65.
96. Fine DH. Microbial identification and antibiotic sensitivity testing, an aid for patients refractory to periodontal therapy. A report of 3 cases. J Clin Periodontol 1994;21:98–106.
97. van Winkelhoff AJ, Winkel EG. Microbiological diagnostics in periodontics: biological significance and clinical validity. Periodontol 2000 2005;39:40–52.
98. Shaddox LM, Walker C. Microbial testing in periodontics: value, limitations and future directions. Periodontol 2000 2009;50:25–38.

Normal Oral Flora and the Oral Ecosystem

Lakshman Samaranayake, DSc, DDS, FRCPath, FDSRCS, FDSRCPS, FRACDS[a,b,*],
Victor H. Matsubara, PhD, DDS, MSc[c]

KEYWORDS

- Oral ecology • Oral microbiome • Dental plaque biofilms • Saliva

KEY POINTS

- The oral ecosystem comprises the oral flora, so-called oral microbiome, the different anatomic microniches of the oral cavity and its bathing fluid, saliva.
- The oral microbiome comprises a diverse group of organisms and includes bacteria, archaea, fungi, protozoa, and viruses.
- The oral microbiome exists either suspended in saliva as planktonic phase organisms or attached to oral surfaces essentially as a plaque biofilm.
- The homeostasis of the plaque biofilm and its symbiotic relationship with the host is critical for oral health.
- The disequilibrium or dysbiosis within the plaque biofilms is the initiating event that leads to major oral diseases, such as caries and periodontal disease.

ORAL MICROBIAL ECOLOGY

The oral cavity is a unique ecosystem. It comprises a wide range of habitats, including teeth, gingival sulcus, tongue, cheeks, hard and soft palate, and tonsils, with their own, intrinsic, unique mini-environmental conditions. The human mouth is lined by stratified squamous epithelium (keratinized and nonkeratinized); however, this is modified in areas according to function (eg, the tongue) and interrupted by other structures, such as teeth and salivary ducts. The gingival tissues form a cuff around each tooth, and there is a continuous exudate of crevicular fluid from the gingival crevice. A thin layer of saliva also bathes the surface of the oral mucosa.

The mouth, being an extension of an external body site, is colonized by virtually billions of bacteria, fungi, and viruses, now called the oral microbiome. The oral

The authors have nothing to disclose.
[a] Faculty of Dentistry, University of Hong Kong, The Deanery, Floor 7, 34, Hospital Road, Hong Kong, China; [b] University of Queensland, Brisbane, Australia; [c] Department of Oral Microbiology, School of Dentistry, University of São Paulo, Av Professor Lineu Prestes, 2227, São Paulo 05508-000, Brazil
* Corresponding author.
E-mail address: lakshman@hku.hk

http://dx.doi.org/10.1016/j.cden.2016.11.002
dental.theclinics.com

microbiome is in broad terms similar in all humans, although each individual has a characteristic "fingerprint" that is unique to himself or herself. This commensal (or indigenous, or resident) flora exists in symbiotic harmony with the host, but disease conditions supervene when the microbial equilibrium is broken, hence called dysbiosis. The predominant dental diseases in humans, caries and periodontal disease, are caused in this manner. In addition to the commensal microflora, there are others (such as coliforms) that survive in the mouth only for short periods (transient flora). This transient flora, including pathogens, cannot get a foothold in the oral environment because of the colonization resistance exerted by the resident flora.

NORMAL ORAL MICROFLORA AND THE ORAL MICROBIOME

The human body is composed of approximately one hundred trillion cells, of which 90% comprise the resident microflora of the host and only 10% are mammalian.[1] Bacteria are by far the predominant group of organisms in the oral cavity, and there are probably some 500 to 700 common oral species or phylotypes of which only 50% to 60% are cultivable. The remaining uncultivable flora is currently being identified using molecular technology, especially those based on 16S ribosomal RNA sequencing, pyrosequencing, and new-generation sequencing (NGS) technology.

The organisms that establish and predominate on particular surfaces vary depending on the biological and physical properties of each site. In the oral cavity, a diverse array of organisms can be found, usually living in harmony, including bacteria, archaea, fungi, mycoplasmas, protozoa, and possibly a viral flora that may persist from time to time. Collectively, the oral microflora has been termed oral microbiota, and more recently, the oral microbiome.[2]

The oral cavity is home to multiple anatomic microniches where physicochemical features, such as pH, oxygen, temperature, or redox potential, influence the settling of microorganisms, thus creating a complex microbiota.[3,4] The oral cavity harbors a unique and selective microbial composition that many organisms commonly isolated from neighboring ecosystems, such as the gut and the skin, are not found in the mouth. Despite the continuous passage of bacteria into the gut via saliva, only few periodontal microbes can be recovered from gastrointestinal and fecal samples.[5]

In recent studies of the structure, function, and diversity of human oral microbiome, evaluated using NGS, it has been clearly shown that the oral microbiome is unique to each individual.[6] Even healthy individuals differ remarkably in the composition of the resident oral microbes. Although much of this diversity remains unexplained, diet, environment, host genetics, and early microbial exposure have all been implicated in the constituent flora of the climax community.

The oral microbiome exists either suspended in saliva as planktonic phase organisms or attached to oral surfaces essentially as a plaque biofilm. Given the high diversity in the salivary microbiome, for instance, within and between individuals, little geographic variations can be noticed. Individuals from different worldwide locations may present with similar salivary microbiota, indicating that host species is the primary determinant of oral microbiome.[7]

Some oral microbes are more closely associated with disease than others, although they commonly lurk within the normal oral flora without harming the oral health. This equilibrium and homeostasis between beneficial and pathogenic organisms are the key factors that contribute to the development of oral diseases. The specific microbes that help restore a natural healthy microbiome in a given habitat are known as probiotics.[8]

The oral cavity is germ free at birth, although it is straight away colonized by distinct species of bacteria. Once established, the oral microbiome is formed by a wide range of gram-positive and gram-negative bacteria species (**Fig. 1**), including obligate anaerobe (metabolize energy anaerobically and are killed by normal atmospheric concentration of oxygen), and facultative anaerobe (obtain energy from aerobic respiration if oxygen is present, but is capable of switching to fermentation or anaerobic respiration in the absence of oxygen). The oral flora is dynamic, and its composition changes as the biology of the oral cavity alters over time.

ACQUISITION OF THE NORMAL ORAL FLORA

The infant mouth is usually sterile at birth, except perhaps for a few organisms acquired from the mother's birth canal. A few hours later, the organisms from the mother's (or nurse's) mouth (vertical transmission), and possibly a few from the environment, are established in the mouth. The main route of transmission is via saliva, although organisms can be also derived from water, food, and other nutritious fluids. These pioneer species are usually streptococci, which bind to mucosal epithelium (eg, *Streptococcus salivarius*, *Streptococcus mitis*, and *Streptococcus oralis*). The metabolic activity of the pioneer community then alters the oral environment to facilitate colonization by other bacterial genera and species, for instance, *S salivarius* produces extracellular polymers from sucrose, to which other bacteria such as *Actinomyces* spp can attach.

Oral flora on the child's first birthday usually consists of streptococci, staphylococci, *Neisseria*, together with some gram-negative anaerobes such as *Veillonella* spp. Less frequently isolated are *Lactobacillus*, *Actinomyces*, *Prevotella*, and *Fusobacterium* species.

The next evolutionary change in this community occurs during and after tooth eruption, when two further niches are provided for bacterial colonization: the nonshedding hard-tissue surface of enamel and cementum, and the gingival crevice. Gram-positive bacteria such as *Streptococcus mutans*, *Streptococcus sanguinis*, *Actinomyces* spp, *Lactobacillus*, and *Rothia* selectively colonize enamel surfaces. In turn, gram-negative organisms including nonpigmenting *Prevotella* spp, *Porphyromonas* spp, *Neisseria*, and *Capnocytophaga*, all preferring anaerobic environments, colonize the crevicular tissues.[9,10]

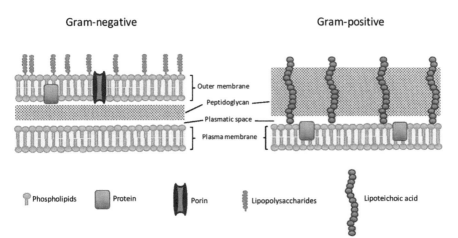

Fig. 1. Gram-positive and gram-negative bacteria based on structural differences of their cell walls.

During puberty, changes in hormone levels also alter the oral microbiome, and a transition to an adult flora composition can be noticed. Spirochaetes, *Veillonella*, *Prevotella*, and black-pigmented *Bacteroides* (eg, *Bacteroides intermedius*) are more frequently isolated during this period of life.[11,12]

The oral microbiome continues to grow in diversity over time until the composition of this complex ecosystem reaches equilibrium between the resident microflora and the local environmental conditions, where a climax community is said to exist. At this stage, the oral flora remains stable, although alteration in critical environment factors at a site due to changes in diet, hormonal levels, and oral hygiene, for instance, can disrupt this "microbial homeostasis" and favor a disease-associated microbiota, so-called dysbiosis.[13] Horizontal transmission of microorganisms, especially periodontal pathogens, may occur through interpersonal contamination.[14] Hence, the normal oral flora mounts an active response, remaining always as a highly dynamic system.

At advanced ages, the direct and indirect effects of senility (**Fig. 2**) affect the microbial homeostasis, facilitating the colonization by exogenous microbes and the imbalances in resident oral microflora.[15] The last major oral bacterial alteration is reached if all teeth are lost. Bacteria that colonize the mouth at this stage are very similar to those in a child before tooth eruption. The introduction of a prosthetic appliance at this stage changes the microbial composition once again. Growth of *Candida* species is particularly increased after the introduction of acrylic (polymethyl methacrylate) dentures, whereas it is now recognized that the prevalence of *Staphylococcus aureus* and lactobacilli is high in those aged 70 years or over.[16]

The acquisition of some bacteria may occur optimally only at certain ages; this phenomenon is termed "window of infectivity." For example, children at the median age of 26 months[17] and 9 months[18] are more susceptible for colonization by mutans streptococci and *Streptococcus sanguinis*, respectively. This window creates the possibility of preventive strategies over these critical periods to reduce the likelihood of colonization of the infant, such as the reduction of mutans streptococci carriage in the mother's mouth for prevention of vertical transmission, thus delaying the onset of dental caries.

BENEFICIAL EFFECTS OF THE RESIDENT ORAL MICROFLORA

The resident microflora contributes directly and indirectly to the normal development of the physiology, nutrition, and defense system of the host. The permanent colonizers act as a barrier to transient/exogenous organisms, some of which are potentially

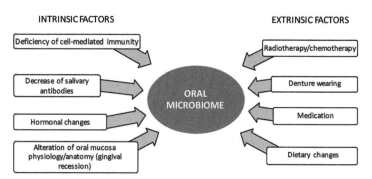

Fig. 2. Intrinsic and extrinsic factors affecting the composition and the homeostasis of the oral microbiome. (*Modified from* Marsh PD, Percival RS. The oral microflora—friend or foe? Can we decide? Int Dent J 2006;56(4 Suppl 1):237; with permission.)

pathogenic. This biofilm property is termed "colonization resistance." The long-term antibiotic treatment is an example of a factor that breaks this resistance because it causes rapid suppression of the resident microflora that leads to overgrowth of drug-resistant minor components of the microflora or exogenous pathogens, which in turn may cause oral diseases.[19] Thus, the resident microflora is considered a part of the innate host defenses. The mechanisms that accomplish the colonization resistance are summarized in **Table 1**. Under normal conditions, therefore, both the host and the microbes mutually benefit from this association.[15]

As mentioned above, the oral cavity offers a multiplicity of micro-habitats and micro-ecosystems or niches for microbial colonization; these are examined in the next section.

ORAL HABITATS

The major oral habitats are buccal mucosa, dorsum of the tongue, tooth surfaces (both supragingival and subgingival), crevicular epithelium, and prosthodontic/orthodontic appliances.[20]

Buccal Mucosa and Dorsum of the Tongue

Special features and niches of the oral mucosa contribute to the diversity of the flora; for instance, the cheek mucosa is relatively sparsely colonized, whereas the papillary surface of the tongue is highly colonized because of the safe refuge provided by the papillae. Epithelial desquamation controls the microbial load on mucosal surfaces, although substantial accumulations of bacteria can develop on the tongue. The epithelial desquamatory process is a constant challenge to microbes that live on the

Table 1
Postulated mechanisms by which the resident oral microbiome evades invading extraneous organisms and thereby eventuates colonization resistance

Mechanism	Effect
Production of inhibitory factors (eg, bacteriocins, hydrogen peroxide)	Affect the viability of invading microbes
Production of metabolic end products (eg, short-chain carboxylic acids)	Lower the pH and create unfavorable conditions for the growth of invading microbes
Production of quorum sensing molecules (eg, homoserine lactone, autoinducers)	Maintains the quality and the quantity of the resident bacteria in biofilms and thereby dissuades colonization of invading bacteria
Competition for essential nutrients and cofactors for microbial growth	Develop environments that are not conducive to the establishment of invading organisms
Competition for receptors for microbial adhesion on mucosal (biotic) and dental and prosthetic (abiotic) surfaces	Saturation of receptor by resident microbiota, preventing the attachment of "latecomers"
Coaggregation with the same species (homotypic) or different species (heterotypic) of bacteria	Development and maintenance of multispecies biofilm that reduce the prevalence of single non-coaggregated cells

Modified from Marsh PD, Percival RS. The oral microflora—friend or foe? Can we decide? Int Dent J 2006;56(4 Suppl 1):234; with permission.

mucosal epithelium. The epithelial squames, loaded with bacteria when dislodged into the oral milieu, is swallowed together with the resident bacteria. Hence, the inhabitants of the oral epithelium need to have effective and efficient mechanisms, mainly chemicals called adhesins, to reattach themselves to the newly exposed, virgin epithelial cells devoid of any organisms. This survival battle for microbes is dynamic, constant, and relentless and works in favor of organisms that have the necessary armamentarium to obtain a quick foothold on the epithelial squames.

Teeth

Microbes and their metabolic products accumulate on tooth surfaces to produce dental plaque biofilm, present in both health and disease. The nature of the bacterial community varies depending on the tooth concerned and the degree of exposure to the environment: smooth surfaces are colonized by a smaller number of species than pits and fissures, whereas subgingival surfaces are more anaerobic than supragingival surfaces. Clearly, the surface topography of the tooth as well as the terrain to which the surface is exposed both dictate the composition of the microbiome of that particular niche.

Crevicular Epithelium and Gingival Crevice

Microbes residing in the crevicular epithelium and the gingival crevice play a critical role in the initiation and the propagation of gingival and periodontal disease, the 2 major afflictions of the human kind. Nevertheless, the crevicular epithelium and the gingival crevice comprise only a small area of the oral epithelium in relative terms. The flow of gingival crevicular fluid (GCF) around the gingival margin provides a source of essential nutrients for many obligate anaerobes. In addition, a spectrum of antibodies, and various chemicals such as lysozyme and lactoferrin in the gingival exudate, plays a crucial role in maintaining the homeostasis of the crevicular microbiome that is found in health.

Prosthodontic and Orthodontic Appliances

Dental appliances may act as inanimate reservoirs of bacteria and yeasts. Yeasts on the fitting surface of full dentures can initiate *Candida*-associated denture stomatitis due to poor denture hygiene.[21]

FACTORS MODULATING MICROBIAL GROWTH

Different microenvironments in the mouth support their own microflora, which differ both qualitatively and quantitatively. The reasons for such variations are complex and include anatomic, salivary, crevicular fluid, microbial factors, and environmental factors, among others (**Fig. 3**).

Anatomic Factors

Bacterial stagnation areas are created as a result of the shape and topography of the teeth (eg, occlusal fissures), malalignment of teeth, poor quality of restorations (eg, fillings and bridges), and nonkeratinized sulcular epithelium. All these factors negatively affect the oral hygiene, favoring the accumulation of dental plaque.

Saliva

Whole (mixed) saliva bathing oral surfaces is derived from the major (parotid, submandibular, and sublingual) and minor (labial, lingual, buccal, and palatal) salivary glands. It is a watery substance with a complex mixture of inorganic ions, including sodium,

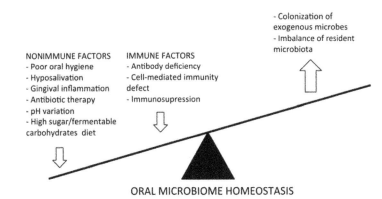

Fig. 3. Dysbiosis of the oral microbiome homeostasis due to immune and nonimmune factors. (*Modified from* Marsh PD, Percival RS. The oral microflora—friend or foe? Can we decide? Int Dent J 2006;56(4 Suppl 1):237; with permission.)

potassium, calcium, chloride, bicarbonate, and phosphate; the concentrations of these ions vary diurnally, and in stimulated and resting saliva. The major organic constituents of saliva are proteins, enzymes, glycoproteins (such as mucin), and antimicrobial agents.

Saliva plays an important role in modulation of bacterial growth. It forms a salivary pellicle on the tooth surface, which is a conditioning film that facilitates bacterial adhesion. The carbohydrates and the proteins of saliva act as a readily available primary source of "food" for bacteria. Growth inhibition of exogenous organisms is also exerted by nonspecific defense factors (eg, lysozyme, lactoferrin, and histatins, which are bactericidal and fungicidal) and specific defense factors (eg, immunoglobulin A, IgA) available in the saliva. The excellent buffering capacity of saliva maintains the pH (6.75–7.25) in optimal conditions for many organisms, besides controlling the local temperature (35–36°C).

Gingival Crevicular Fluid

There is a continuous, although slow flow of crevicular fluid in health, and this increases during inflammatory condition of gingiva (eg, gingivitis). The composition of crevicular fluid is similar to that of serum. The crevicular fluid can influence the ecology of the crevice by flushing microbes out of the crevice (mechanical process) and can act as a primary source of nutrients, like saliva. Proteolytic and saccharolytic bacteria in the crevice use the crevicular fluid to provide peptides, amino acids, and carbohydrates for growth. The GCF also maintains the ideal pH condition for bacteria growth and provides specific and nonspecific defense factors, similar to the serum, with predominance of IgG (IgM and IgA are both present to a lesser extent). The presence of innate immune cells, especially neutrophils, in the gingival crevice helps to protect the periodontal tissue against periodontal pathogens by phagocytosing the microbes or by releasing lysozomal enzymes into the crevicular environment extracellularly.[22]

Microbial Factors

Microbes in the oral environment can interact with each other in both promoting and suppressing the neighboring bacteria using mechanisms described above (see above, section on "Beneficial effects of the resident oral microflora").

Environmental Factors

Various environmental factors, such as temperature, pH, oxidation-reduction (redox) potential, ionic strength, and osmotic pressure, affect the growth and metabolism of microorganisms.[23-27] All these conditions intra oral conditions, especially on tooth surfaces, are not uniform. For instance, the local pH plays an important role in the microbial homeostasis, because many bacteria require a specific pH for growth. The pH of the gingival crevice increases from below neutrality in health to greater than pH 8 in disease,[24] although the acidity of most oral surfaces is regulated by saliva (mean pH 6.7). Depending on the frequency of intake of dietary carbohydrates, the pH of plaque can decrease to as low as 5.0 as a result of bacterial metabolism, changing the composition of the oral microbiome. In turn, the redox potential, is one of the physicochemical parameters characterizing the state of microbial growth. It has great variation in the mouth, and such fluctuations favor the growth of different groups of bacteria. Changes in pH and concentration of the redox active gases (O_2, H_2, and H_2S) are considered to be the major factors governing the growth of microorganisms.[26]

Miscellaneous Factors

During antimicrobial therapy, systemic or topical antibiotics and antiseptics affect the oral flora; for instance, broad-spectrum antibiotics (eg, tetracycline) can wipe out most of the endogenous flora and favor the emergence of yeast species. Thus, candidiasis may supervene after long-term antibiotic therapy.

The host diet is another factor that modulates microbial growth. Diets rich in fermentable carbohydrates promote the growth of acidogenic flora as they act as a major source of nutrients. These carbohydrates are the main class of compounds that alter the oral ecology.

The dentist also interferes with the patient's microbial carriage. Dental procedures, such as dental scaling, can radically alter the composition of the periodontal pocket flora of diseased sites and shift the balance in favor of an oral flora that is associated with health.

Finally, aging has an important influence on the oral microbiome. Conditions inherent to elderly, such as compromised immune systems, reduce salivary flow rate and long-term medications (see **Fig. 2**), may increase their chances of nonoral bacterial contamination (eg, staphylococci and enterobacteria). Hence, a diversity of factors that influence microbial growth affect the complexity of the oral microbiome.

NUTRITION OF THE ORAL MICROBIOME

Oral microorganisms, especially bacteria, use substrates either derived from the host's diet or produced by other bacteria. The pioneer species that colonize oral sites are able to generate end products of metabolism that can then be used by other microorganisms, especially in dense communities such as plaque. **Table 2** summarizes the nutritional resources of oral microflora.

DENTAL PLAQUE BIOFILM

The dental plaque biofilm is a complex, functional community of one or more species of microbes, together with their extracellular products and host compounds mainly derived from the saliva.[28] Note that dental plaque is a biofilm, but not all biofilms are dental plaque.

Table 2	
Nutritional resources available for oral microflora	
Host Resources	**Microbial Resources**
Remnants of the host diet always present in the oral cavity (eg, sucrose, starch)	Extracellular microbial products of the neighboring bacteria
Salivary constituents (eg, glycoproteins, minerals, vitamins)	Intracellular food storage (glycogen) granules
Crevicular exudate (eg, serum proteins and related chemicals, break down products of hemoglobin)	
Inflammatory exudate in periodontal pockets when blood components such as haem are available (mainly for anaerobes)	
Epithelial cell components (byproducts of desquamated epithelial cells may accumulate and may be a source of nutrition)	
Gaseous environment (most require only a very low level of oxygen)	

Distribution

Plaque biofilm is found on dental surfaces and appliances especially in the absence of oral hygiene. In general, it is found in anatomic areas protected from the host defenses and mechanical removal, such as occlusal fissures. Plaque samples are described in relation to their site of origin and are categorized as supragingival, subgingival, or appliance associated (**Table 3**).

Composition

The organisms in dental biofilm are surrounded by an organic matrix, which comprises about 30% of the total volume. The matrix is derived from the products of both the host and the biofilm constituents, and it acts as a food reserve and as a cement, binding organisms both to each other and to various surfaces.[29]

The microbial composition of dental plaque biofilm can vary widely between individuals: some people are rapid plaque-formers; others are slow. Within an individual, there are also large variations in plaque composition (**Table 4**). These variations may occur at different sites on the same tooth, at the same site on different teeth, or at different times on the same tooth site.[30]

Formation

The dental biofilm formation is a complex process comprising several stages. The first step is the pellicle formation, where adsorption of host and bacterial molecules to the

Table 3		
Plaque biofilm distribution		
Supragingival	**Subgingival**	**Appliance-Associated**
Fissure plaque (mainly in molar fissures)	Gingival crevice	Full and partial dentures (denture plaque)
Approximal plaque (contact points of teeth)		Orthodontic appliance-related plaque
Smooth surface (buccal and palatal surfaces)		

Table 4
Composition of dental biofilms at different tooth sites

Bacteria	Dental Sites		
	Fissures	Proximal Surfaces	Gingival Crevice
Streptococcus	+	+	+
Actinomyces	+	+	+
Neisseria	+/−	+	+
Veillonella	+	+	+
Treponema	−	−	+
An G+ rod	+	+	+
An G− rod	+/−	+	+

Abbreviations: +, presence; −, absence; +/−, detected occasionally; An G+ rod, obligate anaerobe gram-positive rods; An G− rod, obligate anaerobe gram-negative rods.
Modified from Fejerskov O, Nyvad B, Kidd E. Biofilms in caries development. Dental caries: the disease and its clinical management. 3rd edition. Wiley-Blackwell; 2015. p. 107–31; with permission.

tooth surface forms an acquired salivary layer. The pellicle formation starts within hours after cleaning the tooth, and it is composed of salivary glycoproteins, phospho-proteins, lipids, and components of gingival crevice fluid. Remnants of cell walls of dead bacteria and other microbial products (eg, glucosyltransferases and glucans) are also part of the pellicle. This stage is essential for the plaque formation, because the oral bacteria do not directly colonize the mineralized tooth surface; they initially attach to this pellicle. Salivary molecules alter their conformation after binding to the tooth surface, exposing receptors for bacteria attachment. These receptors interact with bacterial surface adhesins in a very specific manner that explains the selective adherence of bacterial to enamel.

The transport of bacteria to the vicinity of the tooth surface before attachment occurs by means of either natural salivary flow, Brownian motion, or chemotaxis. The proximity to mineralized surface allows the attachment of pioneer microbes (0–24 hours). This important group of bacteria comprises gram-positive cocci and rods, mainly streptococcal species (*S sanguinis, S oralis,* and *S mitis*), and to a lesser extent, *Actinomyces* spp and gram-negative bacteria (eg, *Haemophillus* spp and *Neisseria* spp).

Initially, interaction between the microbial cell surface and the pellicle-coated tooth involve weak physicochemical forces (van der Waals forces and electrostatic repulsion), which represents a reversible phase of net adhesion. These interactions may rapidly become strong stereochemical reactions between adhesins on the microbial cell surface and receptors on the acquired pellicle. This phase is an irreversible phase in which polymer bridging between organisms and the surface helps to anchor the organism, after which the organisms multiply on the virgin surface. Doubling times of plaque bacteria can vary considerably (from minutes to hours), both between different bacterial species and between members of the same species, depending on the environmental conditions.

After the establishment of initial colonizers, the next stage involves the coadhesion and growth of attached bacteria, leading to the formation of distinct microcolonies (4–24 hours). During this phase, the biofilm is not uniform in thickness, varying from sparsely colonized to almost full surface coverage. The biofilm grows basically by cells division, with the development of columnar microcolonies perpendicular to the tooth surface.[31] Within 1 day, the tooth surface is almost completely covered by a blanket of microorganisms.

Some constituents of the dental plaque produce components of the biofilm matrix, such as polysaccharides. The biofilm matrix, in turn, not only gives support for the structure of the biofilm but also is also biologically involved in retaining nutrients, water, and enzymes within the biofilm.[32]

Between 24 and 48 hours, the biofilm becomes thicker. Adhesins expressed by the secondary colonizers bind to receptors on the cell surface of pioneer microbes, producing a coaggregation or coadhesion of microorganisms. This continuous adsorption of planktonic microbes from saliva, in addition to cell division, contributes to the expansion of the biofilm. In the surface layer, coaggregation of different species creates "corncob" structures.

As the dental biofilm develops, the metabolism of the initial colonizers modifies the environment in the developing biofilm, creating a local condition that is either more attractive to later (secondary) colonizers or increasingly unfavorable to the pioneer group, for example, by making it more anaerobic after their consumption of oxygen or accumulating inhibitory metabolic products.[1]

All these environmental changes lead to a gradual replacement of the initial colonizers by other bacteria more suited to the modified habitat; this process is termed microbial succession (1–7 days). This sequence of events increases species diversity in the dental plaque, concomitant with continued growth of microcolonies.

A progressive shift is observed from mainly aerobic and facultatively anaerobic species (mainly *Streptococcus*) in the early stages of biofilm formation to a situation with predominance of facultatively and obligately anaerobic organisms, gram-negative cocci and rods, fusobacteria, spirochetes, and actinobacteria (especially *Actinomyces*) after 9 days.

A mature biofilm can be found after 1 week or more. The plaque mass reaches a critical size at which a balance between the deposition and loss of plaque bacteria is established, characterizing a climax community. In an old biofilm, structural changes can be seen at the bottom of the dental plaque, for example. The most significant change is the formation of a dense inner layer of pleomorphic *Actinomyces* next to the enamel of root surface. The outer part of a mature biofilm is usually loosely structured with various compositions, from sphere-shape distribution of one type of organism to multispecies outer microflora with parallel distribution.[33]

The bacteria that colonize this climax community may detach and enter the planktonic phase (ie, suspended in saliva) and be transported to new colonization sites, thus restarting the whole cycle.

The colonization of root surfaces follows similar principles to those outlined for enamel surfaces. However, the development of plaque on root surfaces occurs more rapidly due to the uneven surface topography. Despite this difference, regardless of the type of tooth surface, enamel and cementum share the same initial colonizers.

Properties

The oral biofilms function as microbial community and collectively display properties that favor their formation and persistence in the oral cavity (**Table 5**). Many of these properties make the microorganisms within a biofilm more resistant to drugs (antibiotic, antifungals) in comparison to their planktonic counterparts.[34] In the biofilm, microbial cells interact both with each other via cell signaling systems and with other species through conventional synergistic and antagonistic biochemical interactions (see **Table 1**).

Table 5
Properties of dental biofilms

Property	Dental Biofilm Example
Open architecture	Presence of water channel
Protection from host defense	Protection from phagocytosis
Enhanced resistance to antimicrobials	Transfer of resistance genes, mutual protection within the biofilm
Neutralization of inhibitors	Catalase production to protect from hydrogen peroxide
Alteration of gene expression	Increase expression of genes associated with drug resistance
Cell-cell signaling (quorum sensing)	Production of signaling molecules to coordinate gene expression
Broader habitat range	Obligate anaerobes grow in an aerobic environment
More efficient metabolism	Development of microbial food webs
Enhanced virulence	Pathogenic synergism in abscesses

Modified from Fejerskov O, Nyvad B, Kidd E. Biofilms in caries development. Dental caries: the disease and its clinical management. 3rd edition. Wiley-Blackwell; 2015. p. 107–31; with permission.

Cell-cell communication and coordinated population-based behavior among members of a biofilm involve quorum sensing, a system of signaling molecules (eg, homoserine lactone, autoinducers 1) that increases according to the cell density. This ability to send, receive, and process information allows organisms within microbial communities to act as multicellular entities and increases their chances of survival in complex environments.[35]

CALCULUS

Dental calculus is a dental biofilm that suffers a mineralization process due to the precipitation of mineral salts, although not all the biofilm becomes calcified.

Formation

When the plaque biofilm is allowed to grow undisturbed, the degenerating bacteria in a climax community may act as seeding agents of mineralization. Calcium and phosphate ions derived from saliva and GCF may become deposited within deeper layers of dental plaque. The calcification is accelerated by bacterial phosphatases and proteases that degrade some of the calcification inhibitors in saliva (statherin and proline-rich proteins). These processes lead to the formation of insoluble mineral crystals that coalesce to form a highly calcified mass, which is an inorganic content that is similar to bone, dentine, and cementum.[36] The crystals develop initially in the intercellular matrix and on the bacterial surfaces and then finally within the bacteria.[37] The surface of calculus always remains covered by a layer of noncalcified dental plaque biofilm.

Crystal formation establishes a firm adhesion of the calculus to the tooth surfaces. These mineral crystals fill the pits and irregularities of the tooth surface, following the contours of the enamel, cementum, and dentin.[38]

Classification

Calculus, like dental plaque, can be classified as supragingival, which is found coronal to the gingival margin, and subgingival calculus, located apical to the gingival margin, thus not visible on routine clinical examination. The subgingival calculus is affected by hemorrhagic components from the GCF, and the mineralization of anaerobic microorganisms brings the characteristic black pigmentation of this type of calculus. In turn, the supragingival calculus is influenced by saliva, food pigments, and tobacco, presenting a rather claylike consistency.[38] Supragingival calculus is mainly observed on the buccal surfaces of the maxillary molars and the lingual surfaces of the mandibular anterior teeth, as the flow from the salivary gland in these areas favors the deposit of calcium and phosphate ions derived from saliva. By contrast, subgingival calculus is mainly found on the interproximal and lingual tooth surfaces, being randomly distributed throughout the mouth.[36]

Composition

Approximately 80% (dry weight) of calculus is mineralized material (hydroxyapatite) and 20% comprise organic compounds. The inorganic part of both supragingival and subgingival dental calculus consists mainly of calcium phosphate mineral salts, which form crystals of hydroxyapatite, magnesium whitlockite, octacalcim phosphate, and brushite.[38] Supragingival calculus is heterogeneous, with islets of mineralized material and nonmineralized areas within the calculus. Further, the subgingival calculus is somewhat more homogeneously calcified, with a mineralized area within the calculus itself covered by an unmineralized bacterial layer.

The organic compound of calculus includes desquamated epithelial cells, leukocytes, and various types of microorganisms. The predominant flora is cocci, bacilli, and filaments (especially in the outer layers), and occasionally, spiral organisms. The supragingival calculus has more gram-positive organisms; gram-negative species in turn are more present in subgingival calculus. Calculus also has an organic matrix, which is less extensive in subgingival calculus, and consists of proteins, lipids, and carbohydrates. The rough surface and porosity of dental calculus serve as an ideal reservoir for bacterial toxins (eg, lipopolysaccharides) harmful to the periodontium.

The composition and formation of calculus is unique to each individual: heavy, moderate, slight calculus formers, and noncalculus formers can be found throughout the populace. Calculus deposition can also vary from site to site and over time,[39] being influenced by a great variety of variables (**Fig. 4**).[40]

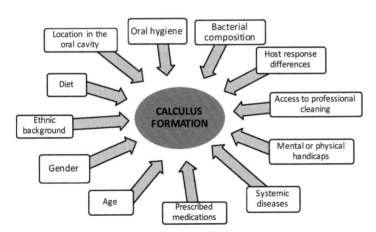

Fig. 4. Factors affecting dental calculus formation.

Box 1	
Proposed mechanisms linking oral infections to secondary systemic disease	
Metastatic infection	Microbes gain entry into the circulatory system through breaches in the oral vascular barrier (bacteremias)
Metastatic injury	Products of bacteria (cytolytic enzymes, exotoxins, and endotoxins) gain access to the cardiovascular system in individuals suffering from periodontitis
Metastatic inflammation	Soluble antigens enter the bloodstream from the oral route, react with circulating specific antibodies, and form macromolecular complexes, leading to immune-mediated disease such as Behçet syndrome (immunologic injury)

Adapted from Parahitiyawa NB, Jin LJ, Leung WK, et al. Microbiology of odontogenic bacteremia: beyond endocarditis. Clin Microbiol Rev 2009;22(1):46–64.

THE ROLE OF ORAL FLORA IN SYSTEMIC INFECTION

The plaque-related oral diseases, especially periodontitis, may alter the course and pathogenesis of several systemic diseases. This relates to a common belief called "focal infection theory" states that localized infection, often asymptomatic, may disseminate microorganisms or their toxins to distant sites within the body and thereby cause disease.

Microbial pathogens associated with periodontal disease have been shown to contribute to atherosclerosis (coronary heart disease) by causing deregulation of the immune system, progressive inflammation, and consequently, disruption of endothelial cell function, one of the earliest indicators of cardiovascular disease.[41] Dental calculus and poor oral hygiene have also been associated with atherosclerosis that led to stroke and death from heart infarction.[42,43]

Bacteria that colonize teeth may cause infective endocarditis.[44] This is because poor oral hygiene and dental disease increase the likelihood for bacteremias during dental procedures, such as tooth extractions, or even tooth-brushing (**Box 1**). Thus, antibiotic prophylaxis and improvements in oral hygiene may reduce the risk of developing infective endocarditis.[45] The aspiration of organism from dental plaque biofilm may also cause bacterial pneumonia, especially in hospitalized patients.[46]

Periodontitis is commonly associated with diabetes mellitus; however, the "2-way relationship" between diabetes and periodontal disease is still unclear. It is thought that proinflammatory mediators, such as interleukin-6 and tumor necrosis factor-α, produced in response to microbial stimulus in periodontal disease sites may reach the systemic circulation and interfere with the function of insulin receptors (see **Box 1**). These events, in turn, would contribute to insulin resistance and impaired glucose homeostasis.[47]

Maternal periodontal disease represents another risk factor, in this case for the baby's health. Pregnancy affected by periodontitis may be more susceptible to preterm birth and low birth weight of neonates.[48] These pregnancy outcomes could potentially be influenced by periodontal disease through indirect mechanisms involving inflammatory cytokines or direct translocation of bacteria and its products to the fetoplacental unit (see **Box 1**).[49]

SUMMARY

The oral ecosystem comprises the oral flora, so-called oral microbiome, the different anatomic microniches of the oral cavity and its bathing fluid, saliva. The oral microbiome comprises a diverse group of organisms and includes bacteria, archaea, fungi, protozoa, and viruses. The oral microbiome exists either suspended in saliva as planktonic phase organisms or attached to oral surfaces essentially as a plaque biofilm. The homeostasis of the plaque biofilm and its symbiotic relationship with the host is critical for oral health. The disequilibrium or dysbiosis within the plaque biofilms is the initiating event that leads to major oral diseases, such as caries and periodontal disease.

REFERENCES

1. Marsh PD. Microbiology of dental plaque biofilms and their role in oral health and caries. Dent Clin North Am 2010;54(3):441–54.
2. Dewhirst FE, Chen T, Izard J, et al. The human oral microbiome. J Bacteriol 2010; 192(19):5002–17.
3. Simon-Soro A, Tomas I, Cabrera-Rubio R, et al. Microbial geography of the oral cavity. J Dent Res 2013;92(7):616–21.
4. Kleinberg I, Jenkins GN. The pH of dental plaques in the different areas of the mouth before and after meals and their relationship to the pH and rate of flow of resting saliva. Arch Oral Biol 1964;9:493–516.
5. Moore WE, Moore LV. The bacteria of periodontal diseases. Periodontol 2000 1994;5:66–77.
6. Ding T, Schloss PD. Dynamics and associations of microbial community types across the human body. Nature 2014;509(7500):357–60.
7. Nasidze I, Li J, Quinque D, et al. Global diversity in the human salivary microbiome. Genome Res 2009;19(4):636–43.
8. Matsubara VH, Bandara HM, Mayer MP, et al. Probiotics as antifungals in mucosal candidiasis. Clin Infect Dis 2016;62(9):1143–53.
9. Marsh PD. Dental plaque as a microbial biofilm. Caries Res 2004;38(3):204–11.
10. Kononen E, Asikainen S, Saarela M, et al. The oral gram-negative anaerobic microflora in young children: longitudinal changes from edentulous to dentate mouth. Oral Microbiol Immunol 1994;9(3):136–41.
11. Moore WE, Burmeister JA, Brooks CN, et al. Investigation of the influences of puberty, genetics, and environment on the composition of subgingival periodontal floras. Infect Immun 1993;61(7):2891–8.
12. Ashley FP, Gallagher J, Wilson RF. The occurrence of Actinobacillus actinomycetemcomitans, Bacteroides gingivalis, Bacteroides intermedius and spirochaetes in the subgingival microflora of adolescents and their relationship with the amount of supragingival plaque and gingivitis. Oral Microbiol Immunol 1988;3(2):77–82.
13. Yang F, Zeng X, Ning K, et al. Saliva microbiomes distinguish caries-active from healthy human populations. ISME J 2012;6(1):1–10.
14. Van Winkelhoff AJ, Boutaga K. Transmission of periodontal bacteria and models of infection. J Clin Periodontol 2005;32(Suppl 6):16–27.
15. Marsh PD, Percival RS. The oral microflora—friend or foe? Can we decide? Int Dent J 2006;56(4 Suppl 1):233–9.
16. Percival RS, Challacombe SJ, Marsh PD. Age-related microbiological changes in the salivary and plaque microflora of healthy adults. J Med Microbiol 1991;35(1): 5–11.
17. Caufield PW, Cutter GR, Dasanayake AP. Initial acquisition of mutans streptococci by infants: evidence for a discrete window of infectivity. J Dent Res 1993; 72(1):37–45.

18. Caufield PW, Dasanayake AP, Li Y, et al. Natural history of Streptococcus sangui-
    nis in the oral cavity of infants: evidence for a discrete window of infectivity. Infect
    Immun 2000;68(7):4018–23.
19. Topoll HH, Lange DE, Muller RF. Multiple periodontal abscesses after systemic
    antibiotic therapy. J Clin Periodontol 1990;17(4):268–72.
20. Marsh PD, Martin MV. Oral microbiology. 5th edition. London: Butterworth-Heine-
    mann; 2009.
21. Samaranayake LP, Ellepola ANB. Studying Candida albicans adhesion. In: An Y,
    Freidman RJ, editors. Handbook of bacterial adhesion: principles, methods and
    applications. New York: Humana Press; 2000. p. 527–40.
22. Socransky SS, Haffajee AD. Microbial mechanisms in the pathogenesis of
    destructive periodontal diseases: a critical assessment. J Periodontal Res
    1991;26(3 Pt 2):195–212.
23. Fey A, Conrad R. Effect of temperature on carbon and electron flow and on the
    archaeal community in methanogenic rice field soil. Appl Environ Microbiol
    2000;66(11):4790–7.
24. McDermid AS, McKee AS, Marsh PD. Effect of environmental pH on enzyme ac-
    tivity and growth of Bacteroides gingivalis W50. Infect Immun 1988;56(5):
    1096–100.
25. Lloret J, Bolanos L, Lucas MM, et al. Ionic stress and osmotic pressure induce
    different alterations in the lipopolysaccharide of a Rhizobium meliloti strain.
    Appl Environ Microbiol 1995;61(10):3701–4.
26. Oktyabrskii ON, Smirnovaa GV. Redox potential changes in bacterial cultures un-
    der stress conditions. Microbiology 2012;81(2):131–42.
27. Otto K, Elwing H, Hermansson M. Effect of ionic strength on initial interactions of
    Escherichia coli with surfaces, studied on-line by a novel quartz crystal microbal-
    ance technique. J Bacteriol 1999;181(17):5210–8.
28. Lang NP, Mombelli A, Attstrom R. Dental plaque and calculus. Clinical periodon-
    tology and implant dentistry. 3rd edition. Oxford (United Kingdom): Blackwell
    Munksgaard; 1997.
29. Listgarten MA. The structure of dental plaque. Periodontol 2000 1994;5:52–65.
30. Fejerskov O, Nyvad B, Kidd E. Biofilms in caries development. Dental caries: the
    disease and its clinical management. 3rd edition. Oxford: Wiley-Blackwell; 2015.
    p. 107–31.
31. Dige I, Nilsson H, Kilian M, et al. In situ identification of streptococci and other
    bacteria in initial dental biofilm by confocal laser scanning microscopy and fluo-
    rescence in situ hybridization. Eur J Oral Sci 2007;115(6):459–67.
32. Branda SS, Vik S, Friedman L, et al. Biofilms: the matrix revisited. Trends Micro-
    biol 2005;13(1):20–6.
33. Nyvad B, Kilian M. Microbiology of the early colonization of human enamel and
    root surfaces in vivo. Scand J Dent Res 1987;95(5):369–80.
34. Bowden GH, Hamilton IR. Survival of oral bacteria. Crit Rev Oral Biol Med 1998;
    9(1):54–85.
35. Hooshangi S, Bentley WE. From unicellular properties to multicellular behavior:
    bacteria quorum sensing circuitry and applications. Curr Opin Biotechnol 2008;
    19(6):550–5.
36. Roberts-Harry EA, Clerehugh V. Subgingival calculus: where are we now? A
    comparative review. J Dent 2000;28(2):93–102.
37. Zander HA, Hazen SP, Scott DB. Mineralization of dental calculus. Proc Soc Exp
    Biol Med 1960;103:257–60.

38. Jepsen S, Deschner J, Braun A, et al. Calculus removal and the prevention of its formation. Periodontol 2000 2011;55(1):167–88.
39. Corbett TL, Dawes C. A comparison of the site-specificity of supragingival and subgingival calculus deposition. J Periodontol 1998;69(1):1–8.
40. White DJ. Dental calculus: recent insights into occurrence, formation, prevention, removal and oral health effects of supragingival and subgingival deposits. Eur J Oral Sci 1997;105(5 Pt 2):508–22.
41. Slocum C, Kramer C, Genco CA. Immune dysregulation mediated by the oral microbiome: potential link to chronic inflammation and atherosclerosis. J Intern Med 2016;280(1):114–28.
42. Soder B, Meurman JH, Soder PO. Dental calculus is associated with death from heart infarction. Biomed Res Int 2014;2014:1–5.
43. Dai R, Lam OL, Lo EC, et al. A systematic review and meta-analysis of clinical, microbiological, and behavioural aspects of oral health among patients with stroke. J Dent 2015;43(2):171–80.
44. Parahitiyawa NB, Jin LJ, Leung WK, et al. Microbiology of odontogenic bacteremia: beyond endocarditis. Clin Microbiol Rev 2009;22(1):46–64.
45. Lockhart PB, Brennan MT, Thornhill M, et al. Poor oral hygiene as a risk factor for infective endocarditis-related bacteremia. J Am Dent Assoc 2009;140(10):1238–44.
46. Ewan VC, Sails AD, Walls AW, et al. Dental and microbiological risk factors for hospital-acquired pneumonia in non-ventilated older patients. PLoS One 2015;10(4):e0123622.
47. Gurav AN. Periodontitis and insulin resistance: casual or causal relationship? Diabetes Metab J 2012;36(6):404–11.
48. Ide M, Papapanou PN. Epidemiology of association between maternal periodontal disease and adverse pregnancy outcomes–systematic review. J Clin Periodontol 2013;40(Suppl 14):S181–94.
49. Pitiphat W, Joshipura KJ, Gillman MW, et al. Maternal periodontitis and adverse pregnancy outcomes. Community Dent Oral Epidemiol 2008;36(1):3–11.

Epidemiology of Oral and Maxillofacial Infections

Arvind Babu Rajendra Santosh, BDS, MDS[a],*, Orrett E. Ogle, DDS[b,c,d],
Dwight Williams, DDS[d], Edward F. Woodbine, DDS[e]

KEYWORDS

- Dental caries • Gingivitis • Periodontitis • Odontogenic infections
- Oral mucosal infections • Antibiotic resistance • Microbe-related oral cancer

KEY POINTS

- Educating dentists on the epidemiologic information of dental caries, gingivitis, periodontitis, odontogenic infections, oral mucosal infections, and microbial-related oral cancer.
- Predominant types of microbes associated with periodontal pockets and odontogenic infections.
- Treatment options and prevention strategies of methicillin-resistant *Staphylococcus aureus* for dental and oral surgery practice.
- Human papilloma virus (HPV) -associated oropharyngeal cancer rates in United States population.
- Prevalence of HPV-associated oropharyngeal cancer in human immunodeficiency virus–infected individuals in United States.

INTRODUCTION

Epidemiologic studies usually provide information on determinants, occurrence, and distribution of health and disease in a defined population. The 3 major links in disease occurrence are etiologic agent, method of transmission, and the host. The different epidemiologic methods are descriptive, analytical, and experimental studies. The general factors that influence the occurrence of infectious disease are the following:

1. Pathogenic agent
2. Host

Disclosure Statement: The authors have nothing to disclose.
[a] Dentistry Programme, Faculty of Medical Sciences, The University of the West Indies, Mona Campus, Kingston 7, Jamaica, West Indies; [b] Atlanta, GA, USA; [c] Dentistry Program, The University of the West Indies, Mona, Jamaica, West Indies; [d] Oral and Maxillofacial Surgery, Woodhull Hospital, Brooklyn, NY, USA; [e] Department of Dentistry/Oral and Maxillofacial Surgery, Woodhull Medical Center, 760 Broadway, Brooklyn, NY 11206, USA
* Corresponding author.
E-mail address: arvindbabu2001@gmail.com

Dent Clin N Am 61 (2017) 217–233
http://dx.doi.org/10.1016/j.cden.2016.11.003
dental.theclinics.com

3. Disease transmission
4. Environment

Epidemiology of dental disease is important when trying to understand the clinical and the public health impact of the disease as well as providing data for assessing methods of controlling this disease. To comprehend the disease process and how it affects different groups of society, one needs to know the distribution of the disease in various communities. Dental caries and periodontal diseases are common in industrialized countries and have been increasing worldwide. A fact sheet on oral health published by the World Health Organization (WHO) in 2012 revealed dental health data focused on dental caries, periodontal disease, edentulousness, socioeconomic, and other risk factors. The key facts of WHO are given in **Box 1**. WHO mentioned that the most common oral diseases are dental caries, periodontal disease, oral infectious diseases, oral cancer, trauma from injuries, and hereditary lesions.[1]

This article outlines the epidemiology of oral and maxillofacial infections, such as:

1. Dental caries
2. Gingivitis
3. Periodontitis
4. Odontogenic infections
5. Oral mucosal infections
6. Microbial-related oral cancer

The epidemiology of antibiotics resistance in oral infections and specifically as it relates to methicillin-resistant *Staphylococcus aureus* (MRSA) in dental and oral surgery practice completes the article.

EPIDEMIOLOGY OF DENTAL CARIES

Dental caries is considered the most prevalent oral disease and the main cause for tooth loss among all populations.[2] It is an infectious disease caused by bacterial strains that coexist in the oral cavity, mainly *Streptococcus mutans* and Lactobacillus. Epidemiologic studies have clearly established that social, economic, cultural, ethnic, and environmental factors play an important role in the formation of dental caries and also influence the individual oral microflora related to oral health.[3,4]

The decayed, missing, filled (DMF) index is used as the key measure of caries occurrence in dental epidemiology. Data from the DMF table published by FDI (Federation

---

Box 1
World Health Organization key facts on dental health

- Worldwide, 60% to 90% of school children and nearly 100% of adults have dental cavities.
- Severe periodontal disease is found in 15% to 20% of middle-aged (35–44 years) adults.
- Globally, about 30% of people aged 65 to 74 have no natural teeth.
- Oral disease in children and adults is higher among poor and disadvantaged population groups.
- Risk factors for oral diseases include an unhealthy diet, tobacco use, harmful alcohol use, poor oral hygiene, and social determinants.

From World Health Organization (WHO). Oral health: fact sheet No. 318. April 2012. Available at: http://www.who.int/mediacentre/factsheets/fs318/en/; with permission.

Dental International) World Dental Federation, Cointrin, Switzerland[5] showed DMF values in permanent teeth of 12-year-old children ranging from 0.3 (Rwanda, Tanzania, Togo) to 7.8 (Serbia) with a global average of 2.0. The DMF in the United States for this population was 1.2. There were high DMF indices in most countries of South America (3.0), Northern Europe, and South Asia, whereas a significant proportion of African countries have low rates of caries.[6] One hundred percent of people in China between the years of 5 and 74 have experienced caries (Deyu Hu: Oral presentation: dental caries trends in China from a review of three national health surveys. Chinese Society of Preventive Dentistry, Chinese Stomatological Association, unpublished data, 2008). It should be noted that caries levels tend to increase with age and is a problematic public health issue in adults. The DMF in the US adult population is 6.2 in the 20- to 34-year-old age group, 10.9 in the 35- to 49-year-old age group, and 15.1 in the 50- to 64-year-old age group (National Institutes of Health).

The research studies on caries epidemiology are usually reported by DMFT (ie, decayed-missing-filled teeth) or DMFS (decayed-missing-filled surfaces) method. Most of the prevalence studies are reported based on visual clinical examination of the carious tooth that is extended to the dentino-enamel junction. Few studies reported caries prevalence with both visual clinical examination and radiographic methods. In recent reports, the International Caries Detection and Assessment System is becoming more evident in epidemiologic research. The detection of dental caries is achieved by the following:

1. Stage of the carious process
2. Topography (pit and fissure or smooth surfaces)
3. Anatomy (crown vs roots)
4. Restoration or restorations or sealant status

The assessment of caries teeth is checked by noncavitated or cavitated tooth; activity of the carious tooth is analyzed by active or arrested cavities. The International Caries Detection and Assessment System has been shown to reliable in detecting coronal dental caries; however, assessment of root caries has not yet been tested in epidemiologic or clinical studies.[7]

EPIDEMIOLOGY OF GINGIVITIS

The inflammation of gingival mucosa is termed gingivitis and is characterized by inflammatory changes, such as redness and swelling of associated gingival mucosa, and is often associated with bleeding from the gingival crevice upon mild mechanical stimulus. US Nation Survey data show that gingivitis is found in early childhood, is more prevalent and severe in adolescence, and then tends to level off in older age groups. US National Survey reported that frequency of gingivitis among school children has ranged from 40% to 60%. US National Survey among employed adults in 1985 to 1986 reported 47% of men and 39% of women aged 18 to 64 exhibited bleeding on probing at least one site. In the third National Health and Nutrition Examination Survey (NHANES III, 1988–1994), gingivitis was identified in 50% of adults on at least 3 or 4 teeth.[8] Hispanic Health and Nutrition Examination Survey (2009–2010) showed that Hispanics in the United States had a higher prevalence of gingivitis than Caucasian adults in United States.[9] Plaque deposits are significantly correlated with the association of gingivitis and are considered as cause and effect.[10] Research studies from developing countries also show that gingivitis is correlated with extensive plaque and calculus association and is the norm among the adult population.[11,12]

EPIDEMIOLOGY OF PERIODONTITIS

The WHO fact sheet noted that severe periodontal disease is found globally in 15% to 20% of middle-aged (35–44 years) adults.[1] A study titled, Prevalence of Periodontitis in Adults in the United States: 2009 and 2010, estimates that 47.2%, or 64.7 million adults, had periodontitis, distributed as 8.7%, 30.0%, and 8.5% with mild, moderate, and severe periodontitis, respectively. These data determine that the milder forms of periodontitis (38.7% or 82% of the total) are more common. The more severe manifestations of the disease, those that lead to tooth loss, are less prevalent.[13]

The WHO reports that severe periodontitis, which may result in tooth loss, is found in 5% to 15% of most populations. Juvenile or early-onset aggressive periodontitis, a severe periodontal condition affecting individuals during puberty that leads to premature tooth loss, affects about 2% of youth.[1] In US adults aged 65 and older, prevalence rates increase to 70.1%. Periodontitis was highest in men, Mexican Americans, adults with less than a high school education, and adults below the 100% Federal Poverty Levels.[13] The Centers for Disease Control and Prevention (CDC) estimates high periodontal disease prevalence in the southern states of the United States.

Periodontitis results from a complex interaction between bacterial infection and host response, often modified by behavioral factors.[14] The host response is the key factor in the clinical expression of periodontitis,[15] with only some 20% of periodontal diseases attributed to bacterial infection.[14] Some 50% of periodontal diseases have also been attributed to genetic variance.[14]

It has long been known that gram-negative anaerobes were the primary pathogens in periodontal pockets. More recently, with better microbiological isolation of bacteria, it has been shown that at periodontal disease sites there are several recognized pathogens that are consistently present. The predominant groups of microorganisms associated in periodontal pocket are listed[16–18] in **Box 2**. The presence of specific microbiota, however, does not predict the development or progression of periodontitis in clinical longitudinal studies for up to 3 years.[19]

In industrialized countries, studies show that smoking is a major risk factor for adult periodontal disease, responsible for more than half of the periodontitis cases among the 35 to 44 age group.[1]

EPIDEMIOLOGY OF ODONTOGENIC INFECTIONS

Odontogenic infections are prevalent worldwide with most being secondary to dental caries, periodontal disease (gingivitis and periodontitis), and endodontic infections and associated with local (tooth loss) or systemic implications.

Box 2
Predominant microbes associated with periodontal pockets

Actinomyces actinomycetemcomitans

Bacteroides forsythus (now *Tannerella forsythensis*)

Porphyromonas gingivalis

Prevotella intermedia

Fusobacterium nucleatum

Campylobacter rectus

Treponema denticola

Surveillance data from the United States (1988–1994 and 1999–2002) show that 25% of the adult population older than 60 years of age have complete edentulism, due to periodontal disease in one-half of the population and other half from dental caries.[20]

The microbial species/phylotypes commonly found in odontogenic infections are listed in **Box 3**. These infections can spread beyond the oral cavity and result in potentially life-threatening complications, such as spread of to the deep fascial spaces of the head and neck, airway obstruction, and septicemia. Almost 60% of all nontraumatic dental emergencies are associated with acute apical abscesses and toothaches.[21]

A nationwide Emergency Department survey of 450 hospitals in 27 US states in 2007 showed 302,507 visits attributed to facial cellulitis from dental origin.[22] Another nationwide inpatient sample taken in 2008 from 1056 hospitals in 42 US states showed 4044 hospital discharges with a primary diagnosis of mouth abscess/cellulitis, accounting for $98 million of hospitalization charges at a mean hospital charge of $24,290 per patient.[23]

Despite the progress made in treating dental caries, a great number of untreated caries that lead to dental abscesses persist in deprived low- and middle-income communities within the United States, and to a greater extent in poor developing countries, where people have little access to even the most basic forms of dental care. In many developing countries, access to oral health services is limited and teeth are often left untreated or are extracted because of pain or abscess formation. There are no good reports or estimates, however, on the incidence of dental abscesses. The last decade has seen a notable change in the behavior of odontogenic infections. The severity of these infections is far greater than in the past, with a more rapid and dramatic spread through the fascial planes surrounding the airways. The length of hospitalization for patients with these infections has also increased.[24]

In addition to bacterial organisms, fungal, protozoal, and viral infections also affect the oral cavity. Almost half (40%–50%) of the 35 million people living with human immunodeficiency virus (HIV) suffer from oral fungal, bacterial, or viral infections. Africa and Asia have the highest prevalence of HIV/AIDS, and oral manifestations, mainly Candida infections, are widespread.[1]

EPIDEMIOLOGY OF ANTIBIOTICS RESISTANCE IN ORAL INFECTIONS

Dentists in the United States prescribe between 7% and 11% of all common antibiotics (betalactams, macrolides, tetracyclines, clindamycin, metronidazole).[25] However, the National Centers for Disease Control and Prevention estimates that

Box 3
Predominant type of microbes associated with odontogenic infections
Fusobacterium
Parvimonas
Prevotella
Porphyromonas
Dialister
Streptococcus
Treponema

approximately one-third of all outpatient antibiotic prescriptions are unnecessary.[26] Some of the unnecessary uses of antibiotics were for toothaches, periapical infection, and dry socket, conditions that should be treated with dental interventions rather than with antibiotics. The increasing resistance to antibiotics seen in recent years is thought to be related to overuse or misuse of broad-spectrum antibiotics. Currently, there now are bacterial species that are resistant to several of the antibiotics that previously were used with great success. MRSA is one such bacterium with extensive resistance.

The oral cavity is colonized by more than 700 species of bacteria, fungi, and protozoa, of which only about 10% are regularly isolated using conventional culture techniques, with the α-hemolytic streptococci being among the most frequent isolates. Other bacteria found in the oral commensal flora include coagulase-negative staphylococci, gram-negative cocci belonging to the families Neisseriaceae and Veillonellaceae, lactobacilli, spirochaetes, corynebacteria, and mycoplasmas. Bacteria that are potentially pathogenic and that are occasionally found in the oral cavity include S aureus, Enterococcus faecalis, Streptococcus pyogenes, members of the family Enterobacteriaceae, Haemophilus influenzae, and actinomycetes.[27]

In clinical practice, the penicillins (Pen V, Amoxicillin, Ampicillin) are the first-line antibiotic for the treatment of odontogenic infections. Increasing rates of penicillin resistance and treatment failures have been reported. The highest rates of penicillin resistance have been observed with the members of the genus Bacteroides and Prevotella.[28] Clindamycin, an alternative to the penicillins, has shown a resistance of less than 10% by Prevotella, Fusobacterium, Porphyromonas, and Peptostreptococcus organisms.[29] No resistance has been reported with metronidazole.

Epidemiology of Methicillin-Resistant Staphylococcus aureus in Dental and Oral Maxillofacial Surgery Practice

Beginning in the 1960s with the initial outbreak in Europe, MRSA has been a health challenge within hospitals and affected communities. Infections by MRSA (and methicillin-sensitive Staphylococcus aureus [MSSA]) commonly result in local skin and soft tissue infections (SSTIs), but the increasing prevalence and virulence of these organisms can result in life-threatening infections, so it is imperative that the significance and impact be understood. S aureus, commonly termed Staph, has been identified since the 1880s wherein it has been the primary culprit in SSTIs, such as scalded skin syndrome, boils, impetigo, bacterial pneumonia, and severe life-threatening bloodstream infections. In recent times, up to 40% of the normal population carries S aureus in the anterior nares, and even higher rates in hospitalized patients and their attendants.[30] In 1940, the discovery of penicillin resulted in the formation of penicillin-resistant (beta-lactamase-producing) organisms and subsequent hospital-acquired infections that ultimately have reached nonhospitalized communities. The production of multiple synthetic and semisynthetic derivatives to address this resistance began and methicillin was developed by 1959.[30] By 1961, the first methicillin-resistant strains of S aureus were identified and have since become a part of the health care dilemma all over the world. Microbiologists have isolated the specific resistance mecA gene, which alters the binding of B-lactams to penicillin binding protein 2A and which must be present for a strain of S aureus to be considered resistant to methicillin.[31,32] In addition, a minimum oxacillin-inhibitory concentration of 4µg/mL or greater must be present to confirm resistance. MRSA now accounts for nearly 60% of S aureus strains isolated from intensive care units (ICUs) and approximately 50% of all nosocomial S aureus infections in US hospitals and is increasing in prevalence.[31]

One study of MRSA bacteremia in the United States estimated 94,000 infections and 19,000 deaths in 2005 (standardized infection rate of 31.8/100,000 and standardized mortality rate of 6.3/100,000),[31] which was larger than the report of the CDC that cited 31,400 hospitalizations for MRSA septicemia in 2000.[31] Patients older than 65 years and those of black race were at greatest risk for severe infection and death as well as initial inappropriate antibiotic choice; therefore, a good understanding of the transmission and risk factors leading to MRSA infection is imperative.

To begin, a distinction must be made between MRSA acquired within a health care facility (HA MRSA), community-onset hospital associated, and those acquired within the community (CA MRSA) because they differ in their clinical presentation and on a molecular level.[31]

MRSA acquired >48 hours after hospitalization or within 12 hours following exposure to a health care facility would meet the criteria of HA MRSA. Compared with CA MRSA, this strain is found to be significantly more resistant to a wider array of antibiotics and thus more problematic once it develops. According to the CDC, in the United States, invasive infection with MRSA within health care settings decreased ~54%, with more than 30,000 fewer infections and 9000 fewer deaths from 2005 to 2011.[31] Risk factors for developing HA MRSA include prolonged and/or overuse of antibiotics, elderly patients and those with multiple comorbidities, long-term use of indwelling catheters, and lengthy hospital stays.

On the other hand, CA MRSA is an infection that develops without association with a health care facility. These infections are often the types of infections that would routinely be treated by the oral and maxillofacial surgeons because they are predominantly associated with skin and soft tissue. CA MRSA has also become the predominant causative agent in SSTIs presenting to and treated in Emergency Departments, especially in inner cities. Enhanced virulence is conferred by the presence of the cytotoxin Panton-Valentine leukocidin that has been isolated in as much as 98% of the CA MRSA cases[33]; solace comes from the fact that the CA MRSA for the most part expresses resistance to B-lactams alone, and thus, treatment usually is successful and of minimal financial strain on the health care system when compared with HA MRSA. The resistance to B-lactams alone, however, is slowly changing and is not a hard and fast rule because new isolates have been identified and resistance continues to mount. CA MRSA should always be a part of the differential diagnosis when presented with an SSTI. As much as 33% of one hospital's personnel was noted to be colonized by MRSA,[34] which simply means that they are much more likely to develop infections from MRSA and/or transfer it to others. Within a community, high-risk groups include any and all individuals who share close spaces with others, such as children in daycare, prison populations, sport teams, community living, that is, shelters, and intravenous (IV) drug users.

Prolonged antibiotic use has also been implicated in CA MRSA, particularly cephalosporins, which was found to increase a person's risk of contracting an infection by 3-fold if taken for 5 or more days.[35]

A third category, community-onset health care–associated MRSA, has been recently coined. These are individuals infected within 48 hours of hospital admission or known significant health care contact, such as the following:

- Hospitalization within 90 days in an acute setting
- Dialysis within 30 days
- Resident of a nursing care facility
- Specialized home care

Community-onset health care–associated MRSA usually affects severely ill individuals with multiple comorbidities and has been associated with intravascular catheters placed for long-term use as much as 75%. This finding differs from CA MRSA in that, quite often, healthy individuals will contract CA MRSA. Colonization of individuals with MRSA is a precursor to infection. MRSA and MSSA can be found in the nares, oropharynx, gastrointestinal tract, inguinal area, and skin. Studies have shown that there are 3 patterns of nasal *S aureus* carriage: persistent carriage, intermittent carriage, and noncarriage.[34] Persistent carriers had positive cultures in at least 80% of the swabs taken. Nasal carriers become infected with MRSA at a higher rate than noncarriers, 25.7% versus 4.3%[36]; however, they were also found to have a low mortality when infected. This ability is most likely due to the antibodies present in carriers, mounting an effective response when required. It must be noted that although carriers were found to be at an increased risk for infection by MRSA, the role and degree of increased risk associated with CA MRSA or HA MRSA are not completely understood.

Once a person is found to be colonized with MRSA, a higher susceptibility to an infection is present, more so than those colonized with MSSA tapering when colonization is no longer present.[37] Besides being common transferrable sources such as infected wounds, inanimate surfaces are also a significant risk. Objects such as beds, doorknobs, handrails, and other objects that colonizers contact were found to be culture positive ~59% of the time. With resistance to oxacillin confirmed, it should be concluded that the isolated organism is resistant to other beta-lactam antibiotics.

Even with these 3 categories of MSRA infection, research has also identified MRSA in a wide range of meat products with a prevalence ranging from 0.4% to 12% and as high as 18% in sheep and goat meat in retail markets,[38] highlighting a potential reservoir for transmission from animal product to humans when consumed.

Assessment of Infection and Treatment

A large number of the patients treated in dental and oral surgical practice are healthy children and young people. This population seems to bear the brunt of severe CA MRSA infections, whereas older patients are commonly associated with HA MRSA.[39,40] Dealing with MRSA in children often presents additional complications because children routinely suffer from infections from multiple microbial agents. Initially, one must refrain from making the assumption that an individual previously infected with MRSA has become reinfected, although that is a great possibility. Children tend to present with a variety of skin infections ranging from impetigo, folliculitis, furuncle, carbuncle, skin abscesses, and cellulitis among others, and laboratory evaluation is necessary to identify the offending organism. Wound culture is helpful because it can identify colonization via Gram stain and can guide empiric antibiotic therapy. Susceptibility testing is also useful in distinguishing MRSA from MSSA, leading to more accurate antibacterial coverage. However, blood cultures due to frequent contamination (and 24–48 hours for results) and nasal cultures were not found to be useful in treating MRSA. Incision and drainage is still the primary modality of treatment when dealing with SSTI with moist heat as an adjunct or as primary therapy for smaller soft tissue infections with or without antibiotic therapy. Antibiotic prophylaxis is strongly encouraged in individuals that meet certain criteria, that is, cardiac defects or history of endocarditis before incision and drainage. Individuals with systemic signs and symptoms, multiple comorbidities, multiple sites of infection, increased size of the lesion (>5 cm), and age less than 12 months of age would benefit from adjunctive antibiotic therapy in addition to drainage. A purely cellulitic lesion should be treated with only systemic antibiotic therapy until resolution or a fluctuant collection develops.

Although SSTI are the most common presentation of CA MRSA and MSSA, it is imperative that the possibility of life-threatening complications of these conditions be anticipated. CA MRSA and CA MSSA may cause pulmonary abscesses and necrotizing pneumonia and death.[41] Infections in patients presenting with furunculosis and/or pneumonia (respiratory complaints) are most commonly caused by CA MRSA with the PVL gene[42] and should be treated aggressively. Early treatment with the appropriate antibiotic, such as vancomycin or other non-beta-lactam antibiotics, and awareness of patient's possible exposure to sources of CA MRSA, such as other siblings with skin infections,[43] may improve outcome.

MRSA causing SSTI within the community is relatively susceptible to non-beta-lactam antibiotics such as clindamycin, trimethoprim/sulfamethoxazole, and doxycycline. That being said, one must be aware of the population profile of communities being treated. One study of a children's care center in China over a 12-month period demonstrated a low prevalence (4%) of CA MRSA among their *S aureus* infection and low resistance rates of MSSA to oxacillin and cefuroxime, but high resistance rates to lincosamides, macrolides, and trimethoprim/sulfamethoxazole.[44]

With respect to cellulitis, researchers have a slight preference for clindamycin because of its coverage and penetration, and combination therapy should also be considered when treating empirically. Caution should be taken however when administering antibiotic therapy, because one should not lose sight of the reason we are faced with this dilemma currently. Trimethoprim/sulfamethoxazole when compared with clindamycin was found to have similar efficacy,[45] and clindamycin did not provide any benefit when compared with cephalexin when treating uncomplicated soft tissue infections.[46]

Parenteral therapy, when indicated, usually will consist of clindamycin or vancomycin and occasionally linezolid when laboratory-testing results indicate resistance to clindamycin or vancomycin. Linezolid also has limitations due to cost, bone marrow suppression, optic and peripheral neuropathy, and serotonin syndrome.[47] Ceftaroline was recently approved for treatment of children older than 2 months of age. Its long-term effects are yet to be examined; however, ceftaroline monotherapy cure rate for patients with MRSA soft tissue infections is 93.4%. It is an alternative in situations wherein clindamycin or vancomycin resistance exists or untoward side effects have occurred and is comparable to vancomycin/aztreonam or cefazolin/aztreonam.[48] Daptomycin has been associated with myolysis and does not penetrate well into lung tissue due to binding by surfactant; therefore, it should not be used in cases of pneumonia.

The antibiotics just reviewed should be considered when faced with some unusual complications of SSTI by MRSA. The oral maxillofacial surgeon and dentists must be aware because they are often consulted by other services for facial and oral infection or trauma. Several case reports highlight this: necrotizing pneumonia from lip abscess,[49] several cases of facial abscess,[50] a rare case of sinusitis progressing to facial cellulitis and nasal septum abscess,[51] and a case of mandibular osteomyelitis after traumatic mandibular fracture managed with external open reduction and rigid fixation.[52]

In the critically ill patient, vancomycin combined with nafcillin or oxacillin is recommended to increase coverage for MRSA as well as MSSA. The critically ill patient poses additional concerns, most notably *Clostridium difficile*, which might exacerbate an already fragile state of health. Parenteral therapy should be continued until criteria such as systemic fever if present resolves initially, laboratory susceptibility testing becomes available, and clinical improvements are met. A minimum of 7 days should be completed as recurrence, and/or an increase in original infection can occur when given for shorter courses. Incomplete and inadequate treatment also increases the chance of developing more virulent resistant strains as well. Once diagnosis is made and treatment is instituted, especially if outpatient, a mandatory follow-up within 48 hours should be planned whether or not antibiotic was a part of initial treatment.

Although treatment may be successful, there may be recurrence, especially if there are predisposing factors, either biologic or on inanimate objects seeding the process. The offending organism in a recurrence is usually identical to the initially isolated organism, and treatment tends to follow standard protocol as would initial presentation.

Some current treatment regimens and recommendations for HA MRSA and CA MRSA are reviewed. Before dissecting the various antibiotics that are available to treat MRSA, one should be reminded that the use of beta-lactams and fluoroquinolones as empirical antibiotic therapy should be undertaken with caution. Even the widespread use of cephalosporin antibiotics for prophylaxis, or use when not needed, predisposes to the development and spread of resistant organisms such as MRSA,[53] and thoughtless use will only escalate the problem at hand. Lui and colleagues[54] recommended no antibiotic with uncomplicated abscesses and boils, and incision and drainage was sufficient unless extremes of age, lack of response, or systemic illness or infection.

To further emphasize the point, 88% of CA MRSA and a much higher percentage of HA MRSA cases are not susceptible to cephalexin. Nonetheless, included here are antibiotics, both oral and parenteral route of administration, that have been proven to yield positive results when treating MRSA (**Table 1**).

Vancomycin

Failure in treatment associated with vancomycin includes, but is not limited to, administration of antibiotics greater than 2 days following bacteremia, advanced age greater than 50, preexisting liver disease, and patients with multiple comorbidities. Trough monitoring is the most accurate method of guiding vancomycin dosing to achieve target concentrations.

For MRSA-related septic arthritis, osteomyelitis, and prosthetic joint infections, the recommended therapy is initially surgical debridement and drainage and IV Vancomycin 15 to 20 mg/kg/dose every 8 to 12 hours, and IV Daptomycin 6 mg/kg/dose once daily, IV Trimethoprim/sulfamethoxazole 4 mg/kg/dose twice daily, Linezolid 600 mg twice daily, IV Clindamycin 600 mg every 8 hours, IV rifampin 600 mg daily added for cases of prosthetic joints. Any combination of these antibiotics can be considered.

Efforts should be made to prevent these infections where possible. Simple procedures such as hand washing among caregivers and family members caring for infected or colonized individuals should be performed. Personal protective equipment, such as

Table 1
Recommended oral and parenteral antibiotic therapy for methicillin-resistant *Staphylococcus aureus*

Oral (Recommended Course 5–10 d)	Parenteral Antibiotics (Recommended Course 7–14 d)
• Trimethoprim-sulfamethoxazole: 500 mg orally (PO) twice daily • Clindamycin: 600 mg PO 3 times daily • Oxazolidinones (linezolid) 600 mg PO twice daily (Tedizolid) 200 mg PO and IV once daily × 6 d (new) • Tetracyclines (doxycycline) 100 mg PO twice daily	• Vancomycin 15–20 mg/kg/dose every 8–12 h not to exceed 2 g/dose (adult) • Ceftaroline: 600 mg every 12 h • Aztreonam 2g every 6–8 h × 10–14 d • Daptomycin 4–6 mg/kg every 24 h × 7–14 d • Dalbavancin, Oritavancin, 1500 mg once weekly administration • Telavancin: 10 mg/kg every 24 h (but with a high rate of toxicity)

gown, gloves, and mask with visors, should be used to avoid contamination and possible spread of bacteria to uninfected patients and among health care workers. Cleaning of exposed surfaces of furniture, handrails, and beds can reduce the bacteria inoculum. Recommendations for use of iodine solutions to reduce bacteria colonization on surfaces and over body may be considered. Chlorhexidine gluconate (0.12% gel) has been suggested for nasal application and in one study did reduce nasal colonization over placebo, but recurrent positive nasal cultures increased from time of surgery to discharge.[55] Use of topical mupirocin to eliminate nasal colonization has been used with variable success. Body wash with Chlorhexidine gluconate 2% or 4% used with intranasal mupirocin in patients colonized with MRSA in an ICU was shown to reduce the rate of MRSA infection.[56]

Now most institutions are developing teams to oversee the choice and utilization of antibiotics. Antibiotic stewardship may ultimately be the method by which the further development of resistant strains of organisms is minimized. When faced with patients with SSTI, having a degree of suspicion or a consideration of possible MRSA will aid in swift and effective management and appropriate choice of antibiotic therapy for the best patient outcome.

EPIDEMIOLOGY OF ORAL MUCOSAL INFECTIONS

Epidemiology of oral mucosal infections has been difficult to include in this article because of the different types of infections involving oral mucosa, the different risk groups studied (immunocompetent, immunocompromised, systemic infections, systemic conditions, association with malignancies or involving chemo/radiotherapy) and variation from institution to institution. In current dental literature, most attempts of epidemiologic studies on oral infections were made for human papillomavirus (HPV), HIV, and candidiasis. HPV infections of the oral cavity are the most extensively studied because of the growing number of reports on association with oral cancer formation. HIV infections are also studied in greater number due to the level of morbidity and/or mortality associated. Fungal infections are the most common type of infectious disease that is studied due to the higher competency of dental surgeons to diagnose fungal infections but probably not the bacterial infections of oral mucosa.[57]

NHANES in 2009 to 2010 conducted a cross-sectional study by considering a statistically representative sample of the civilian noninstitutionalized US population and reported that the prevalence rate of oral HPV infection in men and women aged (14–69 Years) was 6.9% and HPV type 16 was identified in 1%. A higher prevalence rate of HPV was identified in men than women, and individuals aged 30 to 34 years and 60 to 64 years.[58] A recent study mentioned that rate of HPV infection among HIV-infected individuals was 38% (sample size: 52 HIV infected individuals)[59] and 28% (sample size: 404 HIV-infected individuals).[60] A recent systematic review that focused on oral fungal infections among patients receiving cancer therapy reported that prevalence of oral fungal infection was 7.5% in pretreatment, 39.1% during treatment, and 32.6% after the end of cancer therapy. The study also mentioned that head and neck chemotherapy and radiotherapy were independently associated with significantly increased risk of oral fungal infections.[61]

EPIDEMIOLOGY OF MICROBIAL CANCER OF ORAL CAVITY

Bacteria, fungi, and viruses found in oral cavity may be altered to substantially mutagenic and predisposing for risk of cancer development. Associations of cancer development were studied in HPV, HIV, human herpesvirus-8 (HHV-8)/Kaposi sarcoma virus, HHV-4/Epstein-Barr virus, and inflammation in periodontal disease. The most common oral cancer is squamous cell carcinoma, which originates from oral mucosal epithelium. Tobacco chewing and alcohol consumption are considered to be the most common etiologic factors associated with oral cancer. However, about 15% of patients with oral cancer have no known risk factors, and infections in these patients can be attributed to HPVs, Epstein-Barr virus, *Candida albicans*, or certain periodontal bacteria.[62,63]

HPV infection is the principal cause of a distinct form of oropharyngeal squamous cell carcinoma that is increasing in incidence among men in the United States. The prevalence of oral HPV infection among men and women aged 14 to 69 years was 6.9% and of HPV type 16 was 1.0%. The prevalence was higher among men than among women. In the study on the prevalence of oral HPV infection in the United States, associations with age, sex, number of sexual partners, and current number of cigarettes smoked per day were independently associated with oral HPV infection in multivariable models.[58]

Most (90%) of the HPV-related oral cancer studies identified HPV-16 as the most common type associated with oral cancer development.[64] Oropharyngeal cancer includes the anatomic areas: base of tongue, pharyngeal tonsils, anterior and posterior pillars, glossotonsillar sulci, anterior surface of soft palate and uvula, and later, posterior pharyngeal walls. Rates of oropharyngeal cancers were higher among white men and women (8.0 and 1.8) compared with blacks (6.9 and 1.5)[65] (**Table 2**). Studies reported that HIV-infected individuals are at higher risk for oral HPV infection and HPV-associated oropharyngeal cancer[66] (**Table 3**). Kaposi sarcoma affects 10% to 20% of HIV-positive patients.[67] Almost 50% of the affected patients show oral lesions and 20% to 25% of these lesions may be the initial site of involvement.[68]

Table 2 Human papillomavirus–associated oropharyngeal cancer rate in United States (2008–2012)	
Subjects (Ethnicity and Gender)	**Age-Adjusted Rate**
White, female	1.8 per 100,000
White, male	8.0 per 100,000
Black, female	1.5 per 100,000
Black, male	6.9 per 100,000
American Indian/Alaska Natives, female	0.9 per 100,000
American Indian/Alaska Natives, male	4.4 per 100,000
Pacific islanders, female	0.6 per 100,000
Pacific islanders, male	2.0 per 100,000
Hispanics, female	0.9 per 100,000
Hispanics, male	4.2 per 100,000
Non-Hispanics, female	1.9 per 100,000
Non-Hispanics, male	8.0 per 100,000

Data from Viens LJ, Henley SJ, Watson M, et al. Human papillomavirus–associated cancers—United States, 2008–2012. MMWR Morb Mortal Wkly Rep 2016;65:661–6.

Table 3
Prevalence rates of microbial linked oropharyngeal cancer in human immunodeficiency virus–infected individuals with the general population, by study

Description	Data (Standardized Incidence Ratios and 95% Confidence Intervals)	Type of Cancer/ Anatomic Site	Study
United States (1990–2006)	1.8 (1.5–2.0)	Oral cavity and pharynx	Simard et al,[59] 2010
United States (1996–2008)	1.4 (0.9–2.1)	Oral cavity and pharynx	Silverberg et al,[69] 2011
United States (1980–2004)	1.6 (1.2–2.1); MSM: 1.1 (0.7–1.8), IDU: 2.1 (1.3–3.2), Hetero: 3.2(1.6–5.7)	Oral cavity and pharynx	Chatervedi et al,[70] 2009

Abbreviations: Hetero, heterosexual; IDU, injection drug user; MSM, men who have sex with men.
Adapted from Beachler DC, D'Souza G. Oral HPV infection and head and neck cancers in HIV-infected individuals. Curr Opin Oncol 2013;25(5):503–10.

SUMMARY

Dental caries and periodontal disease represent a significantly increasing worldwide. Research studies significantly indicate that plaque and calculus are statistically associated with development of gingivitis. Public awareness of the factor responsible of disease may help to reduce the impact of disease and assist dental surgeons to controlling this disease. Knowledge on microbial epidemiology and factors responsible for antibiotic resistance may help the dental surgeon in improving treatment strategies. The constant evolution and identification of new strains of microorganism require continual adjustments and flexibility in the way MRSA is viewed and responded to.

Although epidemiologic evidence for association between the oral microbial disease and cancer was studied, associations have thus far been very limited with limited sample size and study design. Moreover, case reports actually provide an initial insight to association of pathogen with cancer development; it is not possible to determine the exact cancer pathway or carcinogenesis. Characterization of microbial association and cancer development requires further studies with standardized methods focusing on sample collection, sample size, preparation and handling of sampling, methodology selection, and bioinformatics processing of data to provide an evidence-based relationship between microbial organism and oral cancer.

REFERENCES

1. Oral health: Fact sheet N 318. 2012. Available at: http://www.who.int/mediacentre/factsheets/fs318/en/. Accessed September 21, 2016.

2. Lamont R, Jenkinson H. Caries as an infectious disease. In: Lamont RJ, Jenkinson HF, editors. Oral microbiology at a glance. 1st edition. Singapore: Wiley-Blackwell; 2010. p. 1–8.

3. Steinberg D, Eskander L, Zini A, et al. Salivary levels of mutans streptococci and Lactobacilli among Palestinian school children in East Jerusalem. Clin Oral Investig 2014;18(3):979–83.

4. Petersen PE. Sociobehavioural risk factors in dental caries—an international perspective. Community Dent Oral Epidemiol 2005;33:274–9.

5. Beaglehole R, Benzian H, Crail J, et al. The oral health atlas. Brighton (UK): FDI World Dental Federation; 2009. ISBN: 978-0-9539261-6-9.

6. da Silveira Moreira R. Epidemiology of dental caries in the world. In: Virdi M, editor. Oral Health Care – Pediatric, Research, Epidemiology and Clinical Practices. Rijeka, Croatia: InTech; 2012. Available at: http://www.intechopen.com/books/oral-health-care-pediatric-research-epidemiology-and-clinical-practices/epidemiology-of-dental-caries-in-the-world. Accessed December 28, 2016.

7. Ismail AI, Sohn W, Tellez M, et al. The International Caries Detection and Assessment System (ICDAS): an integrated system for measuring dental caries. Community Dent Oral Epidemiol 2007;35:170–8.

8. Oliver RC, Brown LJ, Löe H. Periodontal diseases in the United States population. J Periodontol 1998;69:269–78.

9. Ismail A, Szpunar SM. The prevalence of total tooth loss, dental caries, and periodontal disease among Mexican Americans, Cuban Americans, and Puerto Ricans: findings from HHANES 1982-1984. Am J Public Health 1990;80:66–70.

10. Burt B, Research, Science and Therapy Committee of the American Academy of Periodontology. Position paper: epidemiology of periodontal diseases. J Periodontol 2005;76(8):1406–19.

11. Baelum V, Fejerskov O, Karring T. Oral hygiene, gingivitis, and periodontal breakdown in adult Tanzanians. J Periodontal Res 1986;21:221–32.

12. Baelum V, Fejerskov O, Manji F. Periodontal diseases in adult Kenyans. J Clin Periodontol 1988;15:445–52.

13. Eke PI, Dye BA, Wei L, et al. Prevalence of periodontitis in adults in the United States: 2009 and 2010. J Dent Res 2012;91(10):914–20.

14. Page RC, Offenbacher S, Schroeder HE, et al. Advances in the pathogenesis of periodontitis: summary of developments, clinical implications and future directions. Periodontol 2000 1997;14:216–48.

15. Darveau RP, Tanner A, Page RC. The microbial challenge in periodontitis. Periodontol 2000 1997;14:12–32.

16. Haraszthy VI, Hariharan G, Tinoco EM, et al. Evidence for the role of highly leukotoxic Actinobacillus actinomycetemcomitans in the pathogenesis of localized juvenile and other forms of early-onset periodontitis. J Periodontol 2000;71:912–22.

17. Ximenez-Fyvie LA, Haffajee AD, Socransky SS. Comparison of the microbiota of supra- and subgingival plaque in health and periodontitis. J Clin Periodontol 2000;27:648–57.

18. Hamlet SM, Cullinan MP, Westerman B, et al. Distribution of Actinobacillus actinomycetemcomitans, Porphyromonas gingivalis and Prevotella intermedia in an Australian population. J Clin Periodontol 2001;28:1163–71.

19. Listgarten MA, Slots J, Nowotny AH, et al. Incidence of periodontitis recurrence in treated patients with and without cultivable Actinobacillus actinomycetemcomitans, Prevotella intermedia, and Porphyromonas gingivalis: a prospective study. J Periodontol 1991;62:377–86.

20. Beltrán-Aguilar ED, Barker LK, Canto MT, et al. Surveillance for dental caries, dental sealants, tooth retention, edentulism, and enamel fluorosis–United States, 1988-1994 and 1999-2002. MMWR Surveill Summ 2005;54(3):1–43.

21. Quinonez C, Gibson D, Jokovic A, et al. Emergency department visits for dental care of nontraumatic origin. Community Dent Oral Epidemiol 2009;37:366–71.

22. Kim MK, Allareddy V, Nalliah RP, et al. Burden of facial cellulitis: estimates from the Nationwide Emergency Department Sample. Oral Surg Oral Med Oral Pathol Oral Radiol 2012;114(3):312–7.

23. Kim MK, Nalliah RP, Lee MK, et al. Factors associated with length of stay and hospital charges for patients hospitalized with mouth cellulitis. Oral Surg Oral Med Oral Pathol Oral Radiol 2012;113(1):21–8.

24. Sandor GK, Low DE, Judd PL, et al. Antimicrobial treatment options in the management of odontogenic infections. J Can Dent Assoc 1998;64(7):508–14.

25. Cleveland JL, Kohn WG. Antimicrobial resistance and dental care: a CDC perspective. Dental Abstracts 1998;43:108–10.

26. Swift JQ, Gulden WS. Antibiotic therapy—managing odontogenic infections. Dent Clin North Am 2002;46:623–33.

27. Sweeney LC. Antibiotic resistance in general dental practice—a cause for concern? J Antimicrob Chemother 2004;53(4):567–76.

28. Snydman DR, Jacobus NV, McDermott LA, et al. Update on resistance of Bacteroides fragilis group and related species with special attention to carbapenems 2006-2009. Anaerobe 2011;17:147–51.

29. Aldridge KE, Ashcraft D, Cambre K, et al. Multicenter survey of the changing in vitro antimicrobial susceptibilities of clinical isolates of Bacteroides fragilis group, Prevotella, Fusobacterium, Porphyromonas, and Peptostreptococcus species. Antimicrob Agents Chemother 2001;45(4):1238–43.

30. Takahashi S, Minami K, Ogawa M, et al. The preventive effects of mupirocin against nasotracheal intubation-related bacterial carriage. Anesth Analg 2003; 97:222–5.

31. Brenner EJ, Kayser FH. Growing clinical significance of methicillin resistant Staphylococcus aureus. Lancet 1968;2:741.

32. Wielders CL, Fluit AC, Brisse S, et al. mecA gene is widely disseminated in Staphylococcus aureus population. J Clin Microbiol 2002;40(11):3970–5.

33. Skiest D, Brown K, Cooper T, et al. Prospective comparison of methicillin-susceptible and methicillin-resistant community associated Staphylococcus aureus infections in hospitalized patients. J Infect 2006;54(5):427–43.

34. Maxwell JG, Ford CR, Peterson DE, et al. Long-term study of nasal staphylococci among hospital personnel. Am J Surg 1969;118:849–54.

35. Kemodle DS, Barg NL, Kaiser A. Low-level colonization of hospitalized patients with methicillin-resistant coagulase-negative staphylococci and emergence of the organisms during surgical antimicrobial prophylaxis. Antimicrob Agents Chemother 1988;32(2):202–8.

36. Stenehjem S, Rimland D. MRSA nasal colonization burden and risk of MRSA infection. Am J Infect Control 2013;41(5):405–10.

37. Ellis MW, Hospenthal DR, Dooley DP, et al. Natural history of community acquired methicillin-resistant staphylococcus aureus colonization and infection in soldiers. Clin Infect Dis 2004;39:971–9.

38. Sergelidis D, Papadopoulos T, Komodromos D, et al. Isolation of methicillin resistant staphylococcus aureus from small ruminant and their meat at slaughter and retail level in Greece. Lett Appl Microbiol 2015;61(5):498–503.

39. Zaoutis TE, Toltzis P, Chu J, et al. Clinical and molecular epidemiology of community acquired methicillin-resistant Staphylococcus aureus infections among children with risk factors for health care-associated infection. Pediatr Infect Dis J 2006;24(4):343–8.

40. Crum NF. The emergence of severe, community acquired methicillin Staphylococcus aureus infections. Scand J Infect Dis 2005;37(9):651–6.

41. Centers for Disease Control and Prevention (CDC). Four pediatric deaths from community acquired methicillin resistant staphylococcus aureus—Minnesota

and North Dakota 1997-1999. MMWR Morb Mortal Wkly Rep 1999;48(32): 707–10.

42. Lina G, Plemont Y, Godall-Gamot F, et al. Involvement of Panton-Valentine leucocidin-producing Staphylococcus aureus in primary skin infections and pneumonia. Clin Infect Dis 1999;29(5):1128–32.

43. Johansson PJ, Gustafsson E, Ringberg H. High prevalence of MRSA in household contacts. Scand J Infect Dis 2007;39:764–8.

44. Wu D, Wang Q, Yang Y, et al. Epidemiology and molecular characteristics of community-associated methicillin-resistant and methicillin-susceptible Staphylococcus aureus from skin/soft tissue infections in a children's hospital in Beijing, China. Diagn Microbiol Infect Dis 2010;67(1):1–8.

45. Miller LG, Daum RS, Creech CB, et al. Clindamycin versus trimethoprim-sulfamethoxazole for uncomplicated skin infection. N Engl J Med 2015;372: 1093–103.

46. Chen AE, Carroll KC, Diener-West M, et al. Randomized controlled trial of cephalexin versus clindamycin for uncomplicated pediatric skin infections. Pediatrics 2011;127(3):e573–80.

47. Bishop E, Melvani S, Howden BP, et al. Good clinical outcomes but high rates of adverse reactions during linezolid therapy for serious infections: a proposed protocol for monitoring therapy in complex patients. Antimicrob Agents Chemother 2006;50(4):1599–602.

48. Corey GR, Wilcox M, Talbot G, et al. Integrated Analysis of CANVAS 1 and 2: phase 3 multicenter, randomized, double blind studies to evaluate the safety and efficacy of ceftaroline versus vancomycin plus aztreonam in complicated skin and skin-structure infection. Clin Infect Dis 2010;51(6):641–50.

49. Bruno G, Bruno J, Miyake A. Community-acquired methicillin-resistant Staphylococcus aureus infection with necrotizing pneumonia from lip abscess: a case report. J Oral Maxillofac Surg 2007;65:2350–3.

50. Carter T, Dierks E, Bracis R, et al. Community acquired methicillin-resistant staphylococcus aureus facial abscesses: case reports. J Oral Maxillofac Surg 2005;63: 1021–5.

51. Cheng LH, Kang BH. Nasal septum and facial cellulitis caused by community acquired methicillin-resistant Staphylococcus aureus. J Laryngol Otol 2010;124: 1014–6.

52. Tuzuner-Oncul A, Ungor C, Dede U, et al. Methicillin-resistant Staphylococcus aureus (MRSA) osteomyelitis of the mandible. Oral Surg Oral Med Oral Pathol Oral Radiol Endod 2009;107(6):e1–4.

53. Schentag J, Hyatt JM, Carr JR, et al. Genesis of methicillin-resistant Staphylococcus aureus (MRSA), how treatment of MRSA has selected for vancomycin-resistant Enterococcus faecium, and the importance of antibiotic management and infection control. Clin Infect Dis 1998;26:1204–14.

54. Lui C, Bayer A, Cosgrove SE, et al. Clinical practice guidelines by the infectious disease society of America for the treatment of methicillin-resistant Staphylococcus aureus in adults and children. Clin Infect Dis 2011;52:e18–55.

55. Segers P, Speekenbrink RG, Ubbink DT, et al. Prevention of nosocomial infection in cardiac surgery by decontamination of the nasopharynx and oropharynx with chlorhexidine gluconate: a randomized controlled trial. JAMA 2006;296:2460–6.

56. Sandri AM, Dalarosa MG, Ruschel de Alcantara L, et al. Reduction in incidence of nosocomial methicillin-resistant Staphylococcus aureus (MRSA) infection in an intensive care unit. Role of treatment with mupirocin ointment and chlorhexidine baths for nasal carriers of MRSA. Infect Control Hosp Epidemiol 2006;27:185–7.

57. Dahlen G. Bacterial infections of the oral mucosa. Periodontol 2000 2009;49: 13–38.
58. Gillison ML, Broutian T, Pickard RK, et al. Prevalence of oral HPV infection in the United States, 2009-2010. JAMA 2012;307(7):693–703.
59. Simard EP, Pfeiffer RM, Engels EA. Spectrum of cancer risk late after aids onset in the United States. Arch Intern Med 2010;170(15):1337–45.
60. Kirk GD, Merlo CA, Lung HIV Study. HIV infection in the etiology of lung cancer: confounding, causality, and consequences. Proc Am Thorac Soc 2011;8:326–32.
61. Lalla RV, Latortue MC, Hong CH, et al. A systematic review of oral fungal infections in patients receiving cancer therapy. Support Care Cancer 2010;18(8): 985–92.
62. Scully C. Oral squamous cell carcinoma; from an hypothesis about a virus, to concern about possible sexual transmission. Oral Oncol 2002;38:227–34.
63. Lissowska J, Pilarska A, Pilarski P, et al. Smoking, alcohol, diet, dentition and sexual practices in the epidemiology of oral cancer in Poland. Eur J Cancer Prev 2003;12:25–33.
64. Gillison ML. Human papillomavirus-related diseases: oropharynx cancers and potential implications for adolescent HPV vaccination. J Adolesc Health 2008; 43(4 Suppl):S52–60.
65. Viens LJ, Henley SJ, Watson M, et al. Human papillomavirus–associated cancers—United States, 2008–2012. MMWR Morb Mortal Wkly Rep 2016;65:661–6.
66. Beachler DC, D'Souza G. Oral HPV infection and head and neck cancers in HIV-infected individuals. Curr Opin Oncol 2013;25(5):503–10.
67. Safai B. Kaposi's sarcoma and acquired immunodeficiency syndrome. In: DeVita VT, Hellman JS, Rosenberg SA, editors. AIDS: etiology, diagnosis, treatment and prevention. 4th edition. Philadelphia: Lippincott-Raven; 1997. p. 295–317.
68. Neville BW, Damm DD, Allen CM, et al. Oral and maxillofacial pathology. 2nd edition. Philadelphia: WB Saunders Co; 2002.
69. D'Souza G, Agrawal Y, Halpern J, et al. Oral sexual behaviors associated with prevalent oral human papillomavirus infection. J Infect Dis 2009;199(9):1263–9.
70. Chaturvedi AK, Madeleine MM, Biggar RJ, et al. Risk of human papillomavirus-associated cancers among persons with AIDS. J Natl Cancer Inst 2009;101: 1120–30.

Odontogenic Infections

Orrett E. Ogle, DDS[a,b,c,*]

KEYWORDS

- Dental infections • Dental abscess • Microbiota of dental infections

KEY POINTS

- The pathogenesis of odontogenic infection is polymicrobial, consisting of various facultative and strict anaerobes. The dominant isolates are strictly anaerobic gram-negative rods and gram-positive cocci. The periapical infection is the most common form of odontogenic infection.
- Although odontogenic infections are usually confined to the alveolar ridge vicinity, they can spread into deep fascial spaces.
- Cavernous sinus thrombosis, brain abscess, airway obstruction, and mediastinitis are possible complications of dental infections.
- The most important element in treating odontogenic infections is the elimination of the primary source of the infection with antibiotics as adjunctive therapy.

INTRODUCTION

An odontogenic infection is an infection of the alveolus, jaws, or face that originates from a tooth or from its supporting structures and is one of the most frequently encountered infections. The most common causes of odontogenic infections are dental caries, deep fillings or failed root canal treatment, pericoronitis, and periodontal disease. The infection starts locally around a tooth and may remain localized to the region where it started, or may spread into adjacent or distant areas. The course of the infection depends on the virulence of the bacteria, host resistance factors, and the regional anatomy.

The periapical infection is the most common form of odontogenic infection and is caused by invasion of the root canal system of the tooth by microorganisms. This acute apical infection entails a concomitant infection of the root canal and the periradicular tissues, because the latter is an extension of the former. Once the microorganisms enter the periapical tissues via the apical foramen, they induce an inflammatory process that can lead to the formation of an abscess. In most cases the infection is

The author has nothing to disclose.
[a] Atlanta, GA, USA; [b] Faculty of Medicine, Mona Dental Program, University of the West Indies, Kingston 6, Jamaica; [c] Oral and Maxillofacial Surgery, Woodhull Hospital, 760 Broadway, Brooklyn, NY 11206, USA
* 4974 Golf Valley Court, Douglasville, GA 30135.
E-mail address: oeogle@aol.com

Dent Clin N Am 61 (2017) 235–252
http://dx.doi.org/10.1016/j.cden.2016.11.004
0011-8532/17/© 2016 Elsevier Inc. All rights reserved.

localized intraorally, but in some instances it may spread into distal areas and result in severe complications, such as sinusitis, airway obstruction, cavernous sinus thrombosis, brain abscess, or even death.

Pericoronitis is another common cause of odontogenic infection. The primary cause is the accumulation of bacteria and food debris that gets trapped in the space between the overlapping gum of a partially exposed (erupted) mandibular third molar and the crown of the tooth. Most cases are chronic and consist of a mild persistent inflammation of the mandibular third molar area. Pericoronitis can, however, become a serious infection associated with fever, swelling, and an abscess that has the ability to spread if left untreated. On occasions the symptoms can become severe because of the rapid spread of infection, requiring that the patient be hospitalization for intravenous (IV) antibiotics and possibly extraction of tooth in an operating room under general anesthesia. Because of the close proximity to the pharynx, airway obstruction becomes a strong possibility.

CLINICAL PRESENTATIONS

The clinical presentation of an odontogenic infection is highly variable depending on the source of the infection (anterior teeth vs posterior teeth; maxillary vs mandibular teeth), whether the infection is localized or if it has become disseminated (**Table 1**). Like all infections, the clinical signs and symptoms are pain/tenderness, redness, and swelling. Patients with superficial dental infections present with localized pain, cellulitis, and sensitivity to tooth percussion and temperature. However, patients with deep infections or abscesses that spread along the fascial planes may present with swelling; fever; and sometimes difficulty swallowing, opening the mouth, or breathing (**Fig. 1**). In single space infection cases the most commonly involved fascial space is the buccal space (60%) (**Fig. 2**), followed by canine space (13%) (**Fig. 3**). In

Table 1	
Clinical presentation of odontogenic infections by location	
Type of Infection	**Clinical Presentation**
Dentoalveolar infection	Swelling of the alveolar ridge with periodontal, periapical, and subperiosteal abscess.
Submental space infection	Firm midline swelling beneath the chin. Caused by infection from the mandibular incisors.
Submandibular space infection	Swelling of the submandibular triangle of the neck around the angle of the mandible. Infection is caused by mandibular molar infections. Trismus is typical.
Sublingual space infection	Swelling of the floor of the mouth with possible elevation of the tongue and dysphagia.
Retropharyngeal space infection	Stiff neck, sore throat, dysphagia, raspy voice. These infections are caused by infections of the molars. The retropharyngeal space infection has a high potential to spread to the mediastinum.
Buccal space infection	Swelling of the cheek. Caused by infection of premolar or molar tooth.
Masticator space infection	Swelling on either side of the mandibular ramus and is caused by infection of the mandibular third molar. Trismus is present.
Canine space infection	Swelling of the anterior cheek with loss of the nasolabial fold and possible extension to the infraorbital region.

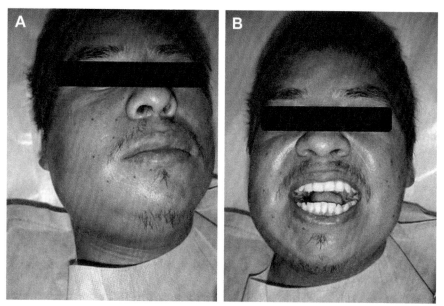

Fig. 1. (A) Buccal and submandibular abscess. (B) Limited jaw opening secondary to dental infection.

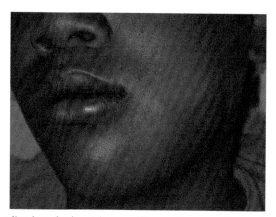

Fig. 2. Abscess localized to the buccal space. The most commonly involved fascial space in single-space infection cases.

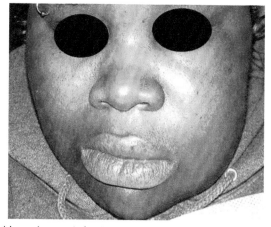

Fig. 3. Canine and buccal space infection.

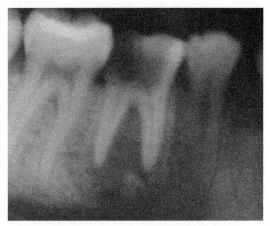

Fig. 4. Bone resorption around the root apex secondary to chronic periapical inflammation. This is manifested on dental radiographs as the typical periapical radiolucency commonly referred to as a PAP.

multiple space infection the submandibular space and the buccal space are the ones most commonly involved[1] (see **Fig. 1**A).

The acute periapical inflammation/infection usually gives rise to signs and symptoms, such as pain and swelling. The chronic inflammatory response is usually asymptomatic and often leads to bone resorption around the root apex that is manifested on dental radiographs as the typical periapical radiolucency (**Fig. 4**). The chronic asymptomatic periapical pathology may flare-up and present as an acute dental infection.

Ludwig Angina

Ludwig angina is a serious and potentially life-threatening infection characterized by brawny boardlike swelling from a rapidly spreading cellulitis (without lymphatic

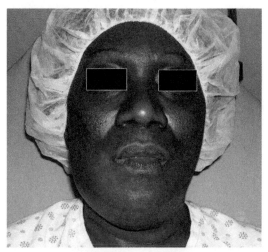

Fig. 5. Ludwig angina: bilateral submandibular swelling, mental space swelling, and bilateral sublingual spaces.

involvement and generally without abscess formation) of the sublingual, submental, and submandibular spaces with elevation and edema of the tongue, drooling, and airway obstruction (**Fig. 5**, **Box 1**).[2,3] The cause of infection in most cases is from infected lower molars or from pericoronitis.

Box 1
Signs and symptoms of Ludwig angina
Rapid swelling of the infected area
Fatigue
Fetid breath
Fever
Trismus
Tongue swelling or protrusion of the tongue out of the mouth
Drooling
Unusual speech
Difficulty swallowing
Neck pain
Neck swelling
Breathing difficulty

Hoarseness, stridor, respiratory distress, decreased air movement, cyanosis, and a "sniffing" position (ie, the characteristic posture assumed by patients with impending upper airway compromise consisting of an upright posture with the neck thrust forward and the chin elevated) are all signs of impending airway catastrophe.[4]

In addition to airway compromise, other reported complications of Ludwig angina include carotid sheath infection and arterial rupture, suppurative thrombophlebitis of the internal jugular vein, mediastinitis, empyema, pericardial and/or pleural effusion, osteomyelitis of the mandible, subphrenic abscess, and aspiration pneumonia.[5,6]

SPREAD OF INFECTION

Odontogenic infections are usually mild and are generally confined to the alveolar ridge or tissues in close proximity (buccal, labial, or lingual vestibule). The infectious process that starts at the apex of the tooth, if left untreated, erodes through the bone (usually through the thinnest portion of the alveolar bone) and spreads to the adjacent tissue. In the mandible, the lingual aspect of the molar region represents the easiest way, whereas in the maxilla the thin buccal plate is the easiest route. How the infection spreads is determined by the relationship of the muscle attachment to the point at which the infection perforates. Most odontogenic infections penetrate the bone in such a way that they become vestibular abscesses. However, if the spread is outside of the muscle attachments, the infection spreads into fascial spaces, resulting in more severe infections. Occasionally, spread beyond the barriers of the fascial spaces may occur, which could result in cavernous sinus thrombosis, brain abscess, airway obstruction, mediastinitis, and endocarditis.

Infections involving the fascial planes of the head and neck spread downward along the cervical fascia, facilitated by gravity, breathing, and negative intrathoracic pressure. Although the pattern of spread varies among patients, a constant trend in the distribution of infection into the spaces is evident.[7,8]

In addition to spread via fascial spaces, infection can also spread via hematogenous or lymphatic routes. Bacteria from an odontogenic infection can enter the bloodstream causing a bacteremia that can have distant effects. In immune-compromised individuals, the bacteremia may progress into septicemia, a more serious blood infection that is accompanied by such symptoms as chills, high fever, rapid heartbeat, severe nausea, vomiting, and mental changes. Hematogenous spread can also occur along the facial, angular, or ophthalmic veins, which lack valves, into the cavernous sinus and into the cranium. These veins that lack valves permit blood flow in either direction depending on the prevailing pressure gradients. This can allow contaminated venous drainage to the cavernous sinus that may lead to cavernous sinus thrombosis (**Fig. 6**). Dental infections, however, accounts for less than 10% of septic cavernous sinus thrombosis cases, and most of these cases are related to maxillary infections.[9] The incidence of cavernous sinus thrombosis has decreased greatly with the advent of effective antimicrobial agents.

The lymphatic system of the head and neck can allow the spread of an odontogenic infection when the organisms enter the lymphatic system and travel in the lymph from a primary node near the infected site to a secondary node at a distal site. The lymphatic fluid flows through tiny tubules with small nodular structures called lymph nodes interconnecting them, finally emptying into the venous system at the junction of the internal jugular and subclavian veins in the neck. After entering the vascular system the infection could spread to other tissues or organs. The lymph nodes produce lymphocytes and act as antimicrobial filters to combat infections that might spread through the lymphatic channels. If the infection is successfully controlled in the

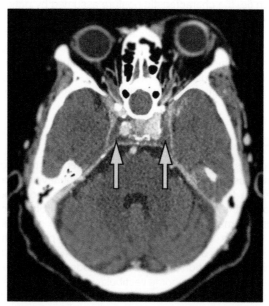

Fig. 6. Computed tomography (CT) showing cavernous sinus thrombosis (*arrows*). (*Adapted from* Sakaida H, Kobayashi M, Ito A, et al. Cavernous sinus thrombosis: linking a swollen red eye and headache. Lancet 2014;384(9946):928; with permission.)

primary node, the infection goes no farther. However, if the infection is severe, it could spread through the primary lymph node or nodes and go on to the next group of nodes. Any group of nodes may overcome the infection if it is not too severe.

MICROBIOLOGY

The pathogenesis of odontogenic infection is polymicrobial, consisting of various facultative anaerobes, such as the streptococci viridans group and the streptococcus anginosus group, and strict anaerobes, especially anaerobic cocci, *Prevotella* and *Fusobacterium* species.[10,11] Recent studies done with careful microbiology techniques under strict anaerobic conditions along with the use of molecular techniques, such as 16S r-RNA gene sequencing and polymerase chain reaction, have identified several difficult-to-culture organisms and have expanded the knowledge of the microflora associated with dental infections.[12] Indeed, datasets from culture and molecular studies have shown that more than 460 unique bacterial taxa belonging to 100 genera and nine phyla have been identified in different types of endodontic infections.[13]

The dominant isolates are strictly anaerobic gram-negative rods and gram-positive cocci, in addition to facultative and microaerophilic streptococci. Anaerobic bacteria outnumber aerobes 3:1.[14] Culture and molecular microbiologic studies have clearly established that the apical abscess microbiota is mixed but overwhelmingly dominated by anaerobic bacteria.[15] Anaerobes (75%) include peptostreptococci, bacteroides, and *Prevotella* organisms, and *Fusobacterium nucleatum*. Aerobes (25%) include α-hemolytic streptococci.

Frequently detected bacterial species in dental infections generally belong to seven different bacterial phyla, and the phyla Firmicutes and Bacteroidetes together contribute to more than 70% of the species found in dental abscesses[15]:

1. Firmicutes: genera *Streptococcus, Dialister, Filifactor,* and *Pseudoramibacter*
2. Bacteroidetes: genera *Prevotella, Porphyromonas,* and *Tannerella*
3. Fusobacteria: genera *Fusobacterium* and *Leptotrichia*
4. Actinobacteria: genera *Actinomyces* and *Propionibacterium*
5. Spirochaetes: genus *Treponema*
6. Synergistetes: genus *Pyramidobacter*
7. Proteobacteria: genera *Campylobacter* and *Eikenella*

Studies have reported various mixtures of bacteria within apical abscess. In one report the most abundant phyla found in acute infections were Firmicutes (52%), Fusobacteria (17%), Bacteroidetes (13%), and other mixed species (18%), whereas the dominant phyla in chronic asymptomatic apical periodontitis infections were Firmicutes (59%), Bacteroidetes (14%), and Actinobacteria (10%). Members of Fusobacteria were much more prevalent in the acute infections but decreased significantly in chronic infections. The bacterial communities in acute abscesses are significantly more diverse than those in chronic infections.[16] In other studies *Prevotella* species have been reported as the most frequent isolates, found in 10% to 87% of dentoalveolar abscesses[13,17] (**Table 2**).

Although in clinical practice practitioners try to find single species or at least a group of major species that is associated with acute odontogenic infections, studies have shown that there is no single pathogen but a set of species, usually organized in multispecies biofilm communities, that is involved and that the cause is heterogeneous.[18] The general profile of bacterial communities is determined by species richness and clinical relevance becomes more evident when bacterial community

Table 2
Bacteria frequently found in dental infections

Gram-Negative Bacteria	Gram-Positive Bacteria
Bacteroides[a]	Firmicutes
Prevotella spp	Streptococcus spp
P intermedia	S anginosus
P nigrescens	S constellatus
P baroniae	S intermedius
P oris	Parvimonas micra (formerly Peptostreptococcus)
Bacteroides forsythus	
Porphyromonas spp	
P endodontalis	
P gingivalis	
Fusobacteria	Actinomyces spp
Fusobacterium	
F nucleatum subsp. nucleatum	
F nucleatum subsp. polymorphum	
F nucleatum subsp. vincentii	
F nucleatum subsp. animalis	
F periodonticum	
Veillonella parvula	Anaerobic lactobacilli
Eikenella corrodens	

[a] Bacteroides melaninogenicus has been reclassified and split into Prevotella melaninogenica and Prevotella intermedia.

Data from Siqueira JF Jr, Rôças IN. Diversity of endodontic microbiota revisited. J Dent Res 2009;88(11):969–81.

profiles are taken into account because there are dominant species in the communities. Culture studies have reported a mean number of species ranging from 2 to 8.5 per pus specimen.[19]

In terms of clinical infection, it is not only the type of bacteria that is significant but also the bacterial load. A high bacterial load is significant because it may result in a heavy bacterial burden that may overwhelm the host defense mechanisms. Total bacterial loads per abscess case have been reported to range from 10^4 to 10^9 cells.[14] An increased bacterial load may increase the diversity of organisms, which may then result in multiple synergistic interactions among the community members and produce an increase in the virulence factor. Interactions between members of a bacterial community can alter the production of virulence factors. In a polymicrobial infection, even species regarded as avirulent and/or in low numbers in the consortium may somewhat affect the virulence of other members of the community.[20] The presence of a virulent strain in high counts may increase the virulence of the whole community and lead to a more serious infection.

Clinical approaches, such as tooth extraction, root canal therapy, incision and drainage, mechanical debridement, and copious irrigation of the infected area are all methods of decreasing the total bacterial load and thus reducing the infectious bioburden on the individual.

ANAEROBES

Anaerobes are involved in almost all dental infections. These are bacteria that require anaerobic conditions to initiate and sustain growth. They usually do not possess

Table 3 Classification of anaerobic organisms frequent in odontogenic infections			
Gram-Positive Cocci	**Gram-Negative Cocci**	**Gram-Positive Bacilli**	**Gram-Negative Bacilli**
Peptostreptococcus	Veillonella	Propionibacterium Actinomyces Lactobacillus	Fusobacterium Prevotella Porphyromonas Bacteroides

catalase, but some can generate superoxide dismutase, which protects them from oxygen. Strict anaerobes are unable to grow if oxygen is greater than 0.5%. Moderate anaerobes are capable of growing between 2% to 8% oxygen. Facultative anaerobes are an organism that is able to grow under aerobic conditions but that develops most rapidly in an anaerobic environment.[21] **Table 3** provides a classification.

The composition of primary odontogenic infections reflects the normal oral microbiota and the method of dissemination. However, because of ecologic interactions and environmental conditions, over time the oral anaerobes eventually become the predominant group in the endodontic and periapical infections.[22] Generally, the presence of gram-negative anaerobic bacilli and anaerobic gram-positive cocci is associated with incidence of acute signs and symptoms: pain, sensitivity to pressure, and cellulitis. Anaerobic infections are characterized by abscess formation, foul-smelling pus, and tissue destruction.

Strict Anaerobes

Dental abscesses caused solely by strict anaerobes occur in only about 20% of cases. Most infections are mixed but strict anaerobes outnumber facultative by a ratio that varies between 1.5 and 3:1.[14] Usually, strictly anaerobic gram-negative rods are more pathogenic than facultative or strictly anaerobic gram-positive cocci (**Box 2**).

Box 2
Strict anaerobes

Streptococci[a]

Fusobacterium: nucleatum and periodonticum

Prevotella: intermedia, nigrescens, and pallens

Porphyromonas: endodontalis and gingivalis

Treponema[b]

Clostridia[b]

[a] Most streptococci are facultative anaerobes but some are obligate (strict) anaerobes.
[b] Not frequent.

Facultative Anaerobes

Facultative anaerobes primarily belong to the viridans group streptococci and the anginosus group streptococci (**Box 3**). *Staphylococcus aureus* has also been found in acute dental abscess.

> **Box 3**
> **Facultative anaerobes**
>
> Viridans group streptococci: mitis, oralis, salivarius, sanguinis, and mutans
>
> Anginosus group streptococci: anginosus
>
> Actinomyces
>
> Lactobacillus

AEROBES

Infections caused only by aerobic bacteria probably account for less than 5% of odontogenic infections.[23] The aerobic bacteria that are involved are primarily invasive *Streptococcus* species that are part of the normal endogenous flora. These aerobic streptococci species may be seen in early stages of the infection resulting in a cellulitic-type of reaction. This quickly changes, however, into a mixed infection that is dominated by anaerobic bacteria. The aerobic bacteria serve as the initiators of the infection, preparing the local environment for anaerobic bacterial invasion as the local tissue condition changes to a more hypoxic state that favors anaerobic growth.

DIAGNOSIS

Oral infections remain among the top reasons for seeking health care in the world.[24] The diagnosis of an odontogenic infection is based on the chief complaint and history of the current problem, clinical signs and symptoms, radiographic examination, and obtaining appropriate material for culture when necessary.

Odontogenic infections can almost always be diagnosed solely from the history along with clinical and radiographic examination. Pain (plus or minus swelling) is generally the major complaint. The offending tooth is tender in most cases of an acute infection. Focus of the history and examination should be location and type of pain; frequency, duration, and onset; and exacerbation and remission (eg, the response to heat or cold).

The number one cause of odontogenic infection is dental caries, with bacteria penetrating the pulp chamber and extending through the root canal system to enter into the periradicular tissues. A carious/nonvital or impacted tooth may be noted on examination. Patients with superficial odontogenic infections may complain of pain localized to one or more teeth and sensitivity to pressure, percussion, and temperature. Patients with deep infections or abscesses that have spread into the fascial planes may have a fever, trismus, and complaints of difficulty swallowing and sometimes breathing.

Acute Apical Abscess

Acute apical abscess is an inflammatory reaction to pulpal infection and necrosis characterized by rapid onset, spontaneous pain, extreme tenderness of the tooth to pressure, pus formation, and swelling of associated tissues. There may be no radiographic signs of destruction and the patient often experiences malaise, fever, and lymphadenopathy.[25]

Chronic Apical Abscess

Chronic apical abscess is an inflammatory reaction to pulpal infection and necrosis characterized by gradual onset, little or no discomfort, and an intermittent discharge of pus through an associated sinus tract. Radiographically, there are typically signs of osseous destruction, such as radiolucency. To identify the source of a draining sinus tract when present, a gutta-percha cone is carefully placed through the stoma or opening until it stops and a radiograph is taken.[25]

Radiographs

The choice of imaging technique depends on the clinical picture.

- A panoramic radiograph of the jaws (**Fig. 7**) is the most ideal screening imaging technique for odontogenic infections. Radiologic signs of the tooth associated with an infection in the supporting bone are extremely common. The panoramic radiograph or a periapical radiograph may reveal the presence of a periapical abscess or in the case of pericoronitis an impacted third molar.
- Computed tomography (CT) is the imaging modality of choice for assessment of deep space infections and is reserved for severe infections with deep space involvement (**Fig. 8**).
- MRI, like CT, is useful for the localization of deep fascial space infections of the head and neck.
- For infections, such as Ludwig angina or infections that have spread into the neck a posterior-anterior and a direct lateral radiograph of the neck may be helpful in identifying compression or deviation of the trachea or the presence of gas within the soft tissues. The same information is obtained from CT scans, but the interpretation may be somewhat more difficult for practitioners who are not familiar with CT scans.

Cultures

Because the microbiology and antibiotic sensitivity of dental infection is well known, it is reasonable to start treatment with one of the known effective antibiotics without performing cultures. The economic cost of culturing all simple odontogenic infections would be astronomical. Furthermore, there is no compelling evidence for routine cultures of simple dental infections and empiric treatment with antibiotics is most often curative. In general, uncomplicated dental infections confined to the alveolar area do not require culturing unless the infection does not respond to initial empiric treatment. With infections that spread to adjacent fascial spaces or in patients with a compromised immune system, needle aspirate or swab culture is indicated for aerobic and anaerobic cultures. Swab cultures, however, may not be productive when

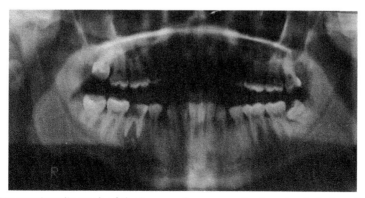

Fig. 7. Panoramic radiograph of the jaws used as a screening imaging technique for odontogenic infections. Radiologic signs of the tooth associated with an infection in the supporting bone can easily be identified.

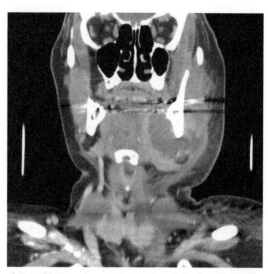

Fig. 8. CT of left submandibular abscess. (*From* Doc 103. Scanner d'un volumineux abcès dentaire (à droite de l'image) sous-mandibulaire de face avec une inflammation importante du tissu cellulo-graisseux sous-cutané. The Free Software Foundation (FSF); Boston, MA, 2010; with permission.)

collecting specimens for anaerobic culture because cotton fibers may be destructive to anaerobes. For an anaerobic culture, the samples should be placed into a special collection tube designed for anaerobic cultures, which often consist of a gassed-out screw top vial that may contain oxygen-free prereduced culture medium that is tightly capped with an effective seal to providing a gas-tight seal for improved stability. For cultures taken from intraoral lesions, contamination by the resident oral flora is inevitable; therefore, where possible, needle aspiration of pus from a loculation within the abscess cavity from an extraoral approach is preferred.

TREATMENT

The decision as to how an odontogenic infection should be treated is based on the source of the infection, severity of the infection, and state of the patient's host defense mechanisms. The first and most important element in treating dental infections is the elimination of the primary source of the infection. This is achieved by extraction of the offending tooth and surgical removal of diseased tissue; or by extirpation of necrotic pulpal tissue and subsequent endodontic therapy. In the case of an acute abscess, incision and drainage to remove accumulated pus (purulence) that contains bacteria is required. The incision and drainage procedure should break up all loculi within the abscess cavity and evacuate as much of the pus as possible. Following the evacuation of the purulent exudate, the use of copious irrigation further dilutes the bacterial population. In a simple periapical abscess, diseased tissue is removed from the pulp chamber and drainage obtained through the root canal.

Odontogenic infections can spread rapidly, therefore initial care is important. Some signs that an infection should be treated by an oral and maxillofacial surgeon are:

- Swelling involving the midface and where the eyelids begin to swell shut
- Swelling that has crossed the lower border of the mandible to involve the submandibular and submental spaces

- Large swelling in the floor of the mouth
- Interincisal opening less than 20 mm
- Difficulty swallowing or breathing
- Swelling or erythema of the neck
- Headache or a stiff neck
- Fever of 102°F (38.9°C) or higher
- Generalized weakness

If the patient has any degree of airway compromise, is systemically unwell (fever, increased pulse, malaise), significant swelling in the submandibular/submental area or in the floor of the mouth, severe trismus, or is unable to take fluids or oral medications, that patient requires hospital admission for IV antibiotics, incision and drainage of the abscess with possible placement of external drains, and extraction of unrestorable teeth. Prolonged nasal intubation or tracheostomy may also be required.

In patients with compromised defense mechanisms their ability to respond normally to an infective challenge is impaired. Their underlying medical condition could make the dental infection progress rapidly, confuse the microbiology, increase the risk of invasive fungal infection and make antimicrobial treatment more complex. The most common immunocompromising situation that the dentist encounters is the patient with diabetes (the rate of type 2 diabetes has quadrupled worldwide between 1980 and 2015),[26] who has an increased susceptibility to become infected and in which the diabetes makes any existing infection worse. Even in patients with well controlled diabetes, moderate to severe dental infections can adversely affect their glycemic control and precipitate a hyperglycemic milieu that favors immune dysfunction with reduced neutrophil activity. Conversely, the metabolic derangements of diabetes may enable and accelerate the infection. It is often necessary, therefore, to aggressively treat the hyperglycemia simultaneously with the infection. Patients with long-standing diabetes tend to have microvascular and macrovascular disease with resultant poor tissue perfusion, which limits the access of phagocytic cells and makes it more difficult for antibiotics to reach the infection site in adequate doses.

When the host immune mechanism is compromised the underlying disease may alter the clinical picture (**Box 4**). Careful monitoring of fever is required because these patients are more prone to bacteremia, which may rapidly lead to septicemia. Consultation with an internist, hematologist, endocrinologist, oncologist, and infectious disease specialist may be necessary. In addition to surgical or endodontic interventions, antibiotics will always be indicated for treating immunocompromized patients. At times, IV antibiotics directed at the oral flora may be required.

Box 4
Some medical conditions that can result in an immunocompromised host

AIDS/human immunodeficiency virus infection

Diabetes

Steroid therapy

Cancer chemotherapy

Elderly

Asplenia

Sickle cell disease

Hypogammaglobulinemia

Hepatitis

Malignancies

Multiple sclerosis

Malnutrition

Ulcerative colitis

Crohn disease

Excessive alcohol

Emotional stress

Physical stressors, such as inadequate sleep

Chronic fatigue syndrome

Autoimmune disorders in general

ANTIBIOTICS

Antibiotics are necessary in many dental infections to hasten complete resolution but they should never be considered as an alternative to dental intervention. Removing the source of the infection remains the major treatment objective and antibiotics are simply adjuncts.

Oral and maxillofacial surgeons have hospital admitting privileges and are trained and credentialed to administer IV antibiotics in the hospital setting. Most dental practitioners, however, use oral antibiotics, which is the focus here. Because the microbiology and antibiotic sensitivity of most pathogens involved in odontogenic infections is well known, it is rational to empirically start treatment with one of the antibiotics that is recognized to be very effective. Culture-dependent antimicrobial tests, particularly for anaerobic bacteria, can take too long to provide results about antibiotic susceptibility and add to the cost of care. For acute infections, penicillin is the drug of choice. In the early stages of clinical symptoms (3–4 days) the facultative streptococci predominates but gram negative obligate anaerobes appear in increasing numbers as time passes without treatment (>4 days). Therefore, in the first 3 to 4 days penicillin V is the antibiotic of choice, and after that clindamycin becomes the drug of choice.[27,28]

Effective, orally administered antibiotics for odontogenic infections are:

- Penicillin
- Amoxicillin
- Clindamycin
- Metronidazole
- Azithromycin
- Moxifloxacin

Penicillin

Penicillin is the drug of choice in treating odontogenic infections because it is effective against the gram-positive aerobes and intraoral anaerobes commonly found in alveolar abscesses. Both aerobic and anaerobic microorganisms are susceptible to penicillin.[29]

Amoxicillin

Amoxicillin is a semisynthetic antibiotic that belongs to the penicillin group of drugs with a broad spectrum of bactericidal activity against many gram-positive and gram-negative microorganisms. Although it has a broader spectrum of activity than penicillin V, it does not seem to provide any better coverage in treating odontogenic infections. Its dosing schedule (twice a day every 12 hours or three times a day every 8 hours) and ability to be taken with food makes it easier for patients to comply and should therefore be the drug of choice in uncooperative individuals.

Clindamycin

Clindamycin has excellent coverage of gram-positive cocci and anaerobic bacteria and is considered the antibiotic of choice for the penicillin-allergic patient and for penicillin-resistant organisms. It inhibits bacterial protein synthesis and is bactericidal at high dosages (300 mg). In the Sanford Guide to Antimicrobial Therapy, clindamycin has replaced penicillin as the recommended antibiotic for the management of odontogenic infections.[30]

Metronidazole

Metronidazole inhibits nucleic acid synthesis by disrupting the DNA of microbial cells. This function only occurs when metronidazole is partially reduced, and because this reduction usually happens only in anaerobic cells, it has little effect on aerobic bacteria.[31] This antibiotic, which is very effective against anaerobes but has absolutely no activity against aerobic bacteria, should be reserved for cases in which only anaerobic bacteria are suspected. However, because anaerobes make up the major constituent of organisms in odontogenic infections its use is effective in clinical practice. In a serious, acute odontogenic infection, it should be combined with penicillin. Some authors have suggested that penicillin in conjunction with metronidazole should now be considered the first-line antibiotic of choice for odontogenic infections because this combination provides excellent bacterial coverage for the mixed organisms usually cultured from dental abscesses.[32]

Azithromycin

Azithromycin is a macrolide antibiotic derived from erythromycin (ie, a second-generation erythromycin drug with better tolerance and better tissue penetration). It is a bacteriostatic agent that inhibits bacterial RNA-dependent protein synthesis. It is lipophilic; has high tissue penetration, particularly to sites of inflammation (usually areas of bacterial infections); and has adequate tissue levels for 7 days with a 3-day treatment regimen. Azithromycin has good activity against aerobic and facultative gram-positive microorganisms (staphylococci and streptococci), anaerobic microorganisms, and many atypical and rapidly growing pyogenic bacteria. The antibacterial activity of azithromycin is excellent for dental infections. This drug is one of two options for patients with type I allergy to penicillin.

Azithromycin would be useful for patients with dental infections for whom other antibiotics have proved ineffective, patients that are intolerant of penicillin, and infections extending into the sinuses. Because azithromycin can be dosed once daily, it improves patient compliance but it should not be considered as first-line therapy in treating odontogenic infections. In pediatric infections, however, azithromycin is an attractive choice because of the short treatment duration, once daily dosing, and acceptable taste.

Moxifloxacin

Moxifloxacin is a broad-spectrum fourth-generation synthetic fluoroquinolone. It is effective against *Eikenella*, *Bacteroides*, *Prevotella*, and most other strains of bacteria that produce β-lactamase. This makes moxifloxacin ideal for infections that did not respond to the penicillins. Although it was reported to have the highest rate of bacterial susceptibility among all antibiotics including penicillin and clindamycin for odontogenic infections,[33,34] it should still be considered as a second-line therapy to penicillin, clindamycin, and metronidazole because of its cost (about $140 for a 7-day course).[35] Moxifloxacin may cause problems with bones, joints, and tissues around joints in children and should not be given to children younger than 18 years old.

SUMMARY

The most common causes of odontogenic infections are dental caries, deep fillings, failed root canal treatment, pericoronitis, and periodontal disease. The periapical infection is the most common form of odontogenic infection and is caused by invasion of the root canal system of the tooth by microorganisms. The pathogenesis of odontogenic infection is polymicrobial, consisting of various facultative anaerobes, such as the streptococci viridans group and the streptococcus anginosus group, and strict anaerobes, especially anaerobic cocci and *Prevotella* and *Fusobacterium* species. The dominant isolates are strictly anaerobic gram-negative rods and gram-positive cocci.

The clinical presentation of an odontogenic infection is highly variable depending on the source of the infection. Patients with superficial dental infections present with localized pain, cellulitis, and sensitivity to tooth percussion and temperature. However, patients with deep infections or abscesses that spread along the fascial planes may present with swelling; fever; and sometimes difficulty swallowing, opening the mouth, or breathing. Although odontogenic infections are usually mild and generally confined to the alveolar ridge or tissues in close proximity, they can spread into deep fascial spaces. Occasionally, spread beyond the barriers of the fascial spaces may occur, which can result in cavernous sinus thrombosis, brain abscess, airway obstruction, mediastinitis, and endocarditis.

The first and most important element in treating dental infections is the elimination of the primary source of the infection with antibiotics as adjunctive therapy.

REFERENCES

1. Santosh AN, Viresh AN, Sharmada BK. Microbiology and antibiotic sensitivity of odontogenic space infection. Int J Med Dent Sci 2014;3(1):303–13.
2. Harwood-Nuss A, Linden C, Luten R, editors. Dental, oral and salivary gland infections. The clinical practice of emergency medicine. 2nd edition. Philadelphia: Lippincott Williams & Wilkins Publishers; 1996. p. 73–7.
3. Kim MK, Allareddy V, Nalliah RP, et al. Burden of facial cellulitis: estimates from the Nationwide Emergency Department Sample. Oral Surg Oral Med Oral Pathol Oral Radiol Endod 2012;114(3):312–7.
4. Lemonick DM. Ludwig's angina: diagnosis and treatment. Hospital Physician; 2002. p. 31–7. Availabe at: http://www.turner-white.com/pdf/hp_jul02_angina.pdf. Accessed December 24, 2016.
5. Barakate MS, Jensen MJ, Hemli JM, et al. Ludwig's angina: report of a case and review of management issues. Ann Otol Rhinol Laryngol 2001;110(5 Pt 1):453–6.
6. Ferrera PC, Busino LJ, Snyder HS. Uncommon complications of odontogenic infections. Am J Emerg Med 1996;14(3):317–22.
7. Zachariades N, Mezitis M, Stavrinidis P, et al. Mediastinitis, thoracic empyema, and pericarditis as complications of a dental abscess: report of a case. J Oral Maxillofacsurg 1988;46(6):493–5.
8. Mihos P, Potaris K, Gakidis I, et al. Management of descending necrotizing mediastinitis. J Oral Maxillofacsurg 2004;62(8):966–72.

9. Yarington CT Jr. The prognosis and treatment of cavernous sinus thrombosis. Review of 878 cases in the literature. Ann Otol Rhinol Laryngol 1961;70(7):263–7.
10. Nair PN. Pathogenesis of apical periodontitis and the causes of endodontic failures. Crit Rev Oral Biol Med 2004;15(6):348–81.
11. Robertson D, Smith AJ. The microbiology of the acute dental abscess. J Med Microbiol 2009;58(2):155–62.
12. Riggio MP, Aga H, Murray CA, et al. Identification of bacteria associated with spreading odontogenic infections by 16S rRNA gene sequencing. Oral Surg Oral Med Oral Pathol Oral Radiol Endod 2007;103(5):610–7.
13. Siqueira JF Jr, Rôças IN. Diversity of endodontic microbiota revisited. J Dent Res 2009;88(11):969–81.
14. Khemaleelakul S, Baumgartner JC, Pruksakorn S. Identification of bacteria in acute endodontic infections and their antimicrobial susceptibility. Oral Surg Oral Med Oral Pathol Oral Radiol Endod 2002;94(6):746–55.
15. Siqueira JF Jr, Rôças IN. Microbiology and treatment of acute apical abscesses. Clin Microbiol Rev 2013;26(2):255–73.
16. Santos AL, Siqueira JF Jr, Rôças IN, et al. Comparing the bacterial diversity of acute and chronic dental root canal infections. PLoS One 2011;6:e28088. Available at: http://journals.plos.org/plosone/article?id=10.1371/journal.pone.0028088.
17. Shweta, Prakash SK. Dental abscess: a microbiological review. Dent Res J (Isfahan) 2013;10(5):585–91.
18. Machado de Oliveira JC, Siqueira JF Jr, Rôças IN, et al. Bacterial community profiles of endodontic abscesses from Brazilian and USA subjects as compared by denaturing gradient gel electrophoresis analysis. Oral Microbiol Immunol 2007; 22(1):14–8.
19. de Sousa EL, Ferraz CC, Gomes BP, et al. Bacteriological study of root canals associated with periapical abscesses. Oral Surg Oral Med Oral Pathol Oral Radiol Endod 2003;96(3):332–9.
20. Peters BM, Jabra-Rizk MA, O'May GA, et al. Polymicrobial interactions: impact on pathogenesis and human disease. Clin Microbiol Rev 2012;25(1):193–213.
21. Mosby's Medical Dictionary. 9th edition. Elsevier; 2013.
22. Gaetti-Jardim E Jr, Landucci LF, de Oliveira KL, et al. Microbiota associated with infections of the jaws. Int J Dent 2012;2012:369751 (8 pages).
23. Mohanty S. Spread of oral infections. In: Saraf S, editor. Textbook of oral pathology. New Delhi (India): Jaypee Brothers Medical Publishers; 2006. p. 190. Chapter 9.
24. Frydman WL, Abbaszadeh K. Diagnosis and management of odontogenic oral and facial infections. Oral Health 2014. Available at: http://www.oralhealthgroup.com/features/diagnosis-and-management-of-odontogenic-oral-and-facial-infections-william-l-frydman-dds-ms-frcd-c/. Accessed March 9, 2016.
25. Glickman GN, Schweitzer JL. Endodontic diagnosis. ENDODONTICS: Colleagues for Excellence. Newsletter from American Association of Endodontists, Chicago, IL 2013. p. 60611–2691. Available at: https://www.aae.org/.../newsletters/. Accessed March 16, 2016.
26. Hackethal V. Type 2 diabetes rates quadruple worldwide since 1980. Medscape Medical News 2016. Available at: http://www.medscape.com/viewarticle/861591#vp_2. Accessed April 9, 2016.
27. Schwartz S. Causes and treatment of odontogenic infections. Continuing Dental Education, Course Number: 336, DentalCare.com. Available at: http://www.dentalcare.com/en-US/dental-education/continuing-education/ce336/ce336.aspx?ModuleName=coursecontent&PartID=4&SectionID=-1. Accessed April 15, 2016.

28. Flynn T, Wiltz M, Adamo A, et al. Predicting length of hospital day and penicillin failure in severe odontogenic infections. Int J Oral Maxillofac Surg 1999;28(Suppl 1):48.
29. Sabiston CB, Gold WA. Anaerobic bacteria in oral infection. Oral Surg Oral Med Oral Pathol 1974;38(2):187–92.
30. Gilbert DN, Moellering RC Jr, Eliopoulos GM, et al, editors. Sanford guide to anti-microbial therapy. 39th edition. Sperryville (VA): Antimicrobial Therapy Inc; 2009.
31. Eisenstein BI, Schaechter M. DNA and chromosome mechanics. In: Engleberg NC, Dermody T, editors. DiRita V Schaechter's mechanisms of microbial disease. Hagerstown (MD): Lippincott Williams & Wilkins; 2007. p. 28.
32. Gregoire C. How are odontogenic infections best managed? JCDA 2010;76(2): 114–6.
33. Warnke PH, Becker ST, Springer I, et al. Penicillin compared with other advanced broad spectrum antibiotics regarding antibacterial activity against oral pathogens isolated from odontogenic abscesses. J Craniomaxillofac Surg 2008; 36(8):462–7.
34. Kuriyama T, Williams DW, Yanagisawa M, et al. Antimicrobial susceptibility of 800 anaerobic isolates from patients with dentoalveolar infection to 13 oral antibiotics. Oral Microbiol Immunol 2007;22(4):285–8.
35. Moxifloxacin Prices, Coupons & patient assistance programs. Available at: www.drugs.com/price-guide/moxifloxacin. Accessed May 13, 2016.

Periodontal Microbiology

John D. Harvey, DDS, MS

KEYWORDS

- Periodontal • Bacteria • Disease • Gingivitis • Periodontitis • Periodontopathogens

KEY POINTS

- Periodontal disease is a mixed bacterial infection that produces inflammatory destruction of the periodontal tissues that surround and support the teeth.
- Periodontal microbiota form a complex ecosystem called dental plaque biofilm, within which pathogens produce virulence factors that allow them to evade host defenses, as well as provoke a host immune response that is damaging to the host tissues.
- Periodontal disease actually results from a disruption of the homeostasis or balance that normally exists between the plaque bacteria, host immune system, and environmental conditions during health.
- The pathogenic bacteria as well as the damaging inflammatory mediators expressed by host immune cells may travel to distant sites through the bloodstream and there induce systemic conditions that could result in heart attacks and strokes.
- Recent advances in molecular biology have enabled the identification of numerous previously undetected bacteria that may themselves play a significant role in the disease.

INTRODUCTION

There are about 700 species of bacteria known to be capable of colonizing the human oral cavity, but only around 200 to 300 of these would be found in the mouth of any one individual.[1] The oral bacteria have long been considered to be mostly commensal with only a small proportion being pathogenic[2] causing either dental caries or periodontal disease, which are among the most prevalent diseases of mankind.[2]

Periodontal disease is essentially a mixed bacterial infection that produces inflammatory destruction of the tissues that surround and support the teeth.[3] It results from a combination of factors, but its primary cause is bacteria found in dental plaque.[2] When left untreated, this disease often results in loss of the affected teeth, thereby accounting for most teeth that are lost during adulthood.[4]

The author has nothing to disclose.
Department of Anatomy, Howard University, College of Medicine, 520 W Street Northwest, Washington, DC 20059, USA
E-mail address: drjhperio@gmail.com

Dent Clin N Am 61 (2017) 253–269
http://dx.doi.org/10.1016/j.cden.2016.11.005
0011-8532/17/© 2016 Elsevier Inc. All rights reserved.

Besides causing tooth loss, periodontal disease also may affect our body's general health.[5] The connection between periodontal disease and overall health is of increasingly greater concern as more evidence emerges linking it with chronic systemic conditions, such as heart disease and respiratory illness,[5,6] as well as with potentially fatal thromboembolic events: myocardial and cerebral infarctions.[5]

The microbiology of periodontal disease cannot be fully appreciated without an understanding of the immunology and the histopathology of the disease because these topics are inextricably interrelated. In our discussion of microbiology, we must also incorporate knowledge from disciplines, such as pharmacotherapeutics and behavioral sciences, in the treatment protocols that we formulate to achieve bacterial or disease control.

TYPES OF PERIODONTAL DISEASE

There are 2 main types of periodontal disease: gingivitis and periodontitis. There are also different types of gingivitis and different types of periodontitis; however, the chronic form of each is the most common.[7,8]

Gingivitis is an inflammation confined to the keratinized mucosa called gingiva that surrounds the neck of the tooth. This inflammation is evidenced by redness and swelling of the soft tissue as well as bleeding from the gingival sulcus (or gingival crevice) on mechanical stimulation[7] with dental instruments or personal hygiene devices, such as a toothbrush or dental floss. Gingivitis is considered a reversible condition.[7,9]

Periodontitis is an irreversible and more serious condition that generally arises out of long-standing gingival inflammation in susceptible individuals.[7] In periodontitis, the inflammatory lesion spreads from the gingiva into the deeper, supportive components of the periodontium, namely, the periodontal ligament, the cementum, and the alveolar bone.[7] Periodontitis causes destruction of these supporting structures of the tooth and, if it is not arrested, may result in looseness of the tooth and, ultimately, tooth loss.[7] Often, when the term *periodontal disease* is used, especially outside of the academic environment, it is almost always referring to periodontitis only and not to gingivitis.

EPIDEMIOLOGY

Even though periodontitis develops from gingivitis, not all cases of gingivitis will progress to become periodontitis.[10] The most recent and most accurate large-scale epidemiologic survey to date indicates that roughly half of the adult population in the United States has periodontitis, whereas the other half has gingivitis.[11] Those patients who demonstrate the progressive attachment loss that characterizes periodontitis can be categorized as disease prone, whereas those who have gingival inflammation that never progresses to attachment loss would be categorized as disease resistant. However, the actual transition to destructive disease in any one individual is thought to depend not only on genetic factors but also on the interplay between genetic (host immune), environmental, and bacterial virulence factors.[7,10]

CHANGES SEEN WITH INFLAMMATION

Healthy gingiva is characterized as pink, firm, stippled, and of knife-edged morphology.[12] Inflammation of the gingiva is triggered by the presence of bacteria in the gingival sulcus and is the body's reaction to what it perceives as an impending bacterial invasion.[13] Clinically, this gingival inflammation is recognized by redness, swelling, a spongy consistency, a shiny smooth surface texture, and bleeding on probing.

Gingival inflammation typically begins in the col: a saddle-shaped depression in the interdental papilla as it loops under the contact point between 2 adjacent teeth.[12] This area under the contact point is the most inaccessible part the healthy tooth for plaque removal. As a consequence, this is usually where one may find the deeper periodontal pockets as well as cratered bone defects in cases of periodontal disease.[14]

A periodontal pocket is a sulcus that has become deepened as a result of inflammation. A normal gingival sulcus ranges from 1 to 3 mm, and any sulcus measurement of 4 mm or greater is, therefore, a pocket. The pocket is called a gingival pocket or pseudopocket if the sulcus deepens because of gingival swelling, as in gingivitis. The pocket is a true periodontal pocket if the sulcus deepens because of the loss of connective tissue attachment to the root.[4,15]

Radiographically, a loss of crestal lamina dura indicates bone deterioration under the col. It is, however, not reliable as a sign of current disease activity but rather a historical record of bone lost by prior disease activity.[16]

Once attachment loss has occurred, cementum gets exposed to the saliva, the crevicular fluid, and the bacteria. This exposure leads to infection and gradual deterioration of the cementum, which eventually becomes necrotic.[15] Histologically, calculus can be found as deep in the tooth as the dentinocemental junction and periodontal bacteria may even be found to have invaded the dentinal tubules of the root after the overlying cementum has been deteriorated.[17]

CAUSE OF PERIODONTAL DISEASE

Periodontal disease is multifactorial, and bacteria are considered to be the main (or primary) etiologic factor.[2] However, there are also several secondary etiologic factors that may play a role in the development of disease in each particular case. Such secondary etiologic factors include plaque-retentive features, such calculus (or tartar), developmental grooves on the root and overhanging restorations; systemic factors, such as hormones and medications; genetic factors, such as congenital immune disorders; and nutritional deficiency, as in scurvy.[10,17–20]

Primary Cause: Bacterial Plaque

Because bacterial plaque is the primary etiologic factor in periodontal disease,[2] a thorough understanding of its formation, its structure, and its biology is fundamental to our efforts to control or combat (prevent) the disease.

The pioneering work of Harald Loe and coworkers[21] published in 1965 confirmed the causal relationship between dental plaque and experimental gingivitis in human subjects. They found that clinically evident chronic gingivitis develops within 7 to 21 days of the cessation of oral hygiene measures and that gingival health is reestablished in 7 to 10 days after oral hygiene is reestablished.[21] They also documented the accompanying shifts in the bacterial population, from predominantly gram-positive and coccoid forms in periodontal health to mostly gram-negative rods and motile forms, such as spirochetes in the diseased state.[22]

IDENTIFICATION OF BACTERIA

Previously, culturing techniques were relied on to help us decipher the microbiota and their relationships within plaque; but advances in technology now enable us to analyze plaque and identify many organisms that we are still unable to culture.[1] The visualization and labeling of individual bacterial cells within plaque, using techniques that employ nucleic acid probes (fluorescence in situ hybridization) or specific antibodies (immunofluorescence) to identify bacteria, and the use of confocal scanning laser microscopy, have yielded much valuable information about the organisms and their relationships within the biofilm, even regarding organisms that have not yet been cultured.[9,23,24]

However, newer techniques for characterizing bacteria based on molecular biology have now become the standard.[1] Through the use of 16S rRNA gene cloning and sequencing, we now know that there are more than 400 periodontal bacterial species, of which less than half have been successfully cultured.[21] Furthermore, many species also have different strains or serotypes.

STRUCTURE AND COMPOSITION OF PLAQUE

In general, gram-positive and facultative organisms are usually associated with periodontal health, and are considered beneficial species, whereas gram-negative and anaerobic bacteria are usually associated with disease. An example of beneficence would be *Streptococcus sanguinis*, which produces hydrogen peroxide[25] that is toxic to *Aggregatibacter actinomycetemcomitans*, a confirmed periopathogen.[26]

Biofilm

Dental plaque is a biofilm: this is an ecosystem in which bacteria form microcolonies that are surrounded by a protective matrix composed of glycoproteins and extracellular polysaccharides. The matrix encloses the plaque microorganisms in a specialized environment that protects them.[9] Bacteria in plaque biofilm are, therefore, 1000 to 1500 times more resistant to antimicrobials than those bacteria existing outside plaque in the same oral environment.[27]

The biofilm is permeated by circulatory channels that allow for inflow of nutrients and outflow of waste products or metabolites. A circulatory system is needed because diffusion would be insufficient to serve the nutritional and respiratory needs of the dense population of organisms.[27,28] Biofilm bacteria also have a means of communication called quorum sensing in which the accumulation of a metabolite beyond a threshold level triggers changes in gene expression throughout the community. This serves to bring about coordinated responses, for instance, in motility or virulence.[29]

Within the biofilm, there are microenvironments that vary in pH and concentrations of various chemicals and metabolites.[28] These variations enable different species with varied metabolic needs to thrive in different microenvironments within the ecosystem, thereby fostering greater diversity among the bacterial population.[9,27] This diversity ensures that the mixed infections caused by dental plaque are more difficult to manage and makes it more difficult to predict the particular organism(s) that are likely to be responsible for each infection.

One clinically important characteristic of dental plaque is that it cannot be removed from the tooth by rinsing or spraying. This characteristic contrasts it with materia alba, a less organized product found in the oral cavity that has relatively far fewer bacteria. Materia alba not physically attached to any surface and, therefore, can be removed with a rinse or spray.[9,27]

Long-standing dental plaque undergoes calcification to form dental calculus or tartar, which becomes more difficult to remove over time. Calculus is plaque retentive and is classified as a secondary etiologic factor in periodontal disease. It usually has a layer of uncalcified plaque on its surface.[9,27]

Plaque Formation

In plaque development, the first layer that forms on a newly cleansed tooth surface is the acquired pellicle. This layer begins to form within seconds by the adsorption of salivary glycoproteins onto tooth enamel, exposed cementum, exposed dentin of the root, or any other hard surface within the oral cavity.[29]

Pellicle formation is quickly followed by the initial attachment of early colonizers to the pellicle. The early colonizers in plaque are predominantly gram positive, facultative and nonmotile, and of the *Streptococcus* (up to 80%) and *Actinomyces* genera.[27,29]

Attachment is a process that involves the recognition of specific receptor molecules in the pellicle by proteins called adhesins that project from bacterial surfaces. One example of attachment occurs between proline-rich proteins of the pellicle and adhesins of *Actinomyces*. The receptor site is called a cryptitope and becomes available only after the adsorbed proline-rich proteins undergo a conformational change to reveal it.[27,29]

Subsequent layers of bacteria attach to those that are already in place, through coaggregation.[28] Certain species of bacteria will only coaggregate with certain other species of bacteria, based on shared characteristics and/or symbiotic relationships.[7] An example of such symbiosis occurs between *Treponema denticola* and *Porphyromonas gingivalis*. *Treponema denticola* produces succinate from amino acid fermentation in subgingival plaque, and *Porphyromonas gingivalis* utilizes succinate. *Porphyromonas gingivalis*, on the other hand, produces certain fatty acids that may stimulate growth of *Treponema denticola*.[25]

Population shifts occur during plaque development.[7,9] As the bacterial population increases within the biofilm by the addition of more layers, the oxygen content becomes depleted, making the environment more suitable for colonization by anaerobic species. This depletion leads to the proliferation of the secondary (or late) colonizers, which are predominantly gram-negative anaerobic rods and filamentous organisms.[9,27] *Fusobacterium* is considered a bridging organism between the early colonizers and the other secondary colonizers because it is uniquely capable of coaggregating with all other species within plaque.[3]

The final group to start proliferating in the biofilm during plaque development is that of the spirochetes, which are motile and tissue invasive.[9,27] It is noteworthy that in the experimental gingivitis of Loe and colleagues,[21] proliferation of spirochetes correlated with the observation of clinical signs, such as gingival redness, swelling, and bleeding on probing.

Supragingival and Subgingival Plaque

In a healthy periodontium, plaque forms in an ongoing basis supragingivally; however, if it is not removed within 2 to 4 days, its increasing volume causes it to extend below the gingival margin and into the sulcus.[17]

Supragingival plaque tends to be associated with calculus formation and root caries if on the root, whereas plaque at the gingival margin tends to be associated with gingivitis. Subgingival plaque is discussed in 2 parts: the part close to the tooth surface is called tooth-associated subgingival plaque and the part further from the tooth surface is called tissue-associated plaque because it contacts the soft tissue of the sulcus or pocket epithelium.[27]

Tooth-associated subgingival plaque is associated with root caries and subgingival calculus formation, whereas tissue-associated subgingival plaque is lacking in matrix, is loosely adherent, has motile organisms, and is associated with periodontitis. Subgingival plaque also exhibits a coronal to apical gradient, in which the further subgingivally that plaque extends, the more anaerobic and gram negative are the bacterial inhabitants found within it.[27] Prominent bacteria found in the plaque sampled from each region are summarized in **Table 1**. The numbers of bacteria in plaque range from 10^3 in a healthy sulcus to 10^8 to 10^{10} in a deep pocket, which represents a substantial challenge to the immune system.[27,31]

Table 1 Distribution of bacterial type by location	
Type of Plaque/By Location	**Distribution of Bacterial Type**
Supragingival plaque	At the tooth surface: mostly gram-positive cocci and short rods At the outer surface: mostly gram-negative rods and filaments as well as spirochetes
Tooth-associated subgingival plaque	Cervically: mostly filamentous organisms, gram-positive rods and cocci, including *Streptococcus spp*, and *Actinomyces spp* Progressing apically: decreasing filaments, and increasing gram-negative rods
Tissue-associated subgingival plaque	Gram-negative rods and cocci, large numbers of filamentous organisms, and motile organisms, including flagellated rods and spirochetes[27,30]

In a landmark publication in 1998, Dr Sigmund Socransky and coworkers[32] from the Forsyth Institute in Boston grouped together specific bacteria that have been found to coaggregate within bacterial plaque.[7] The groups were given names of different colors for convenience: blue, yellow, green, purple, orange, and red. *Aggregatibacter actinomycetemcomitans* serotype b and *Selenomonas* did not cluster with any of the groups.

Of the 6 microbial complexes that were found within subgingival plaque, 2 of them, the orange and red complexes, include organisms that have been closely associated with periodontal pathologic conditions.[7]

The red complex is the group most implicated in active/destructive periodontal disease, being most closely associated with bleeding on probing and often found elevated in plaque located next to periodontal lesions.[7] The red complex comprises *Treponema denticola*, *Porphyromonas gingivalis*, and *Tannerella forsythia*; *Eubacterium nodatum* was added later.

In addition, several noncultivable or poorly cultivable species, identified more recently through advanced techniques, including the gram-positive species *Filifactor alocis* and *Peptostreptococcus stomatitis*, gram-negative species *Dialister*, *Megasphaera*, *Selenomonas*, and species from *Prevotella*, *Desulfobulbus*, and *Synergistes*, have also been found in elevated numbers in diseased sites.[7]

KOCH'S POSTULATES REVISED BY SOCRANSKY

Koch's postulates, used for well more than 100 years to help decide whether a specific human infection is caused by a particular microorganism,[7,27] cannot be directly applied to a mixed infection, such as periodontal disease. For this reason, in 1992 Dr Socransky proposed an alternate set of criteria to be used to implicate an organism in the cause of a particular periodontal disease. Among these is the requirement that the organism should be either absent or present in much smaller numbers in periodontally healthy subjects or subjects with other forms of periodontal disease.[33] This necessary modification of one of the Koch's postulates underscores the change in perspective necessary when it comes to mixed infections.[7]

Plaque Hypotheses

Two long-standing hypotheses have been the subject of much debate over the years to explain the relationship between dental plaque and the development of dental and periodontal disease.[7,27]

On one hand, the nonspecific plaque hypothesis asserted that the disease was caused by the accumulation of dental plaque past the threshold necessary to overwhelm the host defenses. It, however, could not explain why many patients with abundant plaque and calculus never converted from gingivitis to periodontitis. On the other hand, the specific plaque hypothesis proposes that only certain organisms in dental plaque are responsible for particular disease conditions. However, this hypothesis could not account for cases of disease in which these certain organisms or periodontopathogens were not found, and it could not explain the presence of known periodontopathogens in healthy sites or nondestructive lesions.[27]

Marsh and coworkers subsequently devised the ecologic plaque hypothesis, which integrates both of the previous hypotheses into one theory. This newer hypothesis states that both the total amount of plaque as well as specific bacteria within plaque may contribute to the transition from periodontal health to periodontal disease. This hypothesis is more in keeping with the current concept that disease is not caused by a particular organism or amount of plaque but depends on host immune factors, bacterial virulence, and environmental factors and results when homeostasis is disrupted among them.[7,27]

It recognizes the fact that the disease-causing organisms occupy a minor fraction of the total bacteria in plaque and that one or more of these pathogenic species can cause damage and disease when local changes in the plaque microenvironments favor their proliferation beyond their individual thresholds.[7,27]

The true complexity of periodontal disease begins to become apparent when one realizes that each case of active disease, and even perhaps each site of active disease, may have a different species or a different combination of species promoting the disease process at different points in time, depending on the specific conditions that exist in each microenvironment of the biofilm.[3]

IMMUNE RESPONSE

Most of the tissue destruction seen in periodontitis results from the host immune system's response to the periodontal pathogens and involves mechanisms from both innate and adaptive immunity.[34]

Innate Immunity

Innate immunity is an inborn, rapidly activated, nonspecific protective response by our immune system.[34] The classic innate immune response is acute inflammation, characterized by increased vasodilation, increased vascular permeability, and migration of neutrophils to the site of invasion.[35]

It protects the host immediately and through the first few days of a microbial infection. Innate immunity also activates adaptive immunity, which is a learned, more specific, and more long-lasting protection against the infecting organisms.[34]

During an innate immune response, the eukaryotic pattern-recognition receptors present on host cells, such as epithelial cells, fibroblasts, macrophages, and lymphocytes, recognize and interact with the evolutionarily-conserved microbe-associated molecular patterns found in or on the prokaryotic pathogens.[35]

This interaction triggers the host cell to differentiate into a more specialized cell or to increase production of inflammatory mediators, such as enzymes or cytokines. The proinflammatory mediators tumor necrosis factor (TNF)-α, interleukin (IL)-1β, and prostaglandin E2 have long been implicated in the bone loss observed in periodontitis.[34]

Once the proinflammatory mediators have been released, they then provide a positive-feedback loop to the cells that produced them, thereby resulting in a cascade.[34] The local concentrations of inflammatory mediators are greatly amplified by such cascading mechanisms. Fortunately, during the cascade, some of molecules of the proinflammatory mediators will interact with other receptors on host cells, triggering the production of antiinflammatory mediators, such as IL-10 and IL-1 receptor antagonist (IL-ra), that function to limit the extent and duration of the destructive event,[34,35] ideally confining it to a short burst in a local site.

Adaptive Immunity

Adaptive immunity involves the activities of T cells in cell-mediated immunity and B cells and plasma cells in antibody production and subsequent antigen-antibody reactions.[35] It has been found that specially bred severe combined immunodeficiency mice lacking B and T cells have much less bone loss from periodontal inflammation than normal mice. This finding points to the likelihood that adaptive immunity plays a role in periodontal bone destruction.[2]

Regulation of bone resorption occurs via a receptor on osteoclast-precursor cells called RANK (receptoractivator of nuclear factor-κB). RANK is activated by RANK ligand (RANKL) and triggers differentiation into osteoclasts, which then resorb bone.[2,13]

In active periodontitis lesions, B and T cells are the main sources of RANKL that lead to bone destruction. Osteoprotegerin expressed on mesenchymal stem cells, is a RANK receptor inhibitor that is at high levels during health and low levels in periodontitis. RANKL levels are low in health and high in periodontitis.[2,13]

Each subset of T-helper cells can mediate protective as well as harmful responses. The Th17 subset of T-helper cells (CD4+) mediates responses that reinforce innate immunity against extracellular pathogens. However, Th17 cells also produce the cytokine IL-17, which in animal models can cause connective tissue and bone destruction, by inducing matrix metalloproteinases in fibroblasts and polymorphonuclear neutrophils and RANKL in T cells.[2]

Another subset of T-helper cells, the T-regulatory cells (Tregs) have a protective function in inflammation. They produce IL-10, which suppresses induction of RANKL. Tregs promote self-tolerance and downregulate the excessive immune responses to commensal as well as pathogenic microbes, thereby helping to restore homeostasis.[2,10]

B cells in the mucosa-associated lymphoid tissue (MALT) also participate in adaptive immunity in periodontal disease. This process involves dendritic cells in the gingiva, which engulf and process foreign antigen and then present the antigen to naïve T cells in nearby MALT. The naïve T cells become activated and in turn activate B cells to become plasma cells. These plasma cells produce and deposit large quantities of antibodies called secretory immunoglobulin A in the connective tissue subjacent to the site of invasion. The antibodies are transported into the gingival sulcus where they perform functions like preventing adhesion of the pathogenic organisms displaying that specific antigen.[9,36]

These interrelated processes together produce an immune response that ultimately leads to focal destruction of periodontal tissue within active disease sites,[37] hence, the chronic nature of the disease, consisting of long periods of relative quiescence, interrupted by brief periods of destruction when there is disruption in homeostasis, occurring either at random sites or in sites that might have been predisposed by local conditions.[15]

HISTOPATHOLOGY OF PERIODONTAL DISEASE

Gingivitis is reversible and is considered a protective lesion that sequesters the infection without causing loss of support.[7] However, it does have some tissue destruction within it, such as the destruction of collagen within the lamina propria as well as erosions in the sulcular epithelium, giving rise to ulcerations that are responsible for bleeding on probing.[38]

The progression of these events was best described in Page and Schroeder's[39] landmark studies on periodontal pathogenesis (1976), in which they identified 3 histopathologic stages of gingivitis that they named the initial lesion, the early lesion, and the established lesion. These lesions show histologically the progression from a (subclinical) vasculitis to an acute inflammation to a chronic inflammation. The established lesion may remain confined to the marginal gingiva[13] indefinitely.[10]

ATTACHMENT LOSS AND BONE LOSS

If at some point the established lesion is triggered by a loss of homeostasis[2,13] to develop and expand beyond this confined area, the destruction begins to spread laterally and apically[2] to eventually disrupt the collagen that inserts into calcified tooth structure. This disruption is called attachment loss and indicates a transition from gingivitis to periodontitis. Attachment loss is the defining event in periodontitis and is the most significant finding in the fourth histopathologic stage described by Page and Schroeder, the advanced lesion.[10]

Once connective tissue attachment to the root has been disrupted, the inflammatory degradation can then spread to the cementum and also to the alveolar bone The resorption of alveolar bone, orchestrated by the host immune response, occurs ahead of the leading wave of bacterial ingress and is seen as the body's attempt to prevent bacterial invasion of the bone itself.[7,10]

BACTERIA IMPLICATED IN PARTICULAR PERIODONTAL INFECTIONS

The current classification system for periodontal diseases and conditions (Armitage,[40] 1999) lists many diseases and conditions in addition to chronic gingivitis and chronic periodontitis.

Healthy periodontal tissues have bacterial populations consisting mostly of *Streptococcus* and *Actinomyces*, with a small fraction of gram-negative organisms, such as *Prevotella*, *Fusobacterium*, and *Veillonella*.[27] Periodontal infections are associated with wide variety of microbial profiles depending on the type of periodontal disease (**Table 2**).[7]

Bacterial Virulence and Pathogenicity

There is ongoing debate about how we define a periodontal pathogen and also about which organisms would qualify as periodontal pathogens and which would not, because not all bacteria designated as pathogens are virulent and, conversely, some that are considered commensals may include virulent subpopulations.[15]

Certain features of pathogenic bacteria are considered important in enabling them to further the disease process. These virulence factors vary from one group of organisms to another and include cell wall components, such as lipopolysaccharides (LPSs) (gram negative) and lipoteichoic acids (gram positive), capsules, fimbriae and pili, fibrillar layers (fuzzy coats), flagella, vesicles, S layers, and endospores.

The organisms in the red complex, *P gingivalis*, *Tannerella forsythia*, and *Treponema denticola*, are often found elevated in the plaque next to periodontal lesions; hence, they are considered "consensus pathogens."[7]

Furthermore, epidemiologic studies performed in different parts of the world have shown that colonization of the oral cavity by certain species of periodontal bacteria, including *A actinomycetemcomitans*, *P gingivalis*, *Tannerella forsythia*, and *Campylobacter rectus*, makes it highly probable that the individual will have destructive periodontal disease.[7]

Table 2
Microbial profile of various periodontal diseases

Type of Gingival/ Periodontal Infection	Microbial Profile
Gingivitis	1. Plaque-induced (chronic) gingivitis: The bacterial profile is one of near balance, with slightly more facultative organisms than anaerobes but at the same time slightly more gram positives than gram negatives[27] 2. Nonplaque-induced gingivitis: This inflammation is associated with specific infections other than that induced by plaque biofilm or with allergies or with trauma. Those infections that involve organisms other than plaque organisms include gonococcal, syphilitic, and viral and fungal gingival infections.[8]
Chronic periodontitis	This condition is dental plaque-induced and may be modified by chronic illnesses, such as HIV or diabetes, or by environmental conditions, such as smoking. The bacterial profile would be similar to that described for subgingival plaque, particularly the deep subgingival plaque. Predominant bacteria include *Porphyromonas, Prevotella, Tannerella, Campylobacter, Eikenella, Fusobacterium, Parvimonas, Aggregatibacter, Treponema,* and *Selenomonas.*[27]
Aggressive periodontitis	The localized form of this plaque-induced, fast-progressing disease affects first molars and incisors in individuals starting around puberty and is associated with a highly leukotoxic clone of *Aggregatibacter actinomycetemcomitans.*[7] Others also present include *Porphyromonas, Campylobacter, Prevotella, Tannerella,* and spirochetes.[27] The generalized form of aggressive periodontitis affects other permanent teeth in addition to the first molars and incisors, and it usually gets diagnosed in patients' twenties (ie, younger than 30 years). The bacterial profile shows less of *Aggregatibacter* and more of *Porphyromonas, Prevotella, Tannerella, Campylobacter,* and *Treponema.*[27]
Periodontitis as a manifestation of systemic diseases	This condition can be confused with aggressive periodontitis because of the rapid bone loss. It is diagnosed when the systemic condition is the main factor in evidence and significant local irritants are not present.[8] A unique bacterial profile has not been reported but one would expect the general mixed bacterial profile of chronic periodontitis.
Necrotizing periodontal diseases	These conditions are acute inflammatory conditions that arise under conditions of stress, neglect, and immunocompromised states. Other predisposing factors are fatigue, poor nutrition, underlying chronic periodontal disease, and smoking. Hallmarks of the necrotizing diseases are sudden onset, pain, marginal and papillary necrosis of the gingiva, foul odor, and a bacterial profile that features prominently spirochetes, *Fusobacterium nucleatum, Prevotella intermedia,* and *Selenomonas.* Necrotizing periodontal disease can, under conditions of severe malnutrition or in severely immunocompromised patients, extend to cause gangrenous destruction of large areas of soft tissue and bone, a condition called necrotizing ulcerative stomatitis, cancrum oris, or noma.[8,27,41]

(continued on next page)

Table 2 (continued)	
Type of Gingival/ Periodontal Infection	**Microbial Profile**
Abscesses of the periodontium	These infections are acute inflammatory episodes that are usually flareups of chronic conditions. They manifest often as painful fluctuant swellings filled with purulent exudate. Bacteria found are usually gram-negative anaerobes, such as *Fusobacterium* and *Prevotella*.[27]
Periodontitis associated with endodontic lesions	The bacterial populations from both spaces can cross contaminate; however, it is more likely for an endodontic lesion to spread to the periodontium. Infections that start in the pulp are generally mixed anaerobic infections featuring *Fusobacterium*, *Prevotella*, and *Parvimonas*, which are also found in periodontal diseases.[42]
Developmental or acquired deformities and conditions	These conditions include factors such as overhanging restorations (iatrogenic deformities) that lead to exacerbations of the chronic infections of gingivitis and periodontitis, already described earlier; hence, the same bacterial profiles would be expected.[8]
Peri-implant disease	These conditions are inflammatory processes analogous to periodontal disease but occurring around osseointegrated implants. The bacterial profiles are also generally similar to those we find around natural teeth. *Aggregatibacter*, *Porphyromonas*, *Parvimonas*, *Tannerella*, *Treponema*, and *Campylobacter* are among those prominent in periimplantitis.[27]
Halitosis	A clinically and socially significant problem, not listed in Armitage's[40] classification, that can be caused by plaque bacteria is halitosis. The bacteria implicated are those that produce enzymes, such as L-cysteine desulfhydrase, that metabolize sulfur-containing proteins and peptides to produce hydrogen sulfide and other pungent sulfides. This condition may occur with gingivitis-associated bacteria, such as *S sanguinous* and *F nucleatum*, or with periodontitis-associated bacteria, such as *T denticola*, or may even result from the metabolism of tongue bacteria with no accompanying periodontal inflammation.[28]

PERIODONTAL-SYSTEMIC CONNECTION

The tissue destruction caused by plaque-induced inflammation creates ulcers in the pocket epithelium, which gives plaque bacteria and their byproducts as well as inflammatory mediators access to the blood stream. Bacteremias may also occur because of the physical forces that impact gingival tissues, such as tooth brushing and mastication.[7]

LPSs from gram-negative bacteria, such as the periodontal pathogens *P gingivalis*, *Tannerella forsythia*, *A actinomycetemcomitans*, and *Treponema denticola*, activate monocytes/macrophages to release proinflammatory cytokines TNF-a and IL-1b. These cytokines enter the bloodstream and travel to the liver, there inducing production of acute-phase proteins, such as C-reactive protein (CRP). Patients with elevated blood levels of CRP are more likely to develop cardiovascular disease.[7]

LPS and cytokines are such as TNF-a, IL-6 have also been known to provoke atherogenesis in vascular endothelium. When ruptured atheromatous plaques get liberated into circulation, they may eventually block vessels causing infarctions. In this regard, cross-sectional and prospective cohort epidemiologic studies consistently show an association between periodontitis and a higher incidence and prevalence of heart attacks and strokes.[7]

Another mechanism of interest in atherogenesis is the mimicking of a human protein, HSP60, by its bacterial analog GroEL, produced by *P gingivalis*. When we produce antibodies to GroEL, they function like autoantibodies to our own HSP60, leading to apoptosis in vascular endothelial cells which in turn may lead to atherogenesis.[7]

Also, in a recent study, *Streptococcus gordonii* has been found to produce a molecule that mimics human fibrinogen causing formation of blood clots that encase and protect the bacterium within blood vessels. These clots could possibly then lead to endocarditis or infarctions.[43]

Apart from atherogenesis and thromboembolism, evidence also exists that is either suggestive of or corroborates a connection between periodontal disease and each of the following systemic conditions: infectious endocarditis, disseminated intravascular coagulation, diabetes mellitus, preterm low birth weight, and respiratory infections.[7]

PERIODONTAL TREATMENT

Despite our adoption of the ecologic plaque hypothesis, our profession still approaches periodontal therapy more in accordance with the nonspecific plaque hypothesis, with a focus on eliminating plaque and calculus and preventing its buildup.[27]

Mechanical nonsurgical therapy and home care are the main activities used in disease intervention.[7] If infection persists after the initial therapy because of inaccessible bacterial deposits in deep periodontal pockets, then a surgical flap may be used to gain access to the deep deposits; mechanical therapy would be used during the surgery to achieve a more effective removal of deposits.[7] It is important to note that mechanical periodontal therapy has been shown to be beneficial in causing a downregulation of several genes including genes for complement components that would have amplified the inflammatory response.[13]

CHEMOTHERAPEUTICS

Antimicrobial agents are also used against periodontal bacteria as part of therapy. These agents include systemic antibiotics, locally delivered antimicrobials, and over-the-counter as well as prescription mouth rinses.

Systemic Antibiotics

The main indications for systemic antimicrobial therapy would be for patients who are unresponsive to adequate mechanical therapy (refractory periodontitis), patients who present with acute periodontal infections, as prophylaxis for the medically compromised, and as an adjunctive treatment to surgical and nonsurgical therapy. These agents are usually taken by mouth and function either by killing bacteria or stopping them from proliferating.

Thorough medical histories must be elicited from patients in order to minimize the risk of an allergic reaction. Other adverse reactions can occur in patients who may have sensitivity to a particular agent. Common side effects include diarrhea and vaginal candidiasis, both of which result from disruption of normal flora in regions of the body other than the intended target area. Antibiotics may also interact with other medications being taken by patients, producing ineffectiveness or other side effects.

The main antibiotics commonly used in treatment of periodontal disease are amoxicillin, metronidazole, clindamycin, azithromycin, ciprofloxacin, doxycycline, and minocycline[44] (**Table 3**).

Table 3
Antimicrobial medication management of periodontal diseases

Medication	Dosing	Type of Periodontal Disease
Amoxicillin	500 mg, 3 times daily for 8 d; amoxicillin and clavulanate potassium (Augmentin): may be useful against LAP and refractory periodontitis	May be useful against localized and generalized aggressive periodontitis
Metronidazole	500 mg, 3 times daily for 8 d; 500 mg daily for 21 d	May be useful in combination with amoxicillin or amoxicillin and clavulanate potassium (Augmentin) against LAP or refractory periodontitis
Clindamycin	300 mg, 3 times daily for 10 d	Effective against periodontitis that is refractory to tetracyclines
Azithromycin	500 mg, once daily for 4–7 d	Effective against anaerobes and gram-negative bacilli; actively transported to sites of inflammation; may be useful against aggressive periodontitis
Ciprofloxacin	500 mg, twice daily for 8 d	Effective against all strains of *A actinomycetemcomitans* Promotes health-associated flora
Doxycycline	100–200 mg, once daily for 21 d	Once-daily dosing helps compliance; anticollagenase effect, is useful in low (20 mg) dose as host modulation therapy agent Adjunct to scaling and root planing in chronic periodontitis; should not be used when there are developing teeth
Minocycline	100–200 mg, once daily for 21 d	Twice-daily dosing helps compliance; may eliminate spirochetes for up 2 mo; shows improvement in all periodontal parameters
Combination therapy	Metronidazole and amoxicillin: 250 mg of each, 3 times daily for 8 d	Used for refractory periodontitis, as an adjunct in advanced chronic periodontitis and in cases that harbor *A actinomycetemcomitans*
Combination therapy	Metronidazole and ciprofloxacin: 500 mg of each, twice daily for 8 d	Used for refractory periodontitis and as an adjunct in advanced chronic periodontitis

Abbreviation: LAP, localized aggressive periodontitis.

Data from Ciancio S, Mariotti A. Antiinfective therapy. In: Newman MG, Takei HH, Klokkevold PR, et al, editors. Carranza's clinical periodontology. 11th edition. St Louis (MO): Elsevier; 2012. p. 482–91.

Locally Delivered Antimicrobials

The intermicrobial matrix that surrounds and protects the plaque bacteria, makes normal systemic administration of antibiotics ineffective against bacteria within the dental plaque.[27] Special formulations have been made of certain antibiotics for direct

---

Box 1
Locally delivered antimicrobials in periodontal disease

1. Tetracycline-infused fibers

2. Doxycycline (in a bioabsorbable carrier)

3. Minocycline microspheres

4. Chlorhexidine (in bioabsorbable wafers)

5. Metronidazole (in a gel carrier)

---

placement into periodontal pockets.[7] These locally delivered antimicrobials (LDAs) allow for a much greater concentration of medication to be delivered to the site without systemic side effects or risk of toxicity.[13]

These agents are best used as adjunctive therapy during the maintenance phase and in cases whereby there are very few sites that have persistent inflammation despite thorough mechanical nonsurgical therapy or surgical therapy. LDAs that have been used in periodontal disease management are listed in **Box 1**.[44]

PLAQUE CONTROL/ORAL HYGIENE/HOMECARE

Patient-performed oral hygiene is the most important procedure in the long-term maintenance of periodontal health because plaque formation is ongoing. Oral hygiene focuses on the patients' role in disrupting bacterial plaque formation on an ongoing basis.[45] This area is particularly difficult because it most often requires behavior modification and patient compliance. Plaque control should, therefore, be tailored to the patient because each individual may require a different approach to help them translate oral hygiene instructions into new habits.

SUMMARY

Periodontal health can be regarded as a homeostasis between the host and the bacterial community, based on balanced interactions between commensal organisms and the host immune system. Disease manifests when this homeostatic balance is disrupted.[2]

If we consider an analogy in which periodontal disease is represented as a tug of war between the bacteria and the patients' immune system, then the periodontal procedures that we perform on our patients in the office and the oral hygiene procedures performed by patients outside the office should combine to create a stronger pull in favor of the patients' immune system. As our knowledge develops, we should one day be able to restore homeostasis by also correcting the other factors involved apart from the local irritants.

The discussion of the microbiology of periodontal disease is really also a discussion of the overall wellness of patients because our immune system's ability to keep periodontal populations within manageable limits is indeed reflective of our general health.

Therefore, as practitioners we must prioritize patients' periodontal care, as this will enhance their general well-being.

REFERENCES

1. Leys EJ, Griffen AL, Beall C, et al. Isolation, classification, and identification of oral microorganisms. In: Lamont RJ, Hajishengallis GN, Jenkinson HF, editors.

Oral microbiology and immunology. 2nd edition. Washington, DC: ASM Press; 2014. p. 77–81.

2. Hajishengallis G, Kawai T. Immunopathogenic mechanisms in periodontal disease. In: Lamont RJ, Hajishengallis GN, Jenkinson HF, editors. Oral microbiology and immunology. 2nd edition. Washington, DC: ASM Press; 2014. p. 287, 288–290, 295–303.

3. Lamont RJ, Lewis JP, Potempa J. Virulence factors of periodontal bacteria. In: Lamont RJ, Hajishengallis GN, Jenkinson HF, editors. Oral microbiology and immunology. 2nd edition. Washington, DC: ASM Press; 2014. p. 273–5.

4. Natto ZS, Aladmawy M, Alasqah M, et al. Factors contributing to tooth loss among the elderly: a cross sectional study. Singapore Dent J 2014;35:17–22.

5. Fan J, Costalonga M, Ross KF, et al. Systemic disease and the oral microbiota. In: Lamont RJ, Hajishengallis GN, Jenkinson HF, editors. Oral microbiology and immunology. 2nd edition. Washington, DC: ASM Press; 2014. p. 373–90.

6. Mealey B, Klokkevold PR. Impact of periodontal infection on systemic health. In: Newman MG, Takei HH, Klokkevold PR, et al, editors. Carranza's clinical periodontology. 11th edition. St. Louis (MO): Elsevier; 2012. p. 320–30.

7. Papapanou P. Periodontal diseases: general concepts. In: Lamont RJ, Hajishengallis GN, Jenkinson HF, editors. Oral microbiology and immunology. 2nd edition. Washington, DC: ASM Press; 2014. p. 251–9, 261–271.

8. Hinrichs JE, Novak MJ. Classification of diseases and conditions affecting the periodontium. In: Newman MG, Takei HH, Klokkevold PR, et al, editors. Carranza's clinical periodontology. 11th edition. St Louis (MO): Elsevier; 2012. p. 34–64.

9. Scannapieco FA. The oral environment. In: Lamont RJ, Hajishengallis GN, Jenkinson HF, editors. Oral microbiology and immunology. 2nd edition. Washington, DC: ASM Press; 2014. p. 57–62, 66, 72.

10. Preshaw PM, Taylor JJ. Periodontal pathogenesis. In: Newman MG, Takei HH, Klokkevold PR, et al, editors. Carranza's clinical periodontology. 11th edition. St Louis (MO): Elsevier; 2012. p. 194–216.

11. Eke PI, Dye BA, Wei L, et al. Prevalence of periodontitis in adults in the United States: 2009 and 2010. J Dent Res 2012;91:914–20.

12. Fiorellini JP, Kim DM, Uzel NG. Anatomy of the periodontium. In: Newman MG, Takei HH, Klokkevold PR, et al, editors. Carranza's clinical periodontology. 11th edition. St Louis (MO): Elsevier; 2012. p. 12–27.

13. Hajishengallis E, Hajishengallis G. Immunology of the oral cavity. In: Lamont RJ, Hajishengallis GN, Jenkinson HF, editors. Oral microbiology and immunology. 2nd edition. Washington, DC: ASM Press; 2014. p. 217, 218, 222, 224.

14. Takei HH, Carranza FA. Clinical diagnosis. In: Newman MG, Takei HH, Klokkevold PR, et al, editors. Carranza's clinical periodontology. 11th edition. St Louis (MO): Elsevier; 2012. p. 353.

15. Carranza FA, Camargo PM. The periodontal pocket. In: Newman MG, Takei HH, Klokkevold PR, et al, editors. Carranza's clinical periodontology. 11th edition. St Louis (MO): Elsevier; 2012. p. 127–39.

16. Tetradis S, Carranza FA, Fazio RC, et al. Radiographic aids in the diagnosis of periodontal disease. In: Newman MG, Takei HH, Klokkevold PR, et al, editors. Carranza's clinical periodontology. 11th edition. St Louis (MO): Elsevier; 2012. p. 363.

17. Hinrichs JE. The role of dental calculus and other local predisposing factors. In: Newman MG, Takei HH, Klokkevold PR, et al, editors. Carranza's clinical periodontology. 11th edition. St Louis (MO): Elsevier; 2012. p. 134–5, 231.

18. Diehl SR, Chou C-H, Kuo F, et al. Genetic factors and periodontal disease. In: Newman MG, Takei HH, Klokkevold PR, et al, editors. Carranza's clinical periodontology. 11th edition. St Louis (MO): Elsevier; 2012. p. 284.

19. Novak MJ, Novak KF, Preshaw PM. Smoking and periodontal disease. In: Newman MG, Takei HH, Klokkevold PR, et al, editors. Carranza's clinical periodontology. 11th edition. St Louis (MO): Elsevier; 2012. p. 301.

20. Carranza FA, Hogan EL. Gingival enlargement. In: Newman MG, Takei HH, Klokkevold PR, et al, editors. Carranza's clinical periodontology. 11th edition. St Louis (MO): Elsevier; 2012. p. 91.

21. Loe H, Theilade E, Jensen SB. Experimental gingivitis in man. J Periodontol 1965; 36:177.

22. Theilade E, Wright WH, Jensen SB, et al. Experimental gingivitis in man. II. A longitudinal clinical and bacteriological investigation. J Periodontal Res 1966;1:1.

23. Gmür R, Lüthi-Schaller H. A combined immunofluorescence and fluorescent in situ hybridization assay for single cell analyses of dental plaque microorganisms. J Microbiol Methods 2007;69:402.

24. Vartoukian SR, Palmer RM, Wade WG. Diversity and morphology of members of the phylum "synergistetes" in periodontal health and disease. Appl Environ Microbiol 2009;75:3777.

25. Jenkinson HF. General microbiology. In: Lamont RJ, Hajishengallis GN, Jenkinson HF, editors. Oral microbiology and immunology. 2nd edition. Washington, DC: ASM Press; 2014. p. 21–2.

26. Hillman JD, Socransky SS, Shivers M. The relationships between streptococcal species and periodontopathic bacteria in human dental plaque. Arch Oral Biol 1985;30:791.

27. Teughels W, Quirynen M, Jakubovics N. Periodontal microbiology. In: Newman MG, Takei HH, Klokkevold PR, et al, editors. Carranza's clinical periodontology. 11th edition. St Louis (MO): Elsevier; 2012. p. 232–70.

28. Egland PG, Marquis RE. Oral microbial physiology. In: Lamont RJ, Hajishengallis GN, Jenkinson HF, editors. Oral microbiology and immunology. 2nd edition. Washington, DC: ASM Press; 2014. p. 113, 130, 134–138.

29. Jenkinson HF, Lamont RJ. Oral microbial ecology. In: Lamont RJ, Hajishengallis GN, Jenkinson HF, editors. Oral microbiology and immunology. 2nd edition. Washington, DC: ASM Press; 2014. p. 97–102.

30. Dibart S, Skobe Z, Snapp KR, et al. Identification of bacterial species on or in crevicular epithelial cells from healthy and periodontally diseased patients using DNA-DNA hybridization. Oral Microbiol Immunol 1998;13:30.

31. Socransky SS, Gibbons RJ, Dale AC, et al. The microbiota of the gingival crevice area of man. I. Total microscopic and viable counts of specific microorganisms. Arch Oral Biol 1953;8:275.

32. Socransky SS, Haffajee AD, Cugini MA, et al. Microbial complexes in subgingival plaque. J Clin Periodontol 1998;25:134.

33. Socransky SS, Haffajee AD. The bacterial etiology of destructive periodontal disease: current concepts. J Periodontol 1992;63:322.

34. Kirkwood KL, Rossa C Jr. Molecular biology of the host-microbe interaction in periodontal diseases. In: Newman MG, Takei HH, Klokkevold PR, et al, editors. Carranza's clinical periodontology. 11th edition. St Louis (MO): Elsevier; 2012. p. 285–93.

35. Lydyard PM, Cole MF. The immune system and host defense. In: Lamont RJ, Hajishengallis GN, Jenkinson HF, editors. Oral microbiology and immunology. 2nd edition. Washington, DC: ASM Press; 2014. p. 25–49.

36. Fujihashi K, Russell MW, Hajishengallis G. Immunological intervention against oral diseases. In: Lamont RJ, Hajishengallis GN, Jenkinson HF, editors. Oral microbiology and immunology. 2nd edition. Washington, DC: ASM Press; 2014. p. 395.

37. Silva N, Abusleme L, Bravo D, et al. Host response mechanisms in periodontal diseases. J Appl Oral Sci 2015;23(3):329–55.

38. Fiorellini JP, Kim DM, Uzel NG. Clinical features of gingivitis. In: Newman MG, Takei HH, Klokkevold PR, et al, editors. Carranza's clinical periodontology. 11th edition. St Louis (MO): Elsevier; 2012. p. 78.

39. Page RC, Schroeder HE. Pathogenesis of inflammatory periodontal disease. A summary of current work. Lab Invest 1976;33:235–49.

40. Armitage GC. Development of a classification system for periodontal diseases and conditions. Ann Periodontol 1999;4:1.

41. Klokkevold PR. Necrotizing ulcerative periodontitis. In: Newman MG, Takei HH, Klokkevold PR, et al, editors. Carranza's clinical periodontology. 11th edition. St Louis (MO): Elsevier; 2012. p. 165–8.

42. Rosan B, Rossman L, Baumgartner JG. Endodontic microbiology. In: Lamont RJ, Hajishengallis GN, Jenkinson HF, editors. Oral microbiology and immunology. 2nd edition. Washington, DC: ASM Press; 2014. p. 361–71.

43. Society for General Microbiology. Dental plaque bacteria may trigger blood clots. ScienceDaily 2012.

44. Ciancio S, Mariotti A. Antiinfective therapy. In: Newman MG, Takei HH, Klokkevold PR, et al, editors. Carranza's clinical periodontology. 11th edition. St Louis (MO): Elsevier; 2012. p. 482–91.

45. Perry DA. Plaque control for the periodontal patient. In: Newman MG, Takei HH, Klokkevold PR, et al, editors. Carranza's clinical periodontology. 11th edition. St Louis (MO): Elsevier; 2012. p. 452–3.

Microbiology of Acute and Chronic Osteomyelitis and Antibiotic Treatment

 CrossMark

Harry Dym, DDS[a],*, Joseph Zeidan, DMD[b]

KEYWORDS

- Osteomyelitis • Jaw • Mandible • Microbiology • Antibiotic

KEY POINTS

- Osteomyelitis is an inflammation of bone marrow with a tendency for progression, involving the cortical plates and often periosteal tissues, with most cases occurring after trauma to bone or bone surgery or secondary to vascular insufficiency.
- Antimicrobial therapy and surgical débridement are the primary modalities of osteomyelitis treatment, although often it is associated with a prolonged course, requiring a large commitment between patient and clinician as well as sizable health care costs.
- Despite surgical and chemotherapeutic advancements, osteomyelitis remains difficult to treat, and no universally accepted protocol for treatment exists.

Osteomyelitis is an inflammation of bone marrow with a tendency for progression, involving the cortical plates and often periosteal tissues,[1] with most cases occurring after trauma to bone or bone surgery or secondary to vascular insufficiency.[2] Osteomyelitis is also encountered more commonly in tooth-bearing areas[3] and, prior to the advent of antibiotics, osteomyelitis of the mandible was not an uncommon occurrence.[1] With the use of antibiotics, however, osteomyelitis has now become a rare disease.[1] Recently, however, antibiotics have become less effective, presenting therapeutic challenges to surgeons that can result in the loss of teeth or bone.[1] Antimicrobial therapy and surgical débridement are the primary modalities of osteomyelitis treatment, although often it is associated with a prolonged course, requiring a large commitment between patient and clinician as well as sizable health care costs.[2] Despite surgical and chemotherapeutic advancements, osteomyelitis remains difficult to treat, and no universally accepted protocol for treatment exists.[2]

[a] Department of Dentistry and Oral Surgery, The Brooklyn Hospital Center, 121 Dekalb Avenue, Brooklyn, NY 11201, USA; [b] Department of Oral and Maxillofacial Surgery, The Brooklyn Hospital Center, 121 Dekalb Avenue, Brooklyn, NY 11201, USA
* Corresponding author.
E-mail address: HDymdds@yahoo.com

Dent Clin N Am 61 (2017) 271–282
http://dx.doi.org/10.1016/j.cden.2016.12.001   dental.theclinics.com
0011-8532/17/© 2016 Elsevier Inc. All rights reserved.

PATHOGENESIS

Osteomyelitis of the mandible is much more common than of the maxilla due to its dense and poorly vascularized cortical plates along with the vasculature originating from the inferior alveolar neurovascular bundle.[1] Maxillary bone, meanwhile, is much less dense and receives its vasculature from multiple vessels and thus more resistant to developing an osteomyelitis.[1]

Host defenses also play a role in the progression of osteomyelitis. Osteomyelitis has been associated with systemic diseases, such as diabetes mellitus, autoimmune disorders, malignancy, malnutrition, and AIDS.[1] Additional factors that predispose patients to osteomyelitis of the jaws include noncompliant patients who are refractory to health care delivery, patient age, nutritional status, immunosuppression, microvascular disease, and inaccessibility to health care.[4] Medications with roles in osteomyelitis include steroids, chemotherapeutic agents, and bisphosphonates.[1] Local factors that compromise vascularity, such as osteoporosis, bone pathology, and radiation therapy, also increase the possible risk for bony infection.[1]

Osteomyelitis typically occurs as a result of spread of an odontogenic infection or as a result of trauma.[1] The presence of teeth provides a direct pathway to the bone by pulpal or periodontal disease.[3] A hematogenous origin is rare and primarily occurs in young children.[1] The adult process begins with bacteria spreading to the jaw bones, either through extraction of teeth, root canal therapy, or fracture of the jaw bones, resulting in a bacteria-induced inflammatory process.[1] Although commonly self-limiting, there is a potential for progression to a pathologic process.[1] Inflammation leads to hyperemia, increased blood flow, and leukocytes to the affected area.[1] Pus is formed when bacteria and cellular debris cannot be eliminated by the body's natural defense mechanisms.[1] When the pus and inflammatory response occur in the bone marrow, elevated intramedullary pressure is created, which further decreases blood flow to jaw bones.[1] Pus travels via the haversian system and Volkmann canals to spread throughout the medullary and cortical bones, and, as pus perforates the cortical bone, it collects under the periosteum, further compromising the periosteal blood supply.[1] After some time, ultimately the purulence exits the soft tissues via intraoral or extraoral fistulas.[1]

CLASSIFICATION

Many classification systems for osteomyelitis have been presented in the past, such as suppurative or nonsuppurative, hematogenous or secondary to a contiguous focus of infection, and acute or chronic, with the latter becoming the predominant classification system.[1] The differentiation of acute versus chronic is based on the presence of disease for 1 month.[1] Another classification system is based on Zurich, in which chronic osteomyelitis can be divided into suppurative chronic osteomyelitis, osteonecrosis of the jaw, and bisphosphonate-related osteonecrosis of the jaw (BRONJ).[5] Chronic nonsuppurative osteomyelitis of the mandible is also referred to in the literature as primary chronic osteomyelitis (PCO), diffuse sclerosing osteomyelitis (DSO), Garré osteomyelitis, and juvenile mandibular chronic osteomyelitis (JMCO).[6]

Osteomyelitis may be classified into acute and chronic forms.[7] Acute osteomyelitis can be further subdivided into suppurative and nonsuppurative forms as well as progressive or hematogenous forms.[7] Chronic osteomyelitis may be classified by the causative agent or as suppurative or nonsuppurative forms or sclerosing with subclassifications of diffuse or focal disease.[7]

Acute osteomyelitis involves progression from days to a few weeks and is based on acute symptoms, such as fever, leukocytosis, lymphadenopathy, and swelling to the affected area.[3] Cellulitis and trismus may also be present in the acute phase.[4] Acute osteomyelitis may present as a routine infection and may take up to 10 days for bone loss to be radiographically apparent.[7] Acute osteomyelitis is primarily managed medically with antibiotics, with the antibiotic of choice clindamycin because of its effectiveness against streptococci.[7] Patients may require hospital admission for intravenous (IV) antibiotics.[7]

Chronic osteomyelitis is a relapsing and persistent infection spanning months to years with characteristic low-grade inflammation, presence of dead bone, new bone apposition, and fistulous tracts, with treatment requiring (possibly multiple) surgical interventions and long-term broad spectrum antibiotics.[3] Findings include swelling, pain, purulence, intraoral and extraoral draining fistulae, and nonhealing bony and overlying soft tissue wounds.[4] It is often multifactorial in complexity, with complications, such as pathologic fracture or nerve deficits, commonly reported.[3] Its clinical course includes necrosis of mineralized and marrow tissue, suppuration, resorption, sclerosis, and hyperplasia.[3] The primary cause of chronic osteomyelitis is most often the result of odontogenic infection, postextraction complications, trauma, or inappropriate or inadequate antibiotic therapy as well as the virulence of the bacteria (and an immunocompromised host).[3] Management of chronic osteomyelitis can be challenging due to the anatomic location and polymicrobial nature of the disease.[3] Antibiotics, nonsteroidal anti-inflammatory drugs, and steroids are used to control symptoms; however, surgical intervention is usually indicated.[3] Even with appropriate management, treatment may be prolonged and require long-term antibiotic use possibly of an IV nature.[3] Chronic osteomyelitis is not common in developed countries; however, its occurrence is significant in communities with poor socioeconomic conditions and populations with poor standards or oral hygiene.[8] Chronic osteomyelitis is a serious condition requiring prompt hospital admission, antibiotics, and surgical management.[7]

PCO, also known as JMCO, is a rare but well known nonsuppurative inflammatory disease.[9] It exhibits subperiosteal bone formation, mixed radiodense and radiolucent trabecular bone patterns on radiographs, and swelling in the adjacent soft tissues.[6] Restricted mouth opening may be present as well as decreased sensation at the inferior alveolar nerve (Vincent symptom)[9] along with a mild bony expansion may also be present.[10] The absence of pus, fistulas, or sequestration is characteristic of PCO and differentiates primary from acute and secondary chronic osteomyelitis.[9] Inflammatory markers, such as erythrocyte sedimentation rate (ESR) and C-reactive protein (CRP), are frequently increased as well.[6] A white blood cell count, especially in the acute stages, can be useful.[7] Histopathologic findings are consistent with osteomyelitis, but bacterial cultures are often negative, causing controversy as to whether the etiology is infective in nature.[6] Histopathology shows the presence of pagetoid bone formation, lymphocytes, plasma cells that suggest chronic inflammation, and medullary fibrosis.[9] PCO only affects the mandible and occurs without age preference.[9] ESR may not always be reliable because it may be elevated due to fever, dehydration, and antibiotic treatment.[7] CRP may be used to monitor resolution of the infection in response to treatment.[7]

Fungal osteomyelitis is usually seen in immunocompromised patients, the elderly, and patients with diabetes mellitus.[7] Aspergillus species has played an important role in the morbidity and mortality of immunocompromised hosts.[11] Extrapulmonary invasive aspergillosis involving the bones is rare and often neglected, with a paucity of data for risk factors and treatment outcomes.[11] Although rare, invasive aspergillosis causing osteomyelitis has a 25% mortality rate.[11] Amphotericin B is the most commonly used drug to treat Aspergillus osteomyelitis, followed by itraconazole and voriconazole.[11]

MICROBIOLOGY

More than 500 species of bacteria have been identified in the mouth.[1] In the past, staphylococcal species were considered the major pathogen in osteomyelitis of the jaws; however, with refined scientific techniques, further insight into this area has been acquired.[1] In the past, sinus tract cultures were often obtained, often growing *Staphylococcus aureus*, which is a common skin contaminant.[4] Subsequent studies have shown little correlation between surgically obtained cultures and sinus tract isolates.[4] The prime pathogenic species seen in osteomyelitis of the jaw bones are streptococci and anaerobic bacteria, such as *Bacteroides* or *Peptostreptococcus*.[1] In 1 study, the most commonly cultured microorganisms were *Streptococcus*, *Eikenella*, and *Candida*.[3] *Staphylococcus*, *Actinomyces*, *Bacteroides*, *Klebsiella*, *Fusobacterium*, *Lactobacillus*, and *Haemophilus* were also reported.[3]

Infections are often mixed, with several pathogens often seen growing on final culture, leading clinicians to make an empiric antibiotic selection based on the most likely pathogen.[1] Definitive antimicrobial therapy, however, should be based on the final culture and sensitivities.[1]

Culture-directed antibiotic therapy helps avoid multidrug resistance and ensures a more favorable outcome.[3] Antimicrobial agents are routinely administered in chronic osteomyelitis without sufficient bacterial information, however, resulting in treatment failures.[5] Most infections in the oral and maxillofacial region are polymicrobial anaerobes, and not all are amenable to culture.[5]

Goda and colleagues[5] used polymerase chain reaction amplification from 16 patients with chronic osteomyelitis of the jaws. These included patients with osteoradionecrosis, BRONJ, PCO, and suppurative osteomyelitis.[5] Twelve phyla were identified in all samples, which most commonly included *Bacteroides*, *Firmicutes*, *Fusobacteria*, and *Actinobacteria*.[5] It was concluded that chronic osteomyelitis of the jaws is not caused by a single organism but rather a diverse group of bacteria, including aerobic, anaerobic, and unculturable bacteria.[5]

Acute osteomyelitis of the jaws is usually polymicrobial, which includes *Streptococcus*, *Bacteroides*, *Peptostreptococcus*, and other opportunistic pathogens.[4] There is a shift in the predominant flora as the infectious process matures.[4]

Most cases of osteomyelitis of the jaws are associated with endodontic infections, peri-implantitis, lateral periodontitis, and gingivitis.[8] The microbiology of chronic osteomyelitis is influenced by the origin of the infectious process.[8] In cases of hematogenous origin, oxygen-tolerant organisms, such as enteric rods and staphylococci, predominate,[8] whereas osteomyelitis associated with previous odontogenic infections depends on the microorganisms from the previous odontogenic infection, generally producing mixed infections with predominance of oral anaerobes, in particular, *Fusobacterium*, *Porphyromonas*, *Prevotella*, *Parvimonas*, and *Eikenella* that is frequently associated with actinomycetes and staphylococci.[8]

Marx and colleagues[10] reported isolating *Actinomyces* species and *Eikenella corrodens* or *Arachnia* species with *Eikenella corodens* in 26 patients with DSO.

A biofilm is a complex community of sessile microbes attached to a substrate.[2] The organisms, which are often bacteria of fungi, differ from their planktonic or free-floating counterparts, because they function as a community of cells that are attached to a surface, within a matrix of extracellular polymeric substances that are produced to connect and communicate with each other.[2] Organisms within the biofilm exhibit an altered phenotype regarding growth rate, gene transcription, and antimicrobial resistance.[2] Biofilm theory has been used to explain the etiology of infections that constitute between 65% and 80% of microbial diseases treated in the developed world.[2] In long bone osteomyelitis, for example, microbes grow as bacterial biofilms on the bone surface and are resistant to antibiotics and host defenses.[2] Recently, a link between osteomyelitis of the jaws, osteonecrosis of the jaws, and biofilms has been established.[2] Sedghizadeh and colleagues[2] examined bone specimens from patients with osteomyelitis and osteonecrosis of the jaws under scanning electron microscopy for evaluation of biofilms. Results showed that all specimens had biofilms present that were polymicrobial.[2] *Actinomyces* was found consistently in the osteomyelitis samples.[2] Bacterial species in patients with BRONJ included *Fusobacerium, Streptococcus, Actinomyces, Selenomonas*, and *Bacillus*.[2] These organisms are found in the oral cavity and often associated with odontogenic and periodontal infections.[2] In addition, *Candida albicans* was found in all of the BRONJ specimens, however, not in the osteomyelitis ones.[2]

There are many difficulties with traditional screening methods in the analysis of the biofilms associated with osteomyelitis. Screening methods are based on planktonic bacteria growth; however, evolutionarily, bacteria are well adapted to growing in communities and may not grow in vitro as they do in vivo.[2] Culture swabs from the oral cavity also have high rates of contamination and exposure to oxygen may kill many anaerobic bacteria.[2] Moreover, the results of antibiotic sensitivity testing are not applicable to biofilms and can lead to inadequate antibiotic therapy.[2] Susceptibility tests with an in vitro biofilm have shown the survival of osteomyelitis causing biofilms with antibiotics at 1000 times the minimum inhibitory concentration, which are at levels that harm patients (**Box 1**).[2]

ANTIBIOTIC TREATMENT

Treatment is directed to resolution of the infection while maximizing patient function.[7] The predominance of oral anaerobic species in mixed infections in chronic osteomyelitis suggests that ecologic associates are relevant.[8] Because most oral microorganisms are able to form biofilms, treatment of chronic osteomyelitis requires removal of bone sequestration, curettage, débridement, and systemic antibiotics for weeks.[8]

The management of osteomyelitis of the jaws requires both medical and surgical interventions (**Figs. 1–13**).[1] A correct diagnosis is an essential first step, and clinicians must always be aware of possible malignancies that can mimic the presentation of jawbone osteomyelitis until a definitive diagnosis is made by histopathology.[1] Tissues should be sent for Gram stain, culture, sensitivity, and histopathology.[1] Patients should be optimized medically to achieve the best response to antibiotic therapy.[1] Antibiotics should be held preoperatively to obtain more accurate culture and sensitivity results.[3] Empiric antibiotics should be started based on Gram stain because cultures and sensitivities may take several days for a final report.[1] Empiric antibiotics, however, are initiated often with little information on the target bacterial species and are often resistant to conventional antimicrobial therapies.[5] An infectious disease consultation may be of value in selecting the most current antimicrobials.[1] Chronic osteomyelitis may require antibiotics for up to 6 months.[7]

Penicillin remains the empiric antibiotic of choice.[4] Refractory organisms may be treated with metronidazole, clindamycin, ticarcillin and clavulanic acid, cephalosporins, carbapenems, vancomycin in combination with other antibiotics, and

Box 1
Commonly reported microorganisms in acute and chronic osteomyelitis

Actinomyces

Bacteroides

Bacillus

Candida

Eikenella

Firmicutes

Fusobacterium

Haemophilus

Klebsiella

Lactobacillus

Parvimonas

Peptostreptococcus

Porphyromonas

Prevotella

Streptococcus

Selenomonas

Staphylococcus

Data from Refs.[1–5,8,10]

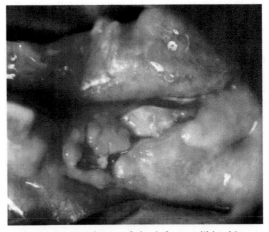

Fig. 1. Exposed necrotic nonhealing bone of the left mandible. (*Courtesy of* H. Dym, DDS, Brooklyn, NY.)

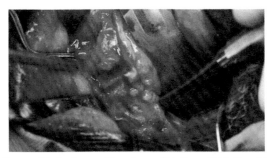

Fig. 2. Necrotic left mandibular bone. (*Courtesy of* H. Dym, DDS, Brooklyn, NY.)

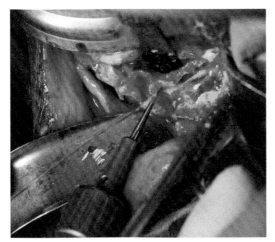

Fig. 3. Ostectomy of the necrotic portion of the mandible. (*Courtesy of* H. Dym, DDS, Brooklyn, NY.)

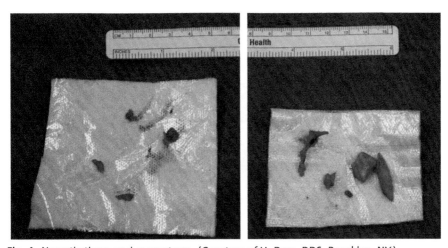

Fig. 4. Necrotic tissue and sequestrum. (*Courtesy of* H. Dym, DDS, Brooklyn, NY.)

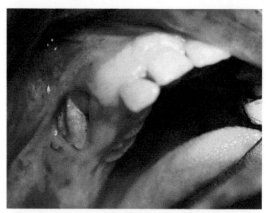

Fig. 5. Necrotic exposed maxillary right alveolar bone. (*Courtesy of* H. Dym, DDS, Brooklyn, NY.)

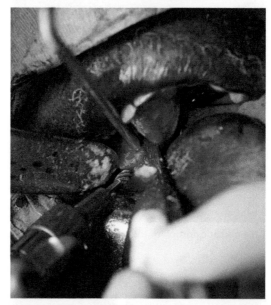

Fig. 6. Débridement of the right maxilla. (*Courtesy of* H. Dym, DDS, Brooklyn, NY.)

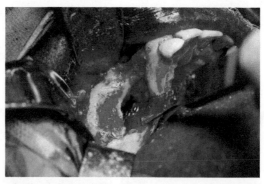

Fig. 7. Completion of débridement of the right maxilla to healthy bleeding bone. (*Courtesy of* H. Dym, DDS, Brooklyn, NY.)

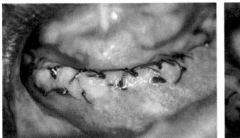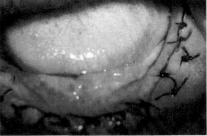

Fig. 8. Mandible, 1 week postoperative. (*Courtesy of* H. Dym, DDS, Brooklyn, NY.)

fluoroquinolones.[4] Common antibiotic regimens include vancomycin 2 g/d to 3 g/d, ertapenem 1 g/d, or Unasyn 1.5 g/d to 3 g/d, administered IV via a peripherally inserted central catheter line.[3] Oral antibiotics can include amoxicillin, clindamycin, Augmentin 875 mg, and doxycycline 100 mg.[3] The duration of antibiotic therapy has been reported with varying recommendations from 4 weeks to 8 weeks or even longer for chronic osteomyelitis.[3] The duration of antibiotics can be based on a patient's compliance, clinical progress, and overall health along with an evaluation of systemic markers of inflammation, such as CRP and ESR.[3] Another

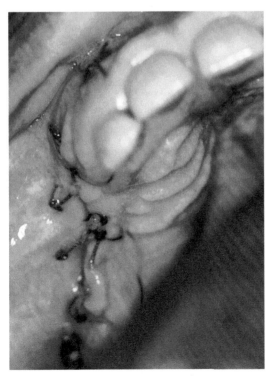

Fig. 9. Right maxilla, 1 week postoperative. (*Courtesy of* H. Dym, DDS, Brooklyn, NY.)

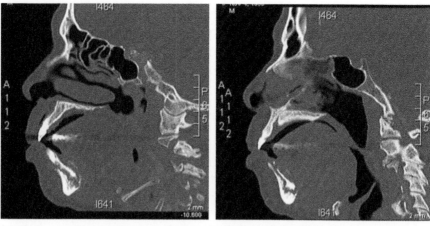

Fig. 10. Preoperative sagittal view CT scan of the left mandible showing necrotic bone and sequestrum. (*Courtesy of* H. Dym, DDS, Brooklyn, NY.)

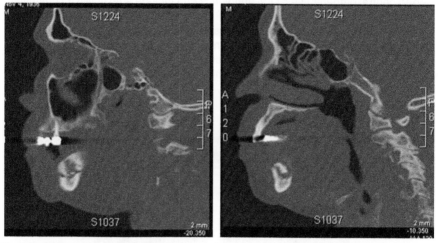

Fig. 11. Postoperative sagittal view CT scan. (*Courtesy of* H. Dym, DDS, Brooklyn, NY.)

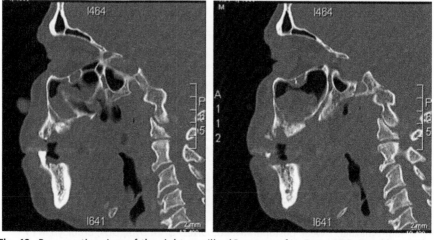

Fig. 12. Preoperative view of the right maxilla. (*Courtesy of* H. Dym, DDS, Brooklyn, NY.)

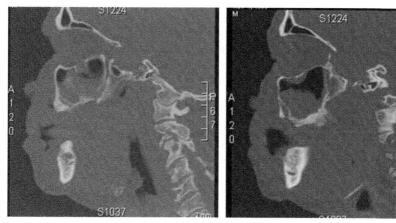

Fig. 13. Postoperative view of the right maxilla. (*Courtesy of* H. Dym, DDS, Brooklyn, NY.)

important aspect in the treatment of osteomyelitis is the ability to provide penetrance via the vascular route.[4] Intra-arterial antibiotic therapy and local implantation of antibiotic-saturated beads have been used with varying results in the literature.[4]

JMCO has reported to have been cured with a 58.3% success rate at a mean follow-up of 4.3 years using a combination of surgical modalities and antibiotic therapy.[6] Oral β-lactam antibiotics were given in doses of 75 to 100 mg/kg in children weighing less than 40 kg, and 2 g to 3 g daily for children weighing more than 40 kg.[6] To avoid diarrhea, amoxicillin plus clavulanate was given at regular doses and supplemented with amoxicillin to achieve a higher daily amoxicillin dose (**Box 2**).[6]

Box 2
Commonly used antibiotics in the treatment of acute and chronic osteomyelitis

Augmentin

Carbapenems

Cephalosporins

Clindamycin

Doxycycline

Ertapenem

Fluoroquinolones

Metronidazole

Penicillin

Ticarcillin and clavulanic acid

Unasyn

Vancomycin in combination with other antibiotics

Data from Refs.[3,4,6]

SUMMARY

Osteomyelitis, although uncommon, continues to be seen and treated by dentists and oral and maxillofacial surgeons. Complete therapy involves both medical and surgical approaches in an effort to achieve total care. Culture-driven antibiotics are critical in the treatment of osteomyelitis, and knowledge of microbiological agents is essential for treating clinicians.

REFERENCES

1. Kushner GM. Osteomyelitis and osteoradionecrosis. In: Miloro M, editor. Peterson's principles of oral and maxillofacial surgery. Lewiston (ME): BC Decker; 2004. p. 300–24.
2. Sedghizadeh PP, Kumar SK, Gorur A, et al. Microbial biofilms in osteomyelitis of the jaw and osteonecrosis of the jaw secondary to bisphosphonate therapy. J Am Dent Assoc 2009;10:1259–65.
3. Baur DA, Altay MA, Flores-Hidalgo A, et al. Chronic osteomyelitis of the mandible: diagnosis and management - an institution's experience over 7 years. J Oral Maxillofac Surg 2014;73:655–65.
4. Hudson JW. Osteomyelitis of the jaws: a 50-year perspective. J Oral Maxillofac Surg 1993;15:1294–301.
5. Goda A, Maruyama F, Michi Y, et al. Analysis of the factors affecting the formation of the microbiome associated with chronic osteomyelitis of the jaw. Clin Microbiol Infect 2013;20:309–17.
6. Renapurkar S, Pasternack MS, Nielsen GP, et al. Juvenile mandibular chronic osteomyelitis: role of surgical debridement and antibiotics. J Oral Maxillofac Surg 2016;74:1–15.
7. Pincus DJ, Armstrong MB, Thaller SR. Osteomyelitis of the craniofacial skeleton. Semin Plast Surg 2009;23:73–9.
8. Gaetti-Jardim E. Microbiota associated with infections of the jaws. Int J Dent 2012;2012:1–8.
9. Agarwal A, Kumar N, Tyagi A, et al. Primary chronic osteomyelitis in the mandible: a conservative approach. BMJ Case Rep 2014;82:1–3.
10. Marx RE, Carlson ER, Smith BR, et al. Isolation of Actinomyces Species and Eikenella corrodens from patients with chronic diffuse sclerosing osteomyelitis. J Oral Maxillofac Surg 1994;52:26–33.
11. Gabrielli E, Fothergill AW, Sutton DA, et al. Osteomyelitis caused by Aspergillus Species: a review of 310 cases. Clin Microbiol Infect 2013;20:559–62.

Oral Mucosal Infections

Insights into Specimen Collection and Medication Management

Arvind Babu Rajendra Santosh, MDS[a],*,
Baddam Venkat Ramana Reddy, MDS[b]

KEYWORDS

- Oral infections • Bacterial pathogen • Microbiologic sampling • Specimen collection
- Specimen transportation • Medication

KEY POINTS

- This article highlights current scientific knowledge on diagnosis and management of bacterial infections of oral cavity, specimen collection and transportation, and medication management of oral microbiological diseases.
- Infections of oral mucosa are an increasing problem in many countries. Increased susceptibility to various types of oral mucosal infections is due to impaired immune response, medications that impair host immune system, increasing age, and sexual intercourse.
- Determining if the lesions are of infectious origin and detection of microorganism type are the most important aspects in the diagnosis and treatment of oral mucosal infections.
- In addition to clinical examination, microscopic examination, and special staining methods, culture techniques and/or molecular methods are considered to be the most important diagnostic approaches for identification of oral mucosal infections.

INTRODUCTION

Infections of the oral mucosa are raising problems in many countries. Impaired host resistance may allow pathogenic organisms to colonize the oral cavity. A pathogenic microorganism is a microbe that can cause disease, whereas a nonpathogenic organism may not cause disease but remains as a part of the normal flora. An infectious disease is caused by a microorganism.[1] An infection is a state in which microorganisms that are not normally present within the host have invaded the host and multiplication of such organisms is occurring. The microbe-host interaction may be transient,

Disclosure Statement: The authors have nothing to disclose.
[a] Dentistry Program, The University of the West Indies, Mona Campus, Kingston 7, Jamaica, West Indies; [b] Department of Oral and Maxillofacial Pathology, SIBAR Institute of Dental Sciences, Takkellapadu, Guntur, Andhra Pradesh 522601, India
* Corresponding author.
E-mail address: arvindbabu2001@gmail.com

commensal, pathogenic, opportunistic, or accidental. A successful pathogen or commensal must be able to enter host tissue, colonize, multiply, acquire nutrients, invade the host system, fight against the immune system, disseminate, and eventually be transmitted to a new susceptible host.[2,3]

The oral flora is diverse and abundant[4] with a reservoir of more than 700 different microorganisms. The first oral flora develops at the time of birth and reaches its climax at puberty.[5] The oral flora can be divided into resident and transient flora. The normal oral flora exists in a state of balance with the host and helps as a defense barrier against pathogenic microorganisms. Oral flora is regulated by a bacterial adhesion mechanism and by epithelial cell desquamation. When the keratinized epithelial surfaces, such as gingiva, palate, and dorsum of the tongue, become hyperkeratinized, they may be able to accommodate opportunistic microorganism such as fungi. Nonkeratinized epithelial surfaces, such as buccal and labial mucosa, may be dominated by dead cells or by cells undergoing apoptosis that may be invaded by bacteria.[6] The tissue-specific microbial differences are evident despite spatial proximity and constant contact between these sites. Bacterial translocation may occur in the presence of cytotoxic drugs, oral cancer, or atrophic epithelium as a result of trauma, chemical injury, or allergic reaction.[7–9] The major source for microbes found in saliva and the major oral site for microbial multiplication is the tongue. Microbial colonization occurs by adhesion of microbe to a host cell (tongue, teeth, or gingiva) or to another microorganism.

Oral microbial infections develop from bacterial, fungal, or viral invasion of the oral mucosa. The observed oral mucosal manifestations of an infectious disease may be due to

1. Local site infection
2. A systemic infection that has oral manifestations
3. An opportunistic infection that causes oral manifestations as a result of systemic or local impairment of immunologic resistance.

Oral infections can have secondary systemic effects through 1 of 3 proposed mechanisms or pathways:

1. Metastatic spread of infection from the oral cavity as a result of transient bacteremia
2. Metastatic injury from the effects of circulating oral microbial toxins
3. Metastatic inflammation caused by immunologic injury induced by oral microorganisms.

Most infections of the oral mucosa appear clinically as localized lesions or a widespread oral manifestation of systemic infection. The symptoms may range from being almost asymptomatic, to mild discomfort, to severe pain. One diagnostic challenge is that oral mucosal infections may be subclinical or chronic, and not accompanied by strong clinical symptoms.[1] This article discusses oral and maxillofacial bacterial infections that are not widely seen in dental practice and not discussed elsewhere in this issue. Specimen collection, transportation, and medication management of oral microbial diseases are presented.

MICROBIOLOGIC SAMPLING METHODS IN ORAL MUCOSAL INFECTIONS

In current dental practice, most attempts of microbial diagnosis are made for fungal infections but not bacterial infections. It is very probable that dental surgeons are competent enough to differentiate fungal mucosal infections from other types of oral mucosal infections although Dahlen[1] has correctly pointed out that bacterial mucosal infections of the oral cavity are more prevalent than fungal infections. Appropriate specimen sampling is an important step in the identification of pathogen. Microbiologic sampling methods include whole saliva, rinsing sample, scraping, swab collection, dental impression, dental plaque, microbiological culture, and aspirate (**Box 1**). Oral rinse and imprint microbiological sampling methods seem to be highly

---

Box 1
List of sampling methods

Whole saliva

Rinsing sample

Scraping

Swab collection

Imprint

Dental impression

Dental plaque

Aspirate

Table 1
Recommended sampling method from various oral mucosal sites

Sampling Site	Recommended Sampling Method	Comments
Lip and perioral skin	Moistened swab	Culture for yeasts and bacteria
	Vesicle fluid, swab	Virus culture and electron microscopy
	Aspirate of abscess	Microscopy and culture
	Serum	Serologic tests for viruses and syphilis
Tongue and oral mucosa	Swab	Culture for yeasts, bacteria, and viruses
	Smear of scrapping	Microscopy for yeasts and bacteria
	Vesicle fluid	Microscopy for yeasts and bacteria
	Tissue biopsy	Culture for bacteria and viruses
		Microscopy for yeasts and suspected infections
	Serum	Culture for bacteria and viruses
		Microscopy for yeasts and suspected infections
Dental abscess or infected cystic lesion	Aspirate	Smear and culture
Infected root canal	Paper point or barbed broach	Aseptic collection, use semisolid transport medium, semiquantitative culture
Dental plaque	Scraping	A variety of sampling tools and procedures available
Gingivae and gingival crevice	Scraping on a sterile sealer	Examine for fusospirochaetal infection, possible viral culture, DNA tests, N Benzoyl-DL-arginine-2-napthylamide tests for periodontal pathogens
Deep dental caries	Saliva	Lactobacillus or streptococcus counts
Prosthesis	Swab and smear	When denture stomatitis is suspected, examine for yeasts

Adapted from Samaranayake LP. Diagnostic microbiology and laboratory methods. In Samaranayake LP, editor. Essential microbiology for dentistry. China: Elsevier; 2012. p. 61; with permission.

correlated. A scraping sample seems to be preferred in mucosal lesions. Molecular methods offer minimal advantage in oral mucosal infections. Microbial cultures are the most used method in oral mucosal infections. Culture studies are important microbiological tests for identification of the pathogen and for antibiotic susceptibility testing because most bacterial pathogens in oral mucosal infections are observed as multiresistant and the availability of effective antibiotic is often limited.[1] The success of treatment outcome of oral mucosal infections depends on selecting the appropriate antibiotic.[1] Thus proper microbiologic sampling method is important when diagnosing and treating oral mucosal infections. Recommended sampling methods[10] from a sampling site in oral mucosal infections are given in **Table 1**.

BACTERIAL INFECTIONS OF THE ORAL CAVITY

The most common bacterial infections of oral cavity are dental caries and periodontal disease. However, other oral bacterial lesions result from either primary site or systemic infection that may have oral manifestations. In general, systemic bacterial infections tend to have signs and symptoms such as headache, malaise, nausea, fever, pain, and enlarged lymph nodes. However, many of these generalized symptoms may not be seen in localized oral mucosal infections. Few primary or systemic bacterial infections of the oral cavity have distinctive clinical signs; instead, ulceration or erythematous areas are noted.

   Box 2 is a comprehensive list of oral and maxillofacial bacterial infections that are covered in this article. Some of the rarer bacterial infections are not covered.

Box 2
Comprehensive list of oral and maxillofacial bacterial infections

1. Tuberculosis

2. Actinomycosis

3. Acute necrotizing gingivitis and periodontitis

4. Leprosy

5. Gonorrhea

6. Syphilis

7. Tetanus

8. Cat-scratch disease

Tuberculosis

Tuberculosis is a chronic infectious disease caused by *Mycobacterium tuberculosis*. Primary tuberculosis usually affects the lungs. Secondary or extrapulmonary tuberculosis manifestations may be seen in the oral cavity. Head and neck lesions in tuberculosis account for 10% to 30%[11] of nonpulmonary lesions. It was also reported that one-third of persons with human immunodeficiency virus (HIV) worldwide are infected with *M tuberculosis* and 8% to 10% develop clinical disease every year.[12]

Pathogenesis

Tuberculosis is primarily transmitted by inhalation of aerosol droplets expelled by infected hosts. Following inhalation, tuberculosis pathogens travel to the lungs and eventually settle in the alveoli. Autoinoculation of tuberculosis pathogen into oral cavity may occur when infected pulmonary mucus interacts with oral ulceration or susceptible area of oral mucosa.[13]

Clinical features

Clinical presentation of active tuberculosis may exhibit persistent and productive cough, night sweats, evening rise of temperature, and weight loss. Oral lesions in tuberculosis are usually rare. However, when presented, the oral manifestation of tuberculosis is usually a painless ulceration with undermined edges on palate, lips, buccal mucosa, or tongue,[14] and usually associated with cervical lymphadenopathy (**Fig. 1**). The palpable cervical lymph nodes in tuberculosis tend to be matted. The differential diagnosis of tuberculous ulceration of oral cavity includes traumatic ulcer, squamous cell carcinoma, aphthous ulcerations, syphilitic ulcer, actinomycosis, Wegener granulomatosis, sarcoidosis, leishmaniosis, zygomycosis, and leprosy.[15] Although oral tuberculosis is rare and often difficult to diagnose, careful consideration of tuberculosis in differential diagnosis of suspicious oral ulcerations is important.

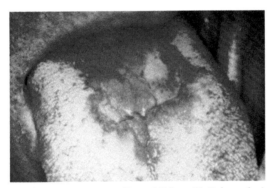

Fig. 1. Deep ulcerative lesion on tongue. (*From* Miziara ID. Tuberculosis affecting the oral cavity in Brazilian HIV-infected patients. Oral Surg Oral Med Oral Path Oral Radiol Endod 2005;100(2):181; with permission.)

Diagnosis

The diagnosis of tuberculosis is usually confirmed by the presence of acid-fast bacilli in the tissue specimen or, more likely, by culture of tuberculous bacilli, sputum examination, chest radiograph, Mantoux test, and bacilloscopy.[16] Special stains, such as Ziehl-Neelsen, are helpful in identifying acid-fast bacilli in granulomatous tissue. Biopsy of oral tuberculous ulcerations is a routine investigation method. Microscopic examination of tuberculous lesions demonstrates granulomatous areas with multinucleated giant cell of Langhans type. The most important diagnostic approaches of oral tuberculosis are careful clinical evaluation, biopsy of oral ulceration or lesion for microscopic observation, acid-fast stain, culture test, immunologic assay, and blood testing.

Management

Tuberculosis is considered an occupationally transmitted disease in dentistry. An outbreak of oral tuberculosis following dental treatment at 2 dental clinics has been reported. A dental surgeon who worked at both clinics was found to have pulmonary tuberculosis and presumably was the source of the infection.[17] Precautions need to be taken to prevent transmission. A face mask, N95 or higher filtering face piece respirator (**Fig. 2**), is designed to protect the health care worker against breathing in very small particle aerosols containing pathogen or viruses that can be generated by an infected person. The Centers for Disease Control and Prevention (CDC) have recommended the use of N95 for dental staff members who work on individuals infected with *M tuberculosis*. The use of a portable high-efficiency particulate arrestance (HEPA) unit is an additional recommendation in dental health facilities that routinely provide care to populations at high risk for tuberculosis disease. Health care workers at risk can be protected by Bacillus Calmette–Guérin (BCG) vaccination.[18] Health care workers considering BCG vaccination should be counseled regarding the risks and benefits associated with both BCG vaccination and treatment of latent tuberculosis infection. Pre-employment tuberculosis screening should be done with a blood test to detect tuberculosis infection. Blood tests, unlike the tuberculin skin test, are not affected by prior BCG vaccination and are less likely to give a false-positive result.[19] The medication management of tuberculosis includes isoniazid and rifampicin. The patient should be referred to pulmonologist for the management of active tuberculosis and consultation for infectious status.

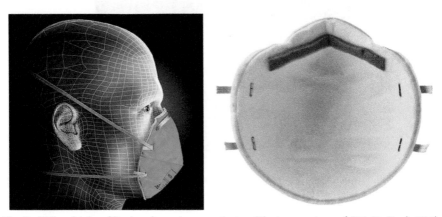

Fig. 2. N95 or higher filtering face piece respirator. (Photos courtesy of 3M, St. Paul, MN.)

Actinomycosis

Actinomycosis is a suppurative and granulomatous chronic bacterial infection caused by *Actinomyces israelii*. Based on the site of infection, actinomycotic infections are classified into cervicofacial, abdominal, and pulmonary types.[20]

Pathogenesis

The exact pathogenesis of actinomycosis remains unclear. A decreased mucosal barrier seems to play a role in entry of pathogenic organism into host tissue. Trauma may play a role in initiating entry of the organism into host tissue, hence postextraction socket, periodontal pocket, or traumatic ulcerated epithelium may act as entry sites for oral cavity infection. Following entry, acute inflammation predominates, followed by a subsequent chronic indolent phase.

Clinical features

The cervicofacial form of actinomycosis is the most common. Clinical presentation of actinomycosis is usually swelling of involved area with induration. The soft tissue swellings eventually develop from underlying jaw infections that tend to discharge pus-containing sulfur granules. The overlying skin demonstrates characteristics of abscess and induration with woody consistency. Cervicofacial actinomycosis usually affects the mandible; however, there are some reports of maxillary involvment[21] (**Figs. 3 and 4**).[22,23] The chronic infection may progress to osteomyelitis of the jaw bone. Untreated osteomyelitis may progress to intracranial infections. Cervicofacial actinomycotic osteomyelitis may also disseminate into the lungs and digestive tract.[24]

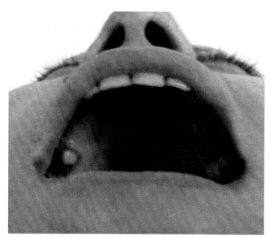

Fig. 3. Actinomycotic sinus tract of the hard palate. (*Modified from* Yadegarynia D, Merza MA, Sali S, et al. A rare case presentation of oral actinomycosis. Int J Mycobacteriol 2013;2(3):188; with permission.)

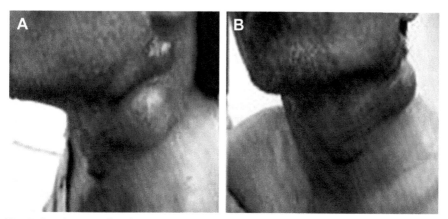

Fig. 4. (*A, B*) Cervicofacial actinomycosis. (*From* Avijgan M, Shakeri H, Shakeri M. A case report of cervicofacial actinomycosis. Asian Pac J Trop Med 2010;3(10):839; with permission.)

Diagnosis

The diagnosis of cervicofacial osteomyelitis is better achieved from surgical biopsy or aspiration of pus. Some literature has suggested that swabs should be avoided. Culture and special staining are helpful in definitive diagnosis. Gram staining of the specimen was reported to be more sensitive than culture, specifically if the patient had started a antibiotic regimen. The microscopic characteristic of actinomycosis is described as colonies of microorganisms appearing to float in a sea of polymorphonuclear leukocytes.[24]

Management

Antibiotic therapy for actinomycosis cannot be standardized. The antibiotic course in actinomycosis depends on the course, clinical presentation, and clinical response. Medicinal treatment of actinomycosis is usually empirical because there has not been uniform success with any antibiotic.[25] Selvin and John[26] reported short-term medicinal management of actinomycosis, including intravenous penicillin G (8 million U per day) for 2 weeks followed by oral penicillin VK (500 mg 4 times a day) for 4 weeks. Surgical drainage of abscess and surgical management of jaw lesions may be indicated based on the jaw involvement.

Leprosy

Leprosy is a chronic granulomatous infectious disease with interpersonal transmission caused by *M leprae*. The microorganism has an affinity primarily for the skin and peripheral nerves. In more advanced stages of leprosy, internal organs and mucous membranes can be affected. Leprosy is prevalent in less developed countries and usually affects populations with low economic status.[27]

Pathogenesis

M leprae is an acid-fast, gram-positive microorganism that shows tropism for cells of reticuloendothelial system and peripheral nervous system, specifically Schwann cells. *M leprae* has affinity to Schwann cells due to specific binding to the G domain of basal lamina of peripheral nerves. The microorganism induces immune suppression by inhibiting the interferon gamma-mediated activation of macrophages.[28]

Clinical features

Orofacial symptoms of leprosy include atrophy of the nasal spine, collapse of the nasal bridge, yellowish or reddish facial spots, loss of eyebrows, auricular spots or nodules, and facial nodules. The oral lesions in leprosy are characterized by tumor-like masses, which may be observed on the tongue, lips, or hard palate. The nonspecific oral lesions in leprosy are gingival hyperplasia, inflammatory papillary hyperplasia, periodontitis, and candidiasis.[29]

Diagnosis

The diagnosis of leprosy is usually achieved by clinical and bacteriologic examination. In 1997, the World Health Organization (WHO) provided 3 cardinal signs for diagnosis of leprosy:

1. Hypopigmented anesthetic skin lesion
2. Thickened peripheral nerve
3. Positive skin smear and/or bacilli observed in biopsy.[30]

Smears can be obtained from nasal mucosa, ear lobe, and/or skin lesions. Ziehl-Neelsen stain is a special staining method used to visualize *M leprae*. Microscopically, leprosy is characterized by a granulomatous nodule with epithelioid histiocytes and lymphocytes in fibrous stroma. Langhans giant cells and vacuolated macrophages (lepra cells) are seen throughout the lesional tissue. The bacilli can be observed readily by acid-fast stains.[31]

Management

In 2012, the WHO stated that paucibacillary presentation of leprosy is managed by rifampicin 600 mg monthly and dapsone 100 mg daily for 6 months. Multibacillary presentation of leprosy is managed by rifampicin 600 mg, clofazimine 300 mg monthly, and clofazimine 50 mg and dapsone 100 mg for 12 months. Single-lesion paucibacillary presentation of leprosy is managed by rifampicin 600 mg, ofloxacin 400 mg, and minocycline 100 mg monthly.[28]

Acute Necrotizing Ulcerative Gingivitis-Periodontitis

Acute necrotizing ulcerative gingivitis-periodontitis is an uncommon periodontal tissue disease that is characterized by necrosis, ulceration, pain, and bleeding. Acute necrotizing ulcerative gingivitis (NUG) and acute necrotizing ulcerative periodontitis (NUP) are considered to be different clinical stages of the same disease process. NUG and NUP are to be termed as necrotizing gingivitis and necrotizing periodontitis because ulceration is not a primary feature but is secondary to necrosis of the gingival margins, whereas necrotizing periodontitis affects the attachment apparatus of the tooth and the term ulcer may not be applicable.[32]

Pathogenesis

Fusobacterium and spirochetes have shown possible association with pathogenesis of necrotizing gingivitis and necrotizing periodontitis.[33] However, a poor immune defense seems to have a role in pathogenesis of necrotizing periodontitis. Poor immune response characterized by leukocyte dysfunction, defective mitogenic lymphocyte reaction, and reduced expression of immunoglobulins is a predisposing factor for necrotizing periodontal disease.[34] Studies also reported a causal relation between necrotizing gingivitis and HIV infection.[32]

Clinical features

Necrotizing gingivitis is clinically characterized as an inflammatory and destructive disease that is often observed with ulcerative and necrotizing papillae. The ulcers are accompanied by a white to gray pseudomembrane that consists of necrotic tissue. Removal of slough or necrotic membrane has a tendency to cause gingival bleeding. Necrotic ulcerations are extremely painful (**Fig. 5**).[35] The pain seems to be the major clinical concern and reason for dental appointments. The transition of necrotizing gingivitis to periodontitis is characterized by crater-like lesions at the interdental region and significant gingival tissue erosion and recession (**Fig. 6**).[36] Lymph node enlargement is seen in advanced stages of necrotizing periodontitis. Few case reports on necrotizing periodontitis presented with oroantral fistula in HIV-infected patients. Overall, oral hygiene is usually poor. Painful gingiva and necrotic ulcerations are

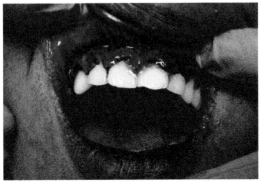

Fig. 5. Necrotic ulcerations of gingiva. (*From* Crystal CS, Coon TP, Kaylor DW. Acute necrotizing ulcerative gingivitis. Ann Emerg Med 2006;47(3):225; with permission.)

distinctive features of necrotizing gingivitis. The clinical signs and symptoms of necro-tizing gingivitis are identical for both HIV-positive and HIV-negative patients.[37]

Diagnosis

The diagnosis of necrotizing gingivitis and necrotizing periodontitis are usually made based on the specific clinical pattern. Necrotizing gingivitis and periodontitis are generally restricted to the interdental papilla and often presented with white pseudo-membrane. Necrotizing disease of gingiva and periodontium are often mistaken for primary herpetic gingivostomatitis.[38]

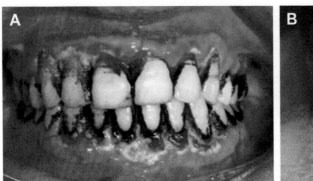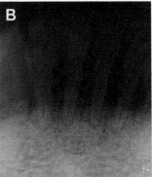

Fig. 6. Acute NUG with periodontal involvement. (*A*) Gingival changes and (*B*) horizontal bone loss in lower anterior region. (*From* Zia A, Andrabi SM, Qadri S, et al. Necrotizing peri-odontitis in a heavy smoker and tobacco chewer – A case report. Singapore Dent J 2015;36:36; with permission.)

Management

Patients are usually managed symptomatically. Debridement under local anesthesia, removal of pseudomembrane using chlorhexidine, nutritional counseling, and smok-ing cessation are a few strategies. Antibiotics are prescribed in the presence of fever or any immunocompromised states. Medication management includes amoxicillin 250 mg 3 times daily for 7 days and/or metronidazole 250 mg 3 times daily for 7 days. Patients are advised on periodontal care for maintenance visits.[37]

SEXUALLY TRANSMITTED BACTERIAL INFECTIONS OF THE ORAL CAVITY
Gonorrhea

Gonorrhea is venereal disease and most often transmitted by sexual intercourse. Gonorrhea is the second most frequent sexually transmitted disease in the United States. CDC in 2013 reported that there were 333,004 cases of gonorrhea reported in the United States of America.[39]

Pathogenesis

Gonorrhea is caused by a gram-negative bacteria, *Neisseria gonorrhea*. The incuba-tion period of the microorganism is 1 to 5 days. *N gonorrhea* is always considered pathogenic and not considered to be normal flora in any instance. Oral manifestations of gonorrhea a usually result of oral-genital contact or inoculation through infected hands. A longitudinal study that investigated incidence of pharyngeal gonorrhea among men who have sex with men (MSM) reported that the pharynx is a common, asymptomatic reservoir for gonorrhea in sexually active MSM.[40]

Clinical features

Gonorrhea is clinically characterized by oral ulcerations that are painful with or without necrosis. Lips, gingiva (**Fig. 7**),[41] tongue and buccal mucosa are frequent sites of oral gonorrhea. Oral lesions are accompanied by fever and regional lymphadenopathy.

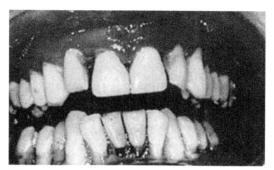

Fig. 7. Edematous inflammation of the gingivae with necrotic interdental papillae associated with oral gonococcal infection. (*From* Terezhalmy GT, Naylor GD. Oral manifestations of selected sexually related conditions. Dermatol Clin 1996; 14(2):305; with permission.)

Diagnosis

The clinical symptoms associated with *N gonorrhea* are typically diagnosed by history and physical examination. Microbiological diagnosis, however, is recommended when clinical diagnosis is in doubt. Nucleic acid amplification testing (NAAT) is the recommended initial microbiological testing for gonorrhea. Other tests, such as antigen test, culture methods, and genetic probing methods, are used in the absence of NAAT. Culture and sensitivity tests are useful in cases in which antibiotic resistance is observed. Routine screening of NAAT is recommended in sexually active patients at high risk of infection and gonorrhea complications. These include HIV-infected men and women, sexually active women who are younger than 25-years-old with multiple sexual partners, MSM, sexually active individuals living in areas of high *N gonorrhea* prevalence, and individuals with other sexually transmitted infections.[42]

Management

Dual therapy is recommended for gonorrheal infections due to a higher prevalence of antimicrobial resistance. Uncomplicated gonorrheal infections are managed by a recommended regimen that includes ceftriaxone 250 mg intramuscularly (IM) in a single dose and azithromycin 1 g orally in a single dose. Clinical reports indicated that ceftriaxone is a safe and effective treatment of uncomplicated gonorrhea at most anatomic sites. A cure rate of 98.9% was reported for pharyngeal infections in gonorrhea patients. Alternative regimens include cefixime 400 mg orally in a single dose and azithromycin 1 g orally in a single dose.[43] For test of cure, culture tests are helpful in identifying antibiotic resistance and are recommended in patients with pharyngeal gonorrhea who are treated with an alternative regimen after 14 days of medicinal treatment. When culture reports are positive for gonorrhea bacteria, then retreatment is recommended and the patient should undergo antimicrobial susceptibility testing.[44]

Syphilis

Syphilis, another sexually transmitted bacterial disease, is caused by *Treponema pallidum*. The manifestations of syphilis are classified into primary, secondary, latent, and tertiary stages. Oral lesions are more prevalent in secondary stage, although other stages can manifest in the oral cavity.

Pathogenesis

T pallidum is sexually transmitted and enters the host tissue via skin and mucous membrane through abrasions during unprotected sexual contact. *T pallidum* can also show vertical transmission via the transplacental route from mother to fetus. Dissemination of the pathogenic organism throughout the body occurs via circulatory system and reticuloendothelial system (lymphatic and lymph node). Entry to central nervous system can occur during any stage of syphilis. Cytotoxins and/or cytolytic enzymes are not associated with the pathogenesis of syphilis. The cytopathic effect of *T pallidum* on cells in culture requires an extraordinarily high number of bacteria. *T pallidum* is able to invade and survive in host tissue, despite lack of metabolic characteristics and sensitivity to oxygen.[45]

Clinical features

The primary stage of syphilis is called chancre and is rarely manifested in oral tissues. The oral ulcerations in primary syphilis may go unnoticed by patients or by unsuspicious clinicians. When the primary stage is manifested in the oral cavity, it is characterized by solitary ulceration that is predominantly seen in the lip (**Fig. 8**) or, rarely, the

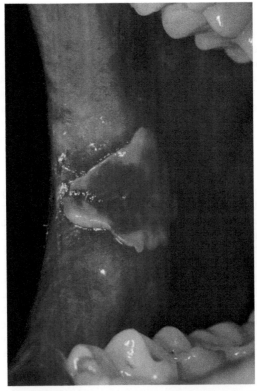

Fig. 8. Ulceration of the right commissure related to primary syphilis. (*From* Hertel M, Matter D, Schmidt-Westhausen AM, et al. Oral syphilis: a series of 5 cases. J Oral and Maxillofac Surg 2014;72(2):342; with permission.)

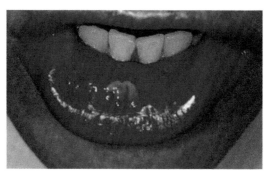

Fig. 9. Ulceration of the lower lip related to secondary syphilis. (*Modified from* Hertel M, Matter D, Schmidt-Westhausen AM, et al. Oral syphilis: a series of 5 cases. J Oral and Maxillofac Surg 2014;72(2):341; with permission.)

tongue. The reflection of secondary syphilis in oral tissue is due to hematogenous spread. Oral manifestations in secondary syphilis (**Fig. 9**) are extensive and/or variable. The signs and symptoms of oral tissue include mucous patches, maculopapular lesions, or nodular lesions. Tertiary syphilis manifestations are observed in one-third of patients who do not receive treatment for secondary syphilis. The oral appearance of tertiary syphilis is gummatous ulcerations and, occasionally, risk of oral squamous cell carcinoma formation. Gummatous ulcerations are usually painless and often seen on the hard palate and tongue. Bone destruction, palatal perforation, and oronasal fistula can be observed in tertiary syphilis patients.[46]

Limited data exist to describe the interaction between syphilis and HIV infection, and the combination of these 2 infections is considered dangerous.[47] A study reported that increased HIV viral load and decreased CD4 counts are increased with syphilis infection.[48,49] It is also worth noting that researchers and clinical experts believe that persistent cerebrospinal fluid abnormalities and clinical neurosyphilis are more common in syphilis patients coinfected with HIV than in those who are not. However, there are few studies with which to draw a conclusion on this.

Diagnosis

Diagnosis of syphilis can be achieved more specifically from lesion exudate or lesion through dark-field examination. Although dark-field examination is considered highly specific and definitive, its accuracy is reported to be limited by the experience of the operator performing the test, the number of live treponemes in the lesion, the presence of pathologic areas or active lesions, and the presence of nonpathologic treponemes in oral and/or anal lesions. No commercial tests are available for *T pallidum*; however, some laboratories provide validated polymerase chain reaction tests for detection of pathogenic organisms in DNA. Presumptive diagnosis of syphilis requires the use of 2 tests: a nontreponemal test (venereal disease research laboratory or rapid plasma reagin) and a treponemal test (fluorescent treponemal antibody absorbed test, *T pallidum* passive particle agglutination, enzyme immune assay, chemiluminescence immunoassays, immunoblots, or rapid treponemal assays).[50,51]

Management

In all stages of syphilis, parenteral administration of penicillin G is preferred for treatment. The dosage and length of treatment usually depend on the stage and clinical manifestation of syphilis. Treatment of latent syphilis and tertiary syphilis requires a longer duration of therapy.[52] The recommended regimen for adults is benzathine penicillin G 2.4 million units IM in a single dose. For infants and children, it is benzathine penicillin G 50,000 units/kg IM, up to the adult dose of 2.4 million units in a single dose. A randomized trial reported that use of additional doses of benzathine penicillin G, amoxicillin, or other antibiotics do not enhance efficacy when used to treat primary and secondary syphilis, regardless of HIV status.[53] The protocol for diagnosis and treatment of syphilis given[54] in **Fig. 10**.

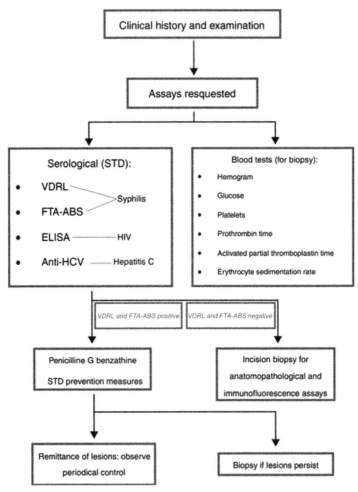

Fig. 10. Protocol for diagnosis and management of syphilis. ELISA, enzyme-linked immunosorbent assay; FTA-ABS, fluorescent treponemal antibody absorbed; HCV, hepatitis C virus; STD, sexually transmitted disease; VDRL, venereal disease research laboratory. (*From* Seibt CE, Munerato MC. Secondary syphilis in the oral cavity and the role of the dental surgeon in STD prevention, diagnosis and treatment: a case series study. Braz J Infect Dis 2016;20(4):395; with permission.)

ORAL MICROBIAL DISEASE SPECIMEN COLLECTION AND TRANSPORTATION
Specimen Collection and Transportation of Bacterial and Fungal Lesions

Appropriate collection of specimen and test for the detection of a pathogenic organism is the most important aspect of microbiological diagnosis. For an oral microbiological disease, the most common specimens collected are aspirated fluid from an abscess area, saliva, or tissue biopsy. The quantity of the specimen may be limited if it is an aspirate content or tissue biopsy, and it may pose a challenge if there is more than 1 microbiological test to be performed. If the microbiological diagnostic test is focused on isolation of a pathogen in culture, care must be taken during the specimen collection period. For example, care must be taken to avoid substances (ie, antimicrobials) that can overgrow or suppress the microorganism. The recommendation for collection of specimen for culture diagnosis is before the administration of antimicrobials to the patient. Transportation of the specimen to the microbiology laboratory is an important aspect in microbiological diagnostic procedures. The clinician should be aware of the time to transport as well as how it should be transported. Aspirate from an abscessed lesion should be transferred to anaerobic vial and the specimen must be tightly capped immediately. The specimen collection methods for bacteria and fungi are almost similar, except that special media is used for specimens that require fungal culture methods. The specimens that require fungal diagnosis may contain substances that suppress bacterial growth. The identification and detection methods of bacteria and fungi are a microbiologist's concern and are briefly presented in **Box 3**.

Box 3
Microbiological detection methods for diagnosis of bacteria and fungi

1. Microscopy
   a. Cytology
   b. Tissue biopsy
   c. Staining (routine, gram staining, differential, and fluorescent stains)

2. Culture
   a. Basic media
   b. Enriched media
   c. Selective and enrichment media
   d. Differential media
   e. Transport media
   f. Anaerobic media
   g. Special media

3. Antigen detection

4. Nucleic acid–based tests
   a. Nonamplified tests
      i. Peptide nucleic acid probes
      ii. DNA and ribosomal RNA (rRNA) target probes
   b. Amplified tests
      i. Polymerase chain reaction

5. Serologic tests

6. Biochemical tests

7. Agglutination tests

8. Genomic and proteomic tests

Specimen Collection and Transportation of Viral Lesions

Collection of specimen for viral diagnosis should be done at the onset of symptoms, except for blood or serologic tests. In serologic diagnosis, blood specimens are collected during the acute phase of disease; that is, the first week of illness. A follow-up serum collection is done 2 weeks later. A generalized request for viral identification from the specimen should not be sent to virology laboratory. When submitting the specimen for viral diagnosis, the clinician should include the most likely pathogenic virus for the patient's signs and symptoms. The dental surgeon can collaborate with an oral medicine dentist, oral and maxillofacial surgeon, oral and maxillofacial pathologist, infectious disease specialist, and/or clinical microbiologist to confirm the details of the appropriate pathogenic virus.[55]

In viral diagnosis, selection of appropriate specimen is based on type of viral pathogen, site of manifestation, onset of disease, and specific diagnostic test. Histopathological, cytologic, or microscopic examination of specimen requires collection of specimen with infected cells to observe cytopathic changes. An antigen test and nucleic acid amplification test can be performed on specimens with cell-free viruses. Clinician should be made aware that anticoagulant heparin can interfere with nucleic acid amplification test because heparin is a nonspecific polymerase inhibitor. Patients under anticoagulant heparin should be consult with a physician before viral culture or other viral diagnostic tests are considered. Collection of blood specimen is determined by the seroconversion period. Specimens collected from active area of oral lesions are suitable for culture method (eg, site of active oral herpetic lesion). The timing for collection of specimen for viral diagnosis is determined by the type of viral infections. In viral infections, such as herpes, measles, and mumps, viral shedding occurs shortly before symptoms appear and then rapidly decrease. Whereas in chronic viral infections, such as HIV, human papilloma virus, and cytomegalovirus, viral shedding can be prolonged or may be short-lived in immunocompetent individuals and persistent in immunocompromised patients. Swab and tissue specimens can be considered for viral diagnosis by culture methods, and the viral transport medium should be considered. The viral transport medium usually contains antibiotics to inhibit the growth of contaminating bacteria and/or fungi. In doubtful clinical conditions (viral, bacteria, or fungal infection), the dental surgeon should collect more than 1 specimen for processing at the microbiology laboratory.

A liquid specimen, such as saliva, should not be diluted in viral transport media. It is also worth noting that wooden shafts or cotton swabs may be toxic for culture methods. Calcium alginate-aluminum shaft swabs also have some chance of interfering with the culture method, immunofluorescence tests, and nucleic amplification tests.[55–57] The identification and detection methods in viral diagnosis are the microbiologist concern are briefly presented in **Box 4**.

Box 4
Microbiological detection methods for viral diagnosis

1. Microscopy
   a. Cytology
   b. Tissue biopsy

2. Viral culture methods

3. Electron microscopy

4. Nucleic acid–based tests

5. Antigen detection methods
6. Serologic tests
   a. Enzyme-linked immunosorbent assay (ELISA)
   b. Immunoassays
   c. Indirect fluorescent antibody tests (IFA)
7. Immunofluorescence tests
8. Polymerase chain reaction test (PCR)

MEDICATION MANAGEMENT OF ORAL MICROBIOLOGICAL DISEASES

Medication management of oral and maxillofacial microbiological disease involves the use of pharmacologic agents to treat, eradicate, and prevent infections. They are classified as antibiotic (bactericidal or bacteriostatic), antifungal, or antiviral. For most oral and maxillofacial infectious diseases, medication management is indicated and, to some extent, surgical therapy is also planned. **Table 2** lists common antimicrobial medications used in bacterial infections of the oral cavity. A few pharmacologic agents used for viral and fungal infections are listed. The choice of antimicrobial therapy for patients with an oral microbiological condition can be complex because several variables must be considered. Factors involved in antimicrobial selection include host-specific factors, pharmacologic factors, and pathogen-specific therapy.

Table 2
Medication management of oral microbiological diseases

Microbiological Disease Category	Disease	Agents Used	Notes
Bacterial infections	Tuberculosis	Isoniazid and rifampicin	• The patient should be referred to pulmonologist for the management of active tuberculosis and consultation for infectious status of patients
	Actinomycosis	Intravenous penicillin G or oral penicillin VK	• Surgical drainage of abscess • Surgical management of the jaw lesion depending on the extent
	Leprosy	Rifampicin, dapsone, clofazimine, ofloxacin, minocycline	• Medication management is determined by presentation (paucibacillary or multibacillary)
	Gonorrhea	Ceftriaxone, azithromycin, cefixime	• Culture tests are recommended to identify antibiotic resistance
	Acute NUG, periodontitis	Amoxicillin, metronidazole, chlorhexidine mouthwash	• Antibiotics are prescribed in the presence of fever or any other immunocompromised conditions
	Syphilis	Benzathine penicillin G	• Randomized trial reported use of additional doses of benzathine penicillin do not enhance efficacy of treatment, regardless of HIV status

(*continued on next page*)

Table 2
(*continued*)

Microbiological Disease Category	Disease	Agents Used	Notes
Viral infections	Recurrent herpes labialis	Acyclovir, penciclovir, famciclovir, valacyclovir	• Must be started at first prodromal sign
	Primary herpes simplex virus infection	Acyclovir, famciclovir, valacyclovir	• Acyclovir is considered gold standard for prophylactic and treatment
	Herpes zoster	Acyclovir, valacyclovir or famciclovir	• Other effective therapies for treatment of postherpetic neuralgia: gabapentin, topical capsaicin, tricyclic antidepressants, opioids, and topical lidocaine patches
	Epstein-Barr virus infection	Supportive therapy is adequate	• Corticosteroid and antiviral medication are usually used in immunocompromised patients
	Cytomegalovirus infection	Infections resolve spontaneously	• Antiviral agents such as ganciclovir, foscarnet, and cidofovir have been effective in the management in immunocompetent patients • Newer drugs in development include maribavir, CMX 001, and AIC246
	Human herpes virus-6 infection	Ganciclovir and foscarnet	• Efficacy of medication is unknown • No randomized trial results available on antiviral therapies in immunocompetent or immunocompromised patients
Fungal infections	Candida	Nystatin, clotrimazole, fluconazole, flucytosine	• Disinfection of non–metal-containing acrylic dentures or removable dental appliance may be achieved by 10 min soak in 0.5% solution of sodium hypochlorite (1 part household bleach mixed with 10 parts of water) • In patients with denture-associated candidiasis, microwave disinfection of non–metal-containing acrylic dentures once per week for 2 treatments was as effective as 14-day course of topical nystatin antifungal treatment • Disinfection of metal-containing dentures is not thoroughly researched; however, researchers proposed the use of chlorhexidine solutions,

(*continued on next page*)

Table 2 (continued)			
Microbiological Disease Category	**Disease**	**Agents Used**	**Notes**
			hydrogen peroxide, and antifungal medication as a means of disinfecting metal-containing dentures and/or dental appliances
	Aspergillosis	Amphotericin B, voriconazole, itraconazole, and caspofungin	• Local irrigation is administered as an adjunct to systemic anti-fungal therapy
	Cryptococcosis	Fluconazole	• In HIV-infected patients, treating cryptococcosis consists of 3 phases: induction, consolidation, and maintenance therapy • Amphotericin B and flucona-zole are recommended
	Histoplasmosis	Itraconazole and amphotericin B	• Electrolyte level, renal func-tion, and blood cell count should be monitored in pa-tients receiving amphotericin B therapy
	Blastomycosis	Amphotericin B deoxycholate, itraconazole	• Patients with central nervous system symptoms are treated by amphotericin B and azole therapy
	Mucormycosis	Liposomal amphotericin B, posaconazole	• Oral fluconazole, itracona-zole, and voriconazole are administered as prophylactic dose in neutropenia and graft-versus-host disease
	Geotrichosis	—	• Responds well to treatment with candidiasis • Amphotericin is most suitable drug
	Rhinosporidiosis	Surgical management	• Surgical removal of growth

SUMMARY

Increased numbers of patients with immunocompromised or debilitating disease are observed in many countries. Impaired host immune systems are frequently associated with increased oral mucosal infections. It is evident that oral mucosal infections are mostly underdiagnosed in dental practices and most attempts for diagnosis of oral mucosal infections are observed with fungal infections and, specifically, candidiasis. Although the clinical picture may not be clear with oral mucosal infections, microbio-logical diagnosis of oral mucosal infections should be frequently considered in dental practice. The literature supports that most cases of oral mucosal infections be subject to microbial culture. It is also worth noting that oral rinse and imprint microbiological methods seem to be effective when generalized oral mucosal lesions are observed. The localized mucosal lesions are sampled by scrapping, swab sample, aspiration, or tissue biopsy. The important diagnostic approaches in oral mucosal infections are

1. To determine whether the lesion of interest is of infectious origin
2. To follow correct microbiological sampling methods
3. To treat the condition based on the investigative report.

The causes of diagnosed oral mucosal condition should be explored. This is because oral mucosal lesions with local causes should be easier to treat than those with systemic causes. In both cases (local or systemic causes), patients should be strictly advised to follow good oral hygiene measures. It is also worth noting that oral mucosal infections are difficult to treat when a patient presents with impaired host defense and antibiotic or drug resistance. The dentist should consider a multidisciplinary approach in managing oral mucosal infection patients with systemic causes. Therefore, the dental surgeon plays an important role in early identification and management of oral mucosal infections. The dental clinician should, therefore, be up to date with clinical presentation, diagnosis, and management of various oral mucosal infections.

REFERENCES

1. Dahlen G. Bacterial infections of the oral mucosa. Periodontol 2000 2009;49: 13–38.
2. Merrell D, Falkow S. Frontal and stealth attack strategies in microbial pathogenesis. Nature 2004;430:250–6.
3. Falkow S. The microbe's view of infection. Ann Intern Med 1998;129:247–8.
4. Aas JA, Paster BJ, Stokes LN, et al. Defining the normal bacterial flora of the oral cavity. J Clin Microbiol 2005;43:5721–32.
5. Marsh PD, Martin MV. Oral microbiology. 4th edition. Oxford (United Kingdom): Wright; 1999.
6. Rudney JD, Chen R. The vital status of human buccal epithelial cells and the bacteria associated with them. Arch Oral Biol 2006;51:291–8.
7. Zhu HW, McMillan AS, McGrath C, et al. Oral carriage of yeast and coliforms in stroke sufferers: a prospective longitudinal study. Oral Dis 2008;14:60–6.
8. Sallberg M. Oral viral infections of children. Periodontol 2000 2009;49:87–95.
9. Samarnayake LP, Keung Leung W, Jin L. Oral mucosal fungal infections. Periodontol 2000 2009;49:39–59.
10. Samaranayake LP. Diagnostic microbiology and laboratory methods. In: Samaranake LP, editor. Essential microbiology for dentistry. China: Elsevier; 2012. p. 61.
11. de Souza BC, de Lemos VM, Munerato MC. Oral manifestation of tuberculosis: a case report. Braz J Infect Dis 2016;20:210–3.
12. Swaminathan S, Padmapriyadarsini C, Narendran G. HIV-associated tuberculosis: clinical update. Clin Infect Dis 2010;50:1377–86.
13. Vaid S, Lee YY, Rawat S, et al. Tuberculosis in the head and neck: a forgotten differential diagnosis. Clin Radiol 2010;65:73–81.
14. Miziara ID. Tuberculosis affecting the oral cavity in Brazilian HIV-infected patients. Oral Surg Oral Med Oral Path Oral Radiol Endod 2005;100:179–82.
15. Hale LT, Tucker CP. Head and neck manifestations of tuberculosis. Oral Maxillofacial Surg Clin N Am 2008;20:635–42.
16. Mignogna MD, Muzio LL, Favia G. Oral tuberculosis: a clinical evaluation of 42 cases. Oral Dis 2000;6:25–30.
17. Smith WHR, Davis D, Mason KD, et al. Intraoral and pulmonary tuberculosis following dental manipulation. Lancet 1982;1:842–3.

18. Lunn JA, Mayho V. Incidence of pulmonary tuberculosis by occupation of hospital employees in the National Health Service in England and Wales 1980-84. J Soc Occup Med 1989;39:30–2.

19. Von Arx DP, Husain A. Oral tuberculosis. Br Dent J 2001;190:420–2.

20. Crossman T, Herold J. Actinomycosis of the maxillae-a case report of a rare oral infection presenting in general dental practice. Br Dent J 2009;206:201–2.

21. Gannepalli A, Ayinampudi BK, Baghirath PV, et al. Actinomycotic osteomyelitis of maxilla presenting as oroantral fistula: a rare case report. Case Rep Dent 2015;689240. http://dx.doi.org/10.1155/2015/689240.

22. Yadegaryniaa D, Merza MA, Salia S, et al. A rare case presentation of oral actinomycosis. Int J Mycobacteriol 2013;2:187–9.

23. Avijgan M, Shakeri H, Shakeri M. A case report of cervicofacial actinomycosis. Asian Pac J Trop Med 2010;3:838–40.

24. Valour F, Sénéchal A, Dupieux C, et al. Actinomycosis: etiology, clinical features, diagnosis, treatment, and management. Infect Drug Resist 2014;7:183–97.

25. Eastridge CE, Prather JR, Hughes FA Jr, et al. Actinomycosis: a 24-year experienc. South Med J 1972;65:839–43.

26. Selvin SS, John JR. Short-term treatment of actinomycosis: two cases and a review. Clin Infect Dis 2004;38:444–7.

27. de Abreu MA, Michalany NS, Wecks LLM, et al. The oral mucosa in leprosy: a clinical and histopathological study. Singapore Dent J 2006;72:312–6.

28. Eichelmann K, Gonzalez Gonzalez SE, Salas-Alanis JC, et al. Leprosy. An update: definition, pathogenesis, classificaiton, diagnosis and treatment. Actas Dermosifilogr 2013;104:554–63.

29. Pereira RM, Silva TS, Thalisson SO, et al. Orofacial and dental conditions in leprosy. Braz J Oral Sci 2013;12:330–4.

30. Britton WJ, Lockwood DN. Leprosy. Lancet 2004;363:1209–19.

31. Ramaprasad P, Fernando A, Madhale S, et al. Transmission and protection in leprosy: indications of the role of mucosal immunity. Lepr Rev 1997;68:310–5.

32. Klotz H. Differentiation between necrotic ulcerative gingivitis and primary herpetic gingivostomatitis. NY State Dent J 1973;39:283–94.

33. Feller L, Lemmer J. Necrotizing gingivitis as it relates to HIV infection: a review of the literature. Perio 2005;2:31–7.

34. Bradley DJ, David E. Acture necrotizing ulcerative gingivitis: a review of diagnosis, etiology and treatment. J Periodontol 1986;57:141–50.

35. Cutler CW, Wasfy MO, Ghaffar K. Impaired bacterial activity of PMN from two brothers with necrotizing ulcerative gingivo-periodontitis. J Periodontol 1994;65:57–63.

36. Crystal CS, Coon TP, Kaylor DW. Acute necrotizing ulcerative gingivitis. Ann Emerg Med 2006;47:225.

37. Zia A, Mukhtar-Un-Nisar Andrabi S, Qadri S, et al. Necrotizing periodontitis in a heavy smoker and tobacco chewer – A case report. Singapore Dent J 2015;36:35–8.

38. Sylvia T, Reema NA. Managing patients with necrotizing ulcerative gingivitis. J Can Dent Assoc 2013;79:d46.

39. Centers for Disease Control and Prevention. Sexually transmitted disease surveillance 2013. Atlanta (GA); 2014.

40. Sheldon RM, Jeffrey DK, Susan PB, et al. Prevalence and incidence of pharyngeal gonorrhea in a longitudinal sample of men who have sex with men: the EXPLORE study. Clin Infect Dis 2006;43:1284–9.

41. Terezhalmy GT, Naylor GD. Oral manifestations of selected sexually related conditions. Dermatol Clin 1996;14:303–17.
42. Workowski KA, Bolan GA, Centers for Disease Control and Prevention. Sexually transmitted diseases treatment guidelines, 2015. MMWR Recomm Rep 2015;64:1.
43. Newman LM, Moran JS, Workowski KA. Update on the management of gonorrhea in adults in the United States. Clin Infect Dis 2007;44:S84–101.
44. Moran JS, Levine WC. Drugs of choice for the treatment of uncomplicated gonococcal infections. Clin Infect Dis 1995;20:S47–65.
45. Peeling RW, Hook EW. The pathogenesis of syphilis: the Great Mimicker, revisited. J Pathol 2006;208:224–32.
46. Leão JC, Gueiros LA, Porter SR. Oral manifestations of syphilis. Clinics (Sao Paulo) 2006;61:161–6.
47. Lynn WA, Lightman S. Syphilis and HIV: a dangerous combination. Lancet Infect Dis 2004;4:456–66.
48. Buchacz K, Patel P, Taylor M, et al. Syphilis increases HIV viral load and decreases CD4 cell counts in HIV-infected patients with new syphilis infections. AIDS 2004;18:2075–9.
49. Hertel M, Matter D, Schmidt-Westhausen AM, et al. Oral syphilis: a series of 5 cases. J Oral Maxillofac Surg 2014;72:338–45.
50. Nandwani R, Evans DT. Are you sure it's syphilis? A review of false positive serology. Int J STD AIDS 1995;6:241–8.
51. Brown DL, Frank JE. Diagnosis and management of syphilis. Am Fam Physician 2003;68:283–90.
52. De Paulo LF, Servato JP, Oliveira MT, et al. Oral manifestations of secondary syphilis. Int J Infect Dis 2015;35:40–2.
53. Rolfs RT, Joesoef MR, Hendershot EF, et al. A randomized trial of enhanced therapy for early syphilis in patients with and without human immunodeficiency virus infection. The Syphilis and HIV Study Group. N Engl J Med 1997;337:307–14.
54. Seibt CE, Munerato MC. Secondary syphilis in the oral cavity and the role of the dental surgeon in STD prevention, diagnosis and treatment: a case series study. Braz J Infect Dis 2016;20:393–8.
55. Murray PR. The clinician and the microbiology laboratory. In: Bennett JE, Dolin R, Blaser MJ, editors. Principles and practice of infectious diseases. 8th edition. Philadelphia: Elsevier Publications; 2015. p. 191–223.
56. Wang JT, Wang TH, Sheu JC, et al. Effects of anticoagulants and storage of blood samples on efficacy of the polymerase chain reaction assay for hepatitis C virus. J Clin Microbiol 1992;30:750–3.
57. Forman MS, Valsamakis A. Specimen collection, transport and processing: virology. In: Murray PR, Baron EJ, Jorgensen J, et al, editors. Manual of clinical microbiology. 9th edition. Washington, DC: American Society for Microbiology; 2007. p. 1284–96.

Oral Bacterial Infections

Diagnosis and Management

Glendee Reynolds-Campbell, BMedSc, MBBS, DM (Medical Microbiology)*,
Alison Nicholson, MBBS, DM (Medical Microbiology),
Camille-Ann Thoms-Rodriguez, BMedSc, MBBS, DM (Medical Microbiology)

KEYWORDS

- Bacteria • Infections • Oral cavity • Microbiology • Microbiome

KEY POINTS

- There are more than 500 bacterial species from several phyla associated with various niches within the oral cavity, as commensals or pathogens.
- It is often difficult to distinguish true pathogens from commensals and this is further exacerbated by the development of polymicrobial infections.
- The diagnosis of oral infections is usually a clinical one but microbiologic diagnosis assists with appropriate therapy and spares unnecessary use of powerful antibiotics.

INTRODUCTION

Normal Flora of the Oral Cavity or the Human Oral Microbiome

The human oral microbiome consists of the microorganisms present within the oral cavity and its adjacent structures extending to the distal third of the esophagus.[1] These structures provide distinct microbial habitats that include the teeth, gingiva, tongue, hard and soft palates, cheeks, and lips. Contiguous structures, such as the tonsils, pharynx, Eustachian tube, middle ear, trachea, lungs, nasal cavity, and sinuses, also provide a niche for various microorganisms.

More than 500 different bacterial species have the capacity to inhabit the oral cavity, but only 280 have been isolated by standard culture methods.[2] These organisms are protective against invasion by other pathogenic species, or are associated with oral and systemic diseases. Molecular studies suggest several phyla to which these organisms belong: Bacteroidetes, Firmicutes, Tenericutes, Actinobacteria, Proteobacteria, Euryarchaeota, Chlamydiae, and Spirochaetes. Commonly isolated species include streptococci, actinomycetes, veillonella, and diphtheroids, and gram-negative anaerobic rods.[3] These organisms are site specific or host specific, transient or resident.[2,3]

Disclosure Statement: The authors have nothing to disclose.
Department of Microbiology, The University of the West Indies, Mona, KGN 7, Jamaica, West Indies
* Corresponding author.
E-mail address: glendee.reynoldscampbell02@uwimona.edu.jm

Common Bacterial Infections of the Oral Cavity

Bacterial infections presenting to dentists include dental caries, gingivitis, periodontitis, and dental abscess.[4] Clinical versus laboratory diagnosis is commonly done, with the latter providing information on susceptibility, which facilitates culture-directed therapy and judicious use of antibiotics.[4,5] The information provided from these tests is used to guide and measure a response to therapy. Rapid point-of-care tests are being developed that will result in clinicians acquiring microbiologic diagnoses in far less time than with conventional tests.[4] Knowledge of the likely implicated pathogen and related antibiograms will prove useful in guiding empiric therapy.

Dental caries refers to tooth decay that occurs postcolonization and adherence to teeth by microorganisms originally a part of the normal flora. Disruption of the balance within the microbiome leads to a breakdown of the tooth enamel.[6]

Such organisms as *Streptococcus mutans*, *Actinomyces* spp, and others usually colonize first (**Table 1**).[7] Secondary colonizers include *Fusobacterium nucleatum* and *Prevotella intermedia* (see **Table 1**). This eventually leads to biofilm and plaque formation. Those at the core tend to be anaerobic and those at the surface, aerobic.[4,7] The acid produced from carbohydrate accumulation erodes teeth enamel, which may initially appear discolored and later develops into a cavity. If the cavitation thus formed is deep enough it may involve the pulp of the tooth.[4]

Table 1	
The microbial characteristics of organisms associated with the development of dental caries	
Characteristics of the Microbial Composition of Caries	
Organism	**Characteristic Features**
Primary colonizers	
Streptococcus spp	Gram-positive; coccoid in shape; facultative anaerobes; most are mesophiles
Actinomyces spp	Gram-positive; individual colonies are rod-shaped but collectively may appear filamentous; most are facultative anaerobes with the exception of *A meyeri*; most are mesophiles
Neisseria spp	Gram-negative; coccoid in shape; some are capnophiles, some are microaerophillic; most are mesophiles
Veillonella spp	Gram-negative; coccoid in shape; obligate anaerobe; mesophile
Secondary colonizers	
Fusobacterium nucleatum	Gram-negative; fusiform rods or spindle-shaped (spindle-shaped rod); anaerobic; able to coaggregate with other species in the oral cavity to form dental plaque; mesophillic
Prevotella intermedia	Gram-negative; rod-shaped; anaerobic; opportunistic pathogen
Capnocytophaga spp	Gram-negative; thin rod-shaped (medium to long rods); gliding ability on agar; facultative anaerobe; capnophile; mesophile
Eikenella corrodens	Gram-negative; rod-shaped; facultative anaerobe; mesophile; bleachy or musty odor; forms pits on chocolate agar
Actinobacillus actinomycetemcomitans	Gram-negative; coccobacillus (curved or straight); capnophile; facultative anaerobe; mesophile
Treponema spp	Gram-negative; spiral-shaped; microaerophillic; mesophile

Data from Refs.[14,15,48]

Microbiologic identification of the causative agents is usually not done because antibiotics are not needed for the management of dental caries.[8] If, however, an abscess develops as a complication of a dental decay then antibiotics may become necessary.[9]

Gingivitis is the inflammation of the gums that can result from the same bacteria present in dental plaque that have been associated with dental caries.[4] Periodontitis is more severe because the gums detach from the teeth and bone loss may occur. The soft tissue and bone supporting the teeth can also become infected. If this is not appropriately managed it may lead to the development of a dental abscess, loss of the tooth, and/or systemic complications through hematologic spread. Even in these instances sample collection for a microbiologic diagnosis is often not sought by dentists.[4] The development of rapid and molecular tests, such as dental probes for detection of plaque organisms, will allow for the more prompt identification of dental pathogens.[4] This may encourage greater use by clinicians given the anticipated reduction in turnaround time. A balance must be achieved between the use of empiric or prophylactic antimicrobial therapy and antibacterial therapy aimed at a specific organism, because this practice may result in the emergence of antibiotic-resistance strains, which is a growing global problem.[5]

PHYLUM: ACTINOBACTERIA

This phylum consists of several genera, such as the actinomycetes, streptomycetes, bifidobacteria and some members of the corynebacteria (diphtheroids). Most are commensals with variable levels of aerotolerance. Anaerobic environments are provided in the crevices of the oral cavity and beneath the layers of plaque and debris resulting from poor oral hygiene. Their morphology tends to be variable ranging from gram-positive rods to branching coccobacillary forms.

Actinomycetes

Many actinomycetes are oral commensals residing in the supragingival and subgingival plaque of healthy individuals. Commonly isolated are *Aggregatibacter naeslundii*, *Aggregatibacter oris*, and *Aggregatibacter johnsonii*. Others include *Aggregatibacter israelii*, *Aggregatibacter gerencseriae*, *Aggregatibacter georgiae*, and *Aggregatibacter odontolyticus*. Disease caused by this genus is commonly referred to as actinomycoses; however, they can also be found in polymicrobial infections. Actinomycotic infection of the craniofacial region generally follows a history of untreated dental caries (involving the root surface), extractions, or trauma that allowed for inoculation of these sulfur granule–producing commensals into deeper tissues. They are also associated with endodontic infections, gingivitis, periodontitis, osteoradionecrosis lesions, odontogenic abscesses, and dental implant–associated infections.[10,11] These infections result in sinus tract formation from which the granules are discharged.

Diagnosis

Contamination from the commensal oral microbiota must be prevented during the sampling process, and although difficult, pure cultures of each isolate should be obtained. Anaerobic culture is done on blood agar plates from samples collected from scrapings or post-dental-extraction/debridement procedures. Purulent material contains the sulfur granules (microcolonies of the organism), which are washed, crushed, and observed microscopically for the characteristic thin-branching non-spore-forming, gram-positive rods. Definitive identification to the species level for all members of this phyla requires the use of commercial biochemical assay kits or molecular study.

Susceptibility and treatment

Clinical and Laboratory Standards Institute (CLSI) guidelines on breakpoints are not available and susceptibility testing is undertaken by reference laboratories using the agar dilution method. Clinically, metronidazole-resistant strains are common, although it was once considered the drug of choice. Newer agents, such as tigecycline and telavancin, have proven much more useful. The newer quinolones, such as moxifloxacin, have proven beneficial.[12]

Bifidobacteria

Of the 32 known species from the genera, 11 have been identified as gut and oral cavity commensals. These include *Bacteroides dentium*, *Bacteroides gallicum*, *Bacteroides bifidum*, *Bacteroides pseudocatenulatum*, and *Bacteroides angulatum*, with *B dentium* being the most common cause of dental caries from this group. This species has also been found in tonsillar samples.[12]

Corynebacteria

Species level identification of members of this genus is only done in serious infections of sterile sites (eg, bloodstream infections), and then only when found in multiple samples and/or if they are the predominant isolate in an aseptically collected sample. They are collectively referred to as coryneform or diphtheroids species. These bacteria rarely cause infections of the oral cavity but may be found as part of a polymicrobial infection making the distinction between their presence as a pathogen versus a commensal a hard one.[13]

Diagnosis

These gram-positive pleomorphic rods tend to assume a club-shaped appearance and smears from cultures exhibit the formation of palisades or clusters that arrange themselves into what is described as Chinese lettering. They are lipophilic and show growth best on agar supplemented by Tween 80. Antigenic assays for distinguishing species is not routine.[13]

Susceptibility and treatment

The CLSI recommends the use of broth microdilution for susceptibility testing for these organisms. Penicillin-based agents, such as ampicillin and amoxicillin/clavulanate, have proven useful in therapy, as have erythromycin, clindamycin, ceftriaxone, ciprofloxacin, and gentamicin.

PHYLUM: PROTEOBACTERIA
Aggregatibacter

Actinobacillus actinomycetemcomitans was renamed *Aggregatibacter actinomycetemcomitans* in recent times. This species is also commonly found in polymicrobial infections with other oral organisms inclusive of *Streptococcus viridans* and both have been implicated as causative agents of infective endocarditis. Although *S viridans* tends to be easily recoverable in blood cultures, this species is associated with culture-negative infective endocarditis because of its slow-growing nature. Its name also speaks to the "concomitant" recovery of this organism with *Actinomyces* spp. It is commonly found in gingival and supragingival crevices and is associated with localized aggressive/juvenile periodontitis, which leads to loss of alveolar bone in the region of the incisors and premolars and hence eventual loss of these teeth. Localized aggressive/juvenile periodontitis and by extension its causative agent is most common in black adolescents.[14]

Diagnosis

Root canal exudates and subgingival plaque serve as suitable specimen for this non-spore-forming anaerobic gram-negative coccobacilli. This facultative anaerobe prefers environments enriched with 5% to 10% CO_2, and growth is stimulated by addition of low-molecular-weight steroid hormones to reagents. Isolated colonies appear rough and crinkled on chocolate or blood agar surfaces within 48 to 72 hours. Studies have shown this appearance to be caused by the organism's ability to tightly adhere to surfaces (agar, glass, plastic). This characteristic is thought to be caused by fibers on the bacterial surface that even allow for similar tight adherence to collagen and fibronectin, components of the surfaces of human cells, increasing the pathogenic potential of the organism. Within 5 to 7 days the colonies appear star-shaped on the agar surface.[15]

Susceptibility and treatment

Actinobacillus actinomycetemcomitans are susceptible to the cephalosporins (with ceftriaxone being the drug of choice for treatment of serious systemic infections), fluoroquinolones, tetracycline, doxycycline, azithromycin, trimethoprim-sulphamethoxazole, rifampin, and aminoglycosides. Treatment of dental disease must, however, be preceded by debridement, scaling, and root planning. Tetracycline, doxycycline, or ciprofloxacin is often used for oral disease or combination therapy with amoxicillin and metronidazole. The latter combination therapy regime has been associated with fewer treatment failure reports, and suppression of subgingival survival of the organism.[15]

Eikenella

This gram-negative anaerobic nonmotile bacillus belongs to the Neisseriaceae family.[16] *Eikenella corrodens* is a common oral commensal, notably transmitted through human bites, which retains the capacity to cause infection at multiple body sites.[17] Along with *A actinomyecetemcomitans* this bacteria is known as one of the HACEK organisms (*Haemophilus, Aggregatibacter, Cardiobacterium, Eikenella,* and *Kingella*), which cause endocarditis. The HACEK organisms are a normal part of the human microbiota, living in the oral-pharyngeal region. *Eikenella* species have also been implicated in infections of the respiratory tract, bones, and wounds.[18,19] In the mouth they are found in the subgingival plaque and participate in polymicrobial infections with gram-positive cocci, causing periodontal tissue inflammation.[20]

Diagnosis

Gram-stained isolates appear as thin pink rods with rounded ends. They grow slowly on blood and chocolate agar supplemented with clindamycin in 5% to 10% CO_2.[17] Distinct 1- to 2-mm pale yellow colonies pit the agar and have spreading edges seen within 48 hours of incubation.[21] *E corrodens* has a musty bleach-like odor.

Susceptibility and treatment

Broad-spectrum penicillins (eg, amoxicillin-clavulanate) and cephalosporins (eg, ceftriaxone and carbapenems) still retain efficacy against this bacterial species. They can be used in combination with aminoglycosides, such as gentamicin and amikacin. Fluoroquinolones can also be used, and vancomycin or macrolides (eg, azithromycin) and tetracyclines (eg, doxycycline).[19,22] Clindamycin and metronidazole, which are usually reserved for treating anaerobic infections, are not effective against this organism.[17]

PHYLUM: CHLAMYDIAE

The Chlamydiae are obligate intracellular parasites with a propensity for the mucous membranes of their host. *Chlamydiae trachomatis* is commonly a pathogen of the genital tract but can cause disease of any mucous membrane with which it comes in contact, including the mucosa of the oral cavity.[23] They can colonize this space without causing disease, ultimately making them a part of the normal flora. Studies have recovered this species from the epithelial lining of diseased and healthy periodontal sites (pocket or sulcus) and from the general mucosa of the tongue and cheeks.[23]

Diagnosis

Oral specimens are collected using periodontal probes and cytobrushes, and such techniques as direct fluorescence assays are used to view these intracellular organisms.[23] Polymerase chain reaction (PCR) techniques can also be used in its identification.

Susceptibility and Treatment

Epithelial cell cultures are done for isolation, which are then exposed to varying concentrations of different antibiotics. The cells are then labeled with fluorescein isothiocyanate antichlamydial antibody and incubated for 48 hours. The culture that contains the lowest concentration of the particular antibiotic capable of inhibiting growth of the organism, is deemed the minimum inhibitory concentration (MIC).[24] This is noted by lack of inclusion formation, hence no fluorescence would be seen. Treatment options include the fluoroquinolones (eg, ofloxacin), macrolides (eg, azithromycin), and tetracyclines (eg, doxycycline). Although resistance is rare, it has been noted with each of these classes of antibiotics and with agents, such as rifampicin.[25]

PHYLA: FIRMICUTES AND TENERICUTES

The Firmicutes include several commensals inclusive of the gram-positive facultative anaerobic cocci from the staphylococcal and streptococcal genera and the gram-negative anaerobic cocci from the genus *Veillonella*. The Tenericutes were renamed the Mollicutes and include the cell wall–lacking species, such as mycoplasma.

Staphylococci

These non-spore-forming species are commensals of the human skin and mucous membranes. The coagulase *Staphylococcus aureus* is the most pathogenic strain of the genus and in the oral cavity has been associated with parotitis and cases of white sponge nevus infections.[26,27] Several of the coagulase-negative staphylococci, such as *Streptococcus epidermidis*, have been found in samples from the subgingival sulci, or around dental implants. They tend to be transient residents of the oral cavity that may remain in the crevices of the periodontal pockets and later inadvertently become seeded into the bloodstream through microulcerations of the surrounding epithelia or after gingival manipulation from a dental procedure. This may result in serious systemic infections, such as endocarditis, and even provide a potential source of pathogens for patients with prosthetic joints. Their propensity for biofilm formation on foreign bodies also results in dentures being another niche in which they may reside.[28]

Diagnosis

These cocci tend to arrange themselves in clusters of cells and are mainly catalase-positive and oxidase-negative. Staphylococci grow well on blood agar with some species of *S aureus* showing pigmented cream to yellow colonies within 18 to 24 hours.

They reserve the capacity to tolerate high salt concentrations of up to 10% NaCl and grow best between 18°C and 40°C. Molecular testing is usually reserved for identification of resistance genes in this genus versus identification of the organisms.[26]

Susceptibility and treatment

All collections or abscesses require incision and drainage for successful treatment. The penicillinase-resistant β-lactams, such as cloxacillin, or the β-lactam–β-lactamase inhibitor combination of amoxicillin-clavulanate (once oxacillin sensitivity has been ascertained) are the first-line agents. Oxacillin or cefoxitin are used to identify strains of staphylococci that are methicillin-sensitive. Those resistant are resistant to all β-lactams and require treatment with vancomycin for severe systemic infections or other agents, such as clindamycin or erythromycin, for less ominous infections. The quinolones tend to be avoided for staphylococcal infections.[29] Chlorhexidine mouthwash is used to decolonize the mouth of methicillin-sensitive or -resistant strains. Methicillin-resistant *S aureus* is particularly concerning because of difficulty in therapeutic options and pathogenic nature of the organism. Other agents, such as the aminoglycosides, rifampin, and trimethoprim-sulfamethoxazole, have been used successfully against these organisms as a part of combination therapy because resistance tends to develop rapidly to some and others require the synergistic effects of a cell wall active agent.

Streptococci

The viridans group of streptococci make up more than 80% of the oral biofilm bacterial constituents, and most are commensals. The strains found in the mouth are from five main viridans group members (**Fig. 1**).[30] If seeded into the bloodstream, these bacteria are particularly adept at causing systemic infections, such as endocarditis, meningitis, and bacteremia. They are opportunistic causes of dental caries and are found on the

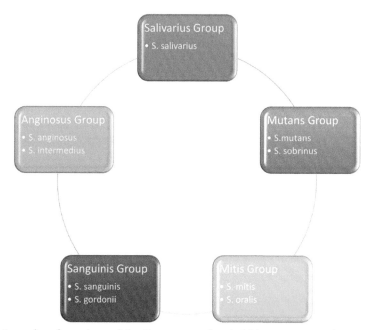

Fig. 1. Examples of members of the five groups of oral viridans streptococci.

tongue, buccal epithelium, within plaque, the palates, and tooth surfaces. This is facilitated by their enhanced binding capacities provided by surface adhesion molecules. *Streptococcus anginosus* group has been noted to cause oropharyngeal abscesses, whereas *S mutans* is the species most often associated with dental caries. This organism is transmissible through oral secretions. It is usually part of a polymicrobial interaction with other bacteria, such as *Veillonella*.[30] This is a symbiotic relationship where streptococcal metabolism provides lactic acid, which is used as a carbon source for nutrition by *Veillonella* spp that in turn detoxify the environment making it suitable for continued growth of *S mutans*. The interspecies biofilm produced is even more antibiotic resistant than single species biofilms. Similar relationships exist between other streptococcal species and *Actinomyces*, *Fusobacterium*, *Porphyromonas*, and *Aggregatibacter* species.[30]

Diagnosis

These gram-positive cocci, which appear in chains, are catalase-negative and approximately 2 μm in size. Their metabolic requirements dictate that growth is best on blood agar. This method also allows for assessment of their hemolytic characteristics. They are facultative anaerobes; however, it has been observed that members of the viridans group thrive best in air supplemented with 5% CO_2. Various biochemical tests are used to differentiate streptococci with the same hemolytic patterns. The Voges-Proskauer test, which determines the bacterial strain's ability to ferment glucose and produce acetoin, is positive for the β-hemolytic *S anginosis* group but negative for the β-hemolytic *Streptococcus mitis* group. *S mutans* is also capable of hydrolyzing mannitol, whereas other members of the oral viridans group cannot. Analytical profile index (API) tests offer more definitive identification based on biochemistry; however, molecular testing is the most definitive method.[30]

Susceptibility and treatment

Increasing rates of penicillin-resistant *S mitis* and *Streptococcus salivarius* strains have been observed. However, penicillin-based antibiotics have remained the treatment of choice. Macrolides, such as erythromycin, can be substituted.[30]

Veillonella

Veillonella species, another common commensal of the mouth, has been implicated in infections of the meninges, lungs, and intervertebral disks after being seeded into the bloodstream (bacteremia). They are gram-negative anaerobic cocci. The species associated with the oral cavity include *Veillonella parvula*, *Veillonella atypical*, *Veillonella dispar*, *Veillonella montpellierensis*, *Veillonella denticariosi*, and *Veillonella rogosae*.[31] They have been identified in fissures and buccal tooth surfaces, and from occlusal caries lesions. In dental plaque they are often accompanied by streptococcal species with which they have metabolic interactions.[32]

Diagnosis

Culture and isolation of this genus is difficult. Saliva and plaque samples are plated onto agar containing blood and vancomycin. Colonies are identified presumptively based on the fact that colonies fluoresce red at 365-nm wavelength. PCR can also be applied for species-level identification.[33]

Susceptibility and treatment

Penicillins (eg, amoxicillin/clavulanate), cephalosporins, clindamycin, metronidazole, and carbapenems have maintained efficacy against *Veillonella*; however, resistance has been noted with vancomycin, tetracycline, aminoglycosides, and ciprofloxacin.[34,35]

Mycoplasma

This genus contains the smallest free-living bacteria. Oral species include *Mycoplasma salivarius*; *Mycoplasma ovale*; and less commonly *Mycoplasma buccale*, *Mycoplasma faucium*, *Mycoplasma pneumoniae*, and *Mycoplasma hominis*.[36] They have also been implicated in recurrent oral ulcerations and have been isolated in samples of saliva, biopsies of buccal mucosae, and buccal mucosal swabs from areas of ulceration in affected individuals. These ulcerations may be related to mucositosis spectrum seen mainly in children with Stevens-Johnson syndrome.[37,38]

Diagnosis

Stuart transport medium or ideally broth-based media, such as SP4 or Shepard 10 B broth, are used.[39] Penicillin is added as a decontaminant to these broths to impede growth bacteria with cell walls. Gram staining is only used to exclude other contaminating bacteria because mycoplasma would not be visualized. Agar plates are incubated are at $37°C$ in 5% to 10% CO_2 for 5 days (up to 3 weeks for *M pneumoniae*). The resulting colonies have a fried egg colonial morphology. Indirect hemagglutination, immunofluorescent antibody assays, complement fixation, enzyme-linked immunosorbent assay techniques, and PCR are applied for identification to the species level.[37,38]

Susceptibility and treatment

Microbroth dilution is the most practical method for MIC determination with this genus. Mycoplasma have intrinsic resistance to all β-lactams, sulphonamides, trimethoprim, and rifampicin. Some species show variable resistance to macrolides and lincosamides. The fluoroquinolones have, however, retained usability against most species.[39]

PHYLUM: BACTEROIDETES AND FUSOBACTERIA

These organisms fall within two phyla, Bacteroidetes and Fusobacteria.[1] The clinically relevant oral pathogens or microflora fall within the following genera, *Bacteroides*, *Prevotella*, *Fusobacterium*, and *Porphyromonas*.[1,40] Many are a part of the normal flora of the mouth but can become opportunistic pathogens if actions, such as brushing the teeth, and prolonged oral infections allow for entry into the bloodstream. This can lead to endocarditis, osteomyelitis, or sepsis.[40]

Although they may share similar characteristics in that most are anaerobic bacilli there are some characteristics that are unique to each genus that allow for their identification.

Bacteroides

These organisms are gram-negative obligate anaerobes.[41] They are nonpigmented and non-spore-forming and are mainly associated with the gut flora, although they can inhabit the mucosal surfaces of the mouth.[8,42] The pathogenic species of this genus are limited to the *Bacteroides fragilis* group and include *Bacteroides fragilis*, *Bacteroides ovatus*, and *Bacteroides thetaiotaomicron*.[40] These anaerobes benefit from polymicrobial communities and hence are implicated in polymicrobial infections.[1,40]

Prevotella

These gram-negative obligate anaerobes form short rods and they are saccharolytic, a feature useful in their identification.[40,43] They are among the dominant organisms in the oral cavity where they can exist as commensals or pathogens involved in most bacterial infections in the oral cavity.[1] For example, *P intermedia* is a secondary colonizer of the tooth and although an opportunistic pathogen it is a component of dental plaque that when formed can lead to caries and it is also a cause of periodontitis and peri-implanatitis. *Prevotella denticola* and *Prevotella tennerae* also are often detected in cavities.[44]

Fusobacteria

The Fusobacterium phylum consists of organisms that are nonmotile pleomorphic and rod-shaped.[40,41] *F nucleatum* and *Fusobacterium necrophorum* are considered the most important species because they relate to clinical infections.[40] They can cause endodontic and periodontal infections, abscesses of the mouth, and peri-implant diseases.[40,45]

Diagnosis

Samples are taken from areas that seem to be infected, avoiding the normal flora of the mucosa in unaffected areas.[40] Suitable specimen include subgingival plaque, aspirates, root canal exudates tissue, aspirates, biopsies, and blood for systemic infections.[40] Swabs are not recommended. Once the anaerobe is sampled it should not be exposed to air and should be delivered to the laboratory within 24 hours.[46] Aspirates of fluids are obtained in a syringe and quickly transferred to cooked meat or other anaerobic system available without delay.[40,41]

Within the laboratory samples must be plated onto solid media, such as nonselective enriched *Brucella* base sheep blood agar plate supplemented with vitamin K and hemin and kanamycin-vancomycin sheep blood agar.[40] A metronidazole disk is added to the plate to aid in the detection of anaerobes most of which, unlike their aerobic counterparts, show susceptibility to metronidazole unless resistance has developed.[40] The plates should be given at least 48 hours of incubation before removal from the anaerobic atmosphere to prevent death of those anaerobes that are extremely sensitive to oxygen exposure.[40] Slow-growing organisms, such as *Porphyromonas* spp and *Biophila* spp, may need a longer incubation period of up to 1 week.[47] Obligate anaerobes only grow on plates incubated in an anaerobic environment. Examination of the Gram stain, colonial morphology, and biochemical characteristics of these organisms can lead to a diagnosis.[40] An analysis of the pattern of carbohydrate fermentation and the production of indole, catalase, and α-fucosidase is used to identify several different *Bacteroides* spp.[40] A presumptive identification of *F nucleatum* is made based on its speckled iridescent bread-crumb-like appearance, the pattern of hemolysis, the production of pigment, and susceptibility to certain antibiotics.[40] A definitive identification of the isolates from sterile sites must be obtained.

Biochemical testing is performed using commercially prepared kits, such as the API 20A (BioMérieux Inc, Durham, NC), and automated methods, such as the Vitek 2 (BioMérieux Inc, Durham, NC), the matrix-assisted laser desorption/ionization-time of flight mass spectrometry (MALDI-TOF MS, BioMérieux Inc, Durham, NC), and PCR.[40] Automated methods are faster; however, they have their limitations. MALDI-TOF MS and PCR are used to detect specific resistance mechanisms but the extent to which this can be done is limited.[40]

Susceptibility and treatment

Methods used include the Kirby Bauer Disc Diffusion method, the E-test, and broth microdilution.[40] Antimicrobial agents thought to have anaerobic activity include penicillin, amoxicillin-clavulanate, piperacillin-clavulanate, cefoxitin, doripenem, ertapenem, imipenem, meropenem, tigecycline, clindamycin metronidazole, and chloramphenicol.[40] Resistance to some of these agents has been documented. Most (96%–100%) of the organisms in the *B fragilis* group show resistance to penicillin.[47]

A significant proportion of *Prevotella* spp show resistance to clindamycin, moxifloxacin, and penicillin.[47] Amoxicillin-clavulanate, piperacillin-tazobactam, metronidazole, and chloramphenicol show good activity against *Prevotella* and *Fusobacteria* spp.[40] Anaerobic culture and susceptibility testing is often only performed in reference laboratories.[40]

Capnocytophaga

These are gram-negative facultative anaerobes of the phylum Bacteroidetes; they are also capnophiles and mesophiles. They are slow-growing, thin cylindrical-shaped bacteria isolated on blood or chocolate agar after about 2 to 4 days incubation with pink to orange pigmented colonies capable of gliding across the agar surface.[40,48]

Capnocytophaga are opportunistic pathogens rarely encountered in infections of the oral cavity.[41,49] They are found in the dental plaque of 14% of persons older than age 60 with dental caries. In most cases they are harmless bystanders forming a part of the normal microflora of the oral cavity of humans and some animals, such as dogs.[50]

Diagnosis
Several biochemical tests, PCR (eg, rapid Micro-Ident, Hain Life-science GmbH, Hamburg, Germany), or MALDI-TOF MS techniques are used for identification.[50] The identification of some of these organisms to the species level often demands the use of molecular techniques, such as 16S rRNA gene analysis.[51]

Susceptibility and treatment
There are no European or CLSI guidelines available for these organisms.[49] Antibiotics that are thought to have activity against *Capnocytophaga* spp include amoxicillin-clavulanate, cefoxitin, linezolid, clindamycin, and fluoroquinolones, such as ciprofloxacin.[40]

PHYLUM: SPIROCHAETES

This phyla contains thin helical gram-negative bacteria from three families and 13 genera.[41] Most spirochaetes found within the oral cavity belong to the genus *Treponema* and many have not been isolated by culture.[41,52] *Treponema pallidum*, the causative agent of syphilis, a sexually transmitted infection, has oral manifestations seen mainly in the second (snail track ulcers) and third (gumma formation with bony destruction) stages of disease, which may predispose to oral squamous carcinoma.[41] Other oral treponemal infections include gingivitis, periodontitis, root canal infections, endodontic abscesses, and acute necrotizing ulcerative gingivitis. *Treponema denticola* in particular has been implicated as a causative agent of gingivitis, having been detected in dental plaque.[41]

Diagnosis

This is usually based on clinical presentation and treatment is usually empiric. The treponemes are very small (0.1–0.5 × 5–20 μm) requiring dark field microscopy for visualization from fresh living samples.[42] They are difficult to culture, hence direct fluorescent antibody tests and serology is applied.[42] Future diagnostic procedures may include molecular tests and analyses that detect a specific trypsin-like enzyme produced by the organism.[4]

Susceptibility and Treatment

Penicillin is the drug of choice and most treponemes have remained susceptible to this antibiotic.[42] Alternatives include the macrolides; however, resistance to these agents has been reported.[51]

SUMMARY

Bacteria causing infections in the mouth are numerous with varying characteristics and nuances. Some are uncultivable and clinical diagnosis and subsequent therapy is applied. Advancements in diagnostic technology have increased the ability to detect, diagnose, and treat infections caused by these organisms in a timelier manner. Accessibility to such tests is important and arms clinicians with the information necessary to give more suitable therapy. Bacteria have emerged that have developed antimicrobial resistance. As a result the treatment of these bacterial infections warrants the selection of the appropriate antimicrobial agent, which is guided by susceptibility testing. This decreases the emergence of antibiotic resistance, an increasing global problem with dire consequences that threatens to usher in the postantibiotic era.

REFERENCES

1. Dewhirst FE, Chen T, Izard J, et al. The human oral microbiome. J Bacteriol 2010; 192:5002–17.
2. Aas J, Paster B, Stokes L. Defining the normal bacterial flora of the oral cavity. J Clin Microbiol 2005;43(11):5721–32.
3. Majumdar S, Singh A. Normal microbial flora of oral cavity. J Adv Med Dental Sci Res 2014;2(4):62–6.
4. Loesche WJ. Microbiology of dental decay and periodontal disease. In: Baron S, editor. Medical microbiology. 4th edition. Galveston (TX): University of Texas Medical Branch at Galveston; 1996. Chapter 99. Available at: http://www.ncbi.nlm.nih.gov/books/NBK8259/.
5. Bal AM, Gould IM. Antibiotic stewardship: overcoming implementation barriers. Curr Opin Infect Dis 2011;24(4):357–62.
6. Centers for Disease Control and Prevention. Water, sanitation & environmentally-related hygiene. Atlanta (GA): CDC; 2014. Available at: http://www.cdc.gov/healthywater/hygiene/disease/dental_caries.html.
7. Avila M, Ojcius DM, Yilmaz O. The oral microbiota: living with a permanent guest. DNA Cell Biol. 2009;28(8):405–11.
8. Zero DT, Fontana M, Martinez-Mier EA, et al. The biology, prevention, diagnosis and treatment of dental caries. J Am Dent Assoc 2009;140:255–345.
9. Mayo Clinic. (n.d.). Tooth abscess. 2016. Available at: http://www.mayoclinic.org/diseases-conditions/tooth-abscess/diagnosis-treatment/treatment/txc-20185957. Accessed June 29, 2016.
10. Sarkonen N, Kononen E, Eerola M, et al. Characterization of *Actinomyces* species isolated from failed dental implant fixtures. Anaerobes 2005;11:231–7.
11. Munson MA, Banerjee A, Watson TF, et al. Molecular analysis of the microflora associated with dental caries. J Clin Microbiol 2004;42:3023–9.
12. Wade W, Kononen E. 10th edition. Propionibacterium, lactobacillus, actinomyces, and other non-spore forming anaerobic gram-positive rods. Manual of clinical microbiology, vol. 1. Washington, DC: ASM Press; 2011.
13. Funke G, Bernard K. 10th edition. Coryneform gram-positive rods. Manual of clinical microbiology, vol. 1. Washington, DC: ASM Press; 2011.
14. Henderson B, Sharp L, Ward JM. Actinobacillus actinomycetemcomitans. J Med Microbiol 2002;51:1013–20.
15. Versalovic J, Carroll KC, Funke G, et al. Manual of clinical microbiology. Washington, DC: ASM Press; 2011.

16. Garrity GM, Bell JA, Lilburn TG. Taxonomic outline of the archaea and bacteria. In: Garriety GM, Bell JA, Lilburn TG, editors. Bergey's manual of systemic bacteriology, vol. 2, 2nd edition. New York: Springer; 2005.

17. Paul K, Patel SS. *Eikenella corrodens* infections in children and adolescents: case reports and review of the literature. Clin Infect Dis 2001;33:54–61.

18. Sheng WS, Hseuh PR, Hung CC, et al. Clinical features of patients with *Eikenella corrodens* infections and microbiological characteristics of the causative isolates. Eur J Clin Microbiol Infect Dis 2001;20:231–6.

19. Udaka T, Hiraki N, Shiomori T. *Eikinella corrodens* in head and neck infections. J Infect 2007;54:343–8.

20. Furcht C, Esrich K, Merte K. Detection of *Eikenella corrodens* and *Actinobacillus actinomycetemcomitans* by use of the polymerase chain reaction (PCR) in vitro and in subgingival plaque. J Clin Periodontol 1996;23:891–7.

21. Zbinden R, Von Graevenitz A. 10th edition. *Actinobacillus*, *Capnophaga*, *Eikenella*, *Kingella*, *Pasturella* and other fastidious or rarely encountered gram-negative rods. Manual of clinical microbiology, vol. 1. Washington, DC: ASM Press; 2011.

22. Merriam CV, Citron DM, Tyrell KL, et al. In vitro activity of azithromycin and nine comparator agents against 296 strains of oral anaerobes and 31 strains of *Eikenella corrodens*. Int J Antimicrob Agents 2006;28:244–8.

23. Reid S, Lopatin D, Foxman B, et al. Oral *Chlamydia trachomatis* in patients with established periodontitis. Clin Oral Investig 2000;4(4):226–32.

24. Suchland RJ, Geisler WM, Stamm WE. Methodologies and cell lines used for antimicrobial susceptibility testing of *Chlamydia* spp. Antimicrob Agents Chemother 2003;47:636–42.

25. Gaydos C, Essig A. 10th edition. Chlamydiaceae. Manual of clinical microbiology, vol. 1. Washington, DC: ASM Press; 2011.

26. Becker K, von Eiff C. 10th edition. *Staphylococcus*, *Micrococcus* and other Catalase positive cocci. Manual of clinical microbiology, vol. 1. Washington, DC: ASM Press; 2011.

27. Marrelli M, Tatullo M, Dipalma G, et al. Oral infection by *S. aureus* in patients affected by white sponge nevus: a description of two cases occurring in the same family. Int J Med Sci 2012;9(1):47–50.

28. Friedlander A. Oral cavity staphylococci are a potential source of prosthetic joint infection. Clin Infect Dis 2010;50(10):1682–3.

29. Patterson DL. "Collateral damage" from cephalosporin or quinolone antibiotic therapy. Clin Infect Dis 2004;38(4):S341–5.

30. Spellerberg B, Brandt C. 10th edition. Streptococcus. Manual of clinical microbiology, vol. 1. Washington, DC: ASM Press; 2011.

31. Arif N, Sheehy EC, Do T. Diversity of *Veillonella* spp. from sound and carious sites in children. J Dent Res 2008;87(3):278–82.

32. Chalmers NI, Palmer RJ, Cisar JO, et al. Characterization of a *Streptococcus* sp.-*Veillonella* sp. community micromanipulated from dental plaque. J Bacteriol 2008; 190(24):8145–54.

33. Guitierrez de Ferro MI, Riuz de Valladares RE, Benito de Cardenas IL. Recovery of veillonella from saliva. Rev Argent Microbiol 2005;37:22–5.

34. Roberts S, Shore K, Paviour S, et al. Antimicrobial susceptibility of anaerobic bacteria in New Zealand: 1999-2003. J Antimicrob Chemother 2006;57(5):992–8.

35. Veillonella: bacterial strain, organism, antimicrobial therapy. 2016. Available at: www.globalrph.com/Veillonella.htm. Accessed June 29, 2016.

36. Shiabata K, Totsuka M, Watanabe T. Phospahtase activity as a criterion for differentiation of oral mycoplasmas. J Clin Microbiol 1986;23(5):970–2.
37. Yachoui R, Kolasinski S, Feinstein D. *Mycoplasma pneumoniae* with atypical Stevens – Johnson syndrome: a diagnostic challenge. Case Rep Infect Dis 2013; 2013:457161.
38. Gordon AM, Dick HM, Mason DK, et al. Mycoplasmas and recurrent oral ulceration. J Clin Pathol 1967;20:865–9.
39. Waites K, Taylor-Robinson D. 10th edition. Mycoplasma and ureaplasma. Manual of clinical microbiology, vol. 1. Washington, DC: ASM Press; 2011.
40. Kononen E, Wade W, Citron M. 10th edition. *Bacteroides, Porphyromonas, Prevotella, Fusobacterium* and other anaerobic gram negative rods. Manual of clinical microbiology, vol. 1. Washington, DC: ASM Press; 2011.
41. Murray PR, Rosenthal KS, Pfaller MA. Medical microbiology. Philadelphia: Elsevier; 2009.
42. Wexler HM. *Bacteroides*: the good, the bad, and the nitty-gritty. Clin Microbiol Rev 2007;20:593–621.
43. Shah HN, Collins DM. *Prevotella*, a new genus to include *Bacteroides melaninogenicus* and related species formerly classified in the genus *Bacteroides*. Int J Syst Evol Microbiol 1990;40:205–8.
44. Kononen E, Paju S, Pussinen PJ, et al. Population-based study of salivary carriage of periodontal pathogens in adults. J Clin Microbiol 2007;45:2446–51.
45. Siquera JF, Rocas IN. The microbiota of acute apical abscesses. J Dent Res 2009;88:61–5.
46. Citron DM, Warren YA, Hudspeth MK. Survival of aerobic and anaerobic bacteria in purulent clinical specimens, maintained in the Copan Venturi Transystem and Becton Dickinson Port-a-Cul transport systems. J Clin Microbiol 2000;38:892–4.
47. Jousimies-Somer HR, Summanen P, Citron DM, et al. Wadsworth-KTL anaerobic bacteriology manual. 6th edition. Belmont (CA): Star Publishing; 2002.
48. Jolivet-Gougeon A. *Capnocytophaga* species. Infect Dis Antimicrob Agents 1988;9(4):170–3. Available at: http://www.antimicrobe.org/b92.asp.
49. Kato Y, Shirai M, Murakami M, et al. Molecular detection of human periodontal pathogens in oral swab specimens from dogs in Japan. J Vet Dent 2011;28:84–9.
50. Bastida MT, Valverde M, Smithson A, et al. Fulminant sepsis due to *Capnocytophaga canimorsus*: diagnosis by matrix assisted laser desorption/ionization time of flight mass spectrometry. Med Clin (Barc) 2014;142:230.
51. de Melo Oliveira MG, Abels S, Zbinden R, et al. Accurate identification of fastidious gram-negative rods: integration of both conventional phenotypic methods and 16S rRNA gene analysis. BMC Microbiol 2013;16(13):162.
52. Dahle UR, Tronstad L, Oslen I. Spirochaetes in oral infections. Endod Dent Traumatol 1993;3:87–94.

Oral Fungal Infections
Diagnosis and Management

David R. Telles, DDS[a,b,c,d,e,]*, Niraj Karki, MD[f,g], Michael W. Marshall, DDS, FICD[b,c,h]

KEYWORDS

- Candidiasis • Oral thrush • Oral fungal infection • Mucormycosis • Histoplasmosis
- Blastomycosis • Aspergillosis • Geotrichosis

KEY POINTS

- Most solitary or primary oral fungal infections are rare with the exception of oral candidiasis.
- Candidiasis is the leading infection that most dental practitioners will see in clinical practice.
- Unless diagnosed early and treated aggressively, mucormycosis can be a locally invasive and disfiguring oral and maxillofacial fungal infection.
- This review includes several oral and maxillofacial fungal infections, including mucormycosis, candidiasis, aspergillosis, blastomycosis, histoplasmosis, cryptococcosis, and coccidioidomycosis.

INTRODUCTION

Fungal infections are of great concern in dentistry. Patients may present with infections that can be superficial or indicative of a more serious systemic illness. This article focuses on fungal infections that can range from primary (superficial) to disseminated infections that have a high mortality. Included in the review are the most common oral and maxillofacial fungal infections, route of spread, diagnosis, treatment as well

The authors have nothing to disclose.
[a] Oral & Maxillofacial Surgery, Herman Ostrow USC School of Dentistry, 925 West 34th, Street, Los Angeles, CA 90089, USA; [b] Oral & Maxillofacial Surgery, Private Practice: Huntington Beach Oral & Maxillofacial Surgery, 7677 Center Avenue, Suite 206, Huntington Beach, CA 92647, USA; [c] Long Beach Memorial Medical Center, 2801 Atlantic Avenue, Long Beach, CA 90806, USA; [d] Orange Coast Memorial Medical Center, 9920 Talbert Avenue, Fountain Valley, CA 92708, USA; [e] Orange County Global Medical Center, 1001 N Tustin Avenue, Santa Ana, CA 92705; [f] Infectious Diseases, Internal Medicine, University of New England College of Osteopathic Medicine, 11 Hills Beach Road, Biddeford, ME 04005, USA; [g] Infectious Diseases, The Aroostook Medical Center, 140 Academy Street, Presque Isle, ME 04769M, USA; [h] Oral & Maxillofacial Surgery, Division of Otolaryngology, UCI School of Medicine, 101 The City Drive South, Orange, CA 92868, USA
* Corresponding author. Oral & Maxillofacial Surgery, Private Practice: Huntington Beach Oral & Maxillofacial Surgery, 7677 Center Avenue, Suite 206, Huntington Beach, CA 92647.
E-mail address: drtelles@hbomfs.com

http://dx.doi.org/10.1016/j.cden.2016.12.004
0011-8532/17/© 2017 Elsevier Inc. All rights reserved.
dental.theclinics.com

as prevention. Although uncommon in a dental practice setting, one may encounter fungal infections, such as candidiasis, mucormycosis, histoplasmosis, blastomycosis, aspergillosis, cryptococcosis, geotrichosis and coccidioidomycosis. **Table 1** is a broader and comprehensive list of potential oral and maxillofacial fungal infections to serve as reference if one encounters an uncommon organism not covered in this article.

CANDIDIASIS

Candida is a dimorphic yeast (fungus) found commonly in the gastrointestinal tract of humans and as normal flora of the skin and mucous membranes. In its normal form, *Candida* is not pathogenic and stays in balance such that it cannot progress to cause infection. Typically, *Candida* infections occur when one of several scenarios happen, including but not limited to, host defenses becoming compromised, a breakdown of the normal skin or mucosal barrier, a disturbance of the host by external factors (such as intake of broad-spectrum antibiotics), or other internal/external risk factors increasing the likelihood of a *Candida* infection. The *Candida* species consists of 2- to 6-μm yeastlike organisms that reproduce through budding.[1] The genus *Candida* includes more than 200 species, most of which are not pathogenic in humans.[2] The most common *Candida* species encountered is *Candida albicans* and accounts for more than 90% of oral cavity isolates.[3,4] Other common *Candida* species encountered with human pathogenicity include *Candida parapsilosis*, *Candida tropicalis*, *Candida glabrata*, *Candida krusei*, *Candida guilliermondii*, and *Candida lusitaniae*.[4] In healthy individuals, *Candida* spp is reported to be present in 25% to 75% of the population in the absence of any lesion caused by *Candida*.[5,6]

Candidiasis can present in several forms of infection depending on how deeply the organism has spread, or if host defenses allow for more substantial infections. The most commonly encountered infection from *Candida* is oral thrush, also known as pseudomembranous candidiasis. This type of infection is typically characterized by a white cottage cheese–like film that clinically can be wiped off to reveal a base that

Table 1
Superficial and deep oral and maxillofacial fungal infections

Superficial mycoses		Deep mycoses	
Candidiasis		Subcutaneous	
Hyperplastic	Stomatitis	Sporotrichosis	Entomophthoromycosis
Erythematous	Median rhomboid glossitis	Lobomycosis	Chromomycosis
Pseudomembranous	Cutaneous	Rhinosporidiosis	
Angular cheilitis	Pneumonia		
Deep systemic mycoses			
Histoplasmosis	Blastomycosis	Coccidioidomycosis	Paracoccidioidomycosis
Cryptococcosis			
Deep opportunistic			
Aspergillosis	Mucormycosis	Geotrichosis	Trichosporon
Penicilliosis	Basidiomycosis	Cephalosporiomycosis	Paecilomycosis
Alternariosis	Cercosporomycosis	Fusariomycosis	

Various potential oral and maxillofacial fungal infections; all bolded are included in the focus of this article.
Courtesy of D.R. Telles, DDS, Huntington Beach, CA.

typically is erythematous and at times bleeds. The plaque that can be removed is typically made up of aggregates of the pseudo-hyphae and hyphae form of the organism and byproducts of epithelial breakdown. This infection occurs in higher-risk populations such as neonates, whose host defenses have yet to develop. In a neonate, typically the transmission can be from either a health care worker or the mother. Because of not having innate immunodefenses, oral thrush in the first several months of life can result. In addition to neonates, oral candidiasis increased in the early to mid-1980s due to the progression of human immunodeficiency virus/acquired immunodeficiency syndrome (HIV/AIDS). During the early years of HIV management, oral thrush began developing in young individuals and became a red flag of HIV infection. With the introduction of highly active antiretroviral therapy (HAART), the advances in management of HIV improved drastically, impacting the incidence of candidiasis and resulting in a significant reduction of thrush worldwide in HIV patients.[7] However, it is important to note that oropharyngeal (ie, esophageal) candidiasis is a clinical predictor of HIV disease progression, and after the initial presentation of oropharyngeal candidiasis, AIDS is typically seen within 1 to 3 years.[8] In contrast, because of the overuse/misuse of oral antibiotics as well as advances in medical management (including organ transplant, stem cell transplantation, parenteral nutrition, advanced surgical procedures, and chemoradiotherapy), there has been an increase in superficial and invasive forms of candidiasis.[9]

With disease progression, there are other forms of candidiasis that affect the maxillofacial complex, including angular cheilitis, median rhomboid glossitis, chronic hyperplastic, atrophic candidiasis/denture stomatitis, chronic mucocutaneous, and chronic multifocal candidiasis. In a patient, when encountered with *Candida*, unless host defenses are compromised, it is rare to see the development and progression of candidal infections. In this article, candidal infections, limited to the oral and maxillofacial complex and the disease progression to deeper or invasive candidiasis, are focused on.

Table 2 shows several different host defenses as well as deficiencies that prevent or expose the host to the development of a *Candida* infection.[10]

Table 2
Host defenses and deficiencies preventing or exposing host to *Candida* infection

Host defenses	Host deficiencies
Skin/mucous membrane barrier	Acquired
Salivary nonimmune defenses	HIV/AIDs
Lysozyme	Uncontrolled diabetes mellitus or other
Lactoferrin	endocrinopathies
Lactoperoxidase	Broad-spectrum antibiotics
Histatins	Chemoradiotherapy
Antileukoprotease	Chronic steroid use
Calprotectin	Long-term indwelling catheterization
B-protein	Fluid and electrolyte disorders
Histidine-rich polypeptides	Organ or bone marrow transplant
Oral immune defenses	Malnutrition with or without chronic
T cell–polymorphonuclear cells	alcoholism
Phagocytosis	Congenital
Augmentation via lymphokines/	Partial or combined immunodeficiencies
interleukins, for example, tumor necrosis	Di George syndrome
factor-α, IL-12	
Salivary IgA	

Data from Scully C. Candidosis (candidiasis). In: Oral and maxillofacial medicine—the basis of diagnosis and treatment. 3rd edition. Philadelphia: Elsevier; 2013. p. 254–63.

Risk Factors

Oral candidiasis and other forms of *Candida* infections occur more commonly in specific sets of patients most at risk. When encountering a *Candida* infection, the practitioner should always consider the etiologic reason for the development of a candidiasis because typically there is a condition or comorbidity associated with such infections. Although not all conditions can be changed, when encountering conditions causing a *Candida* infection, such as hygiene, diabetes, or denture use (**Box 1**), if these conditions can be modified, then this is the most successful way to both treat the Candida infection and prevent recurrence.

Xerostomia

In the oral cavity, xerostomia can result in several problems with the dentition as well as the risk of developing *Candida* infections. Stasis of saliva and diminished salivary gland function result in the patient's inability to produce several defensive antimicrobial mechanisms in the saliva. Saliva contains several defense mechanisms, including "defensins, lactoferrin, sialoperoxidase, lysozyme, histidine-rich polypeptides and anti-*Candida* antibodies."[11] For example, with respect to lactoferrin, the defense mechanism plays a fungicidal role thatch actively kills *Candida* before entering the host tissue. Mucosal saliva acts therefore as the first line of defense against *Candida*, which allows the commensal organisms to stay in balance with other oral biota.

With respect to corticosteroid intake, Alsaeedi and colleagues[12] reviewed 9 clinical trials regarding patients with chronic obstructive pulmonary disease from a total patient pool of 3976, which found that the risk for development of *Candida* infections increased by 2.1 times when taking inhaled forms of corticosteroids. The basis for chronic steroid intake resulting in *Candida* infection is secondary to the decrease in cellular immunity and phagocytosis.

Box 1
Risk factors for development of oropharyngeal candidiasis

Local Factors

Xerostomia (polypharmacy, Sjogren syndrome, dehydration, radiation)

Broad-spectrum antibiotics or steroid intake

High-carbohydrate diet

Leukoplakia/oral cancer

Denture use

Cigarette use

Systemic Factors

Neonate, advanced age

Diabetes

Nutritional deficiencies

Malignancies

Immunosuppression

From Epstein JB. Diagnosis and treatment of oropharyngeal candidiasis. Oral Maxillofacial Surg Clin N Am 2003;15(1):92; with permission.

Denture Use

Denture stomatitis is the classic representation of *Candida* infections typically presented as the atrophic variant noted by denuded, erythematous mucosa only at times presenting with a pseudomembrane (**Fig. 1**). When atrophic candidiasis is seen under a denture, the thought is that this is related to poor denture hygiene, giving *C albicans* the ability to adhere to the intaglio surface of the denture acrylic, thus resulting in its colonization. Because of the immobile nature of the mucosa and lack of salivary flow, the environment optimizes the mucosa for infection. The intaglio aspect of the denture contains a plaque, resulting in the formation of a biofilm, which has been well studied and documented as a causative agent of denture stomatitis (atrophic candidiasis).[13,14] Based on a review by Arendorf and Walker,[15] approximately 67% of existing denture wearers are thought to have *Candida*-associated denture stomatitis.

Along with denture stomatitis, angular cheilitis (**Fig. 2**) can also be seen in denture wearers because of collapsed vertical dimension of occlusion resulting in the collapse of the corners of the mouth. Over time, the collapsed areas become moist, harboring an ideal environment for both *Candida* and *Staph* infections to develop.[16]

General hygiene recommendations were published by the American Dental Association in 2011 regarding the proper management of dentures. Among these recommendations was the key recommendation that all denture wearers who are experiencing denture stomatitis remove their dentures at night. The treatment is 2-fold: treating the patient intraorally with topical antifungals as well as properly cleaning their dentures. According to Felton and colleagues,[17] the following recommendations should be given to the patient:

1. Dentures should be cleansed daily with a nonabrasive denture cleaner
2. Never soak dentures greater than 10 minutes in a sodium hypochlorite bleach mixture
3. Store dentures overnight in water
4. Ultrasonic cleaning by a licensed dental practitioner is encouraged to reduce biofilm buildup
5. Denture adhesives and other debris should be completely removed from the denture daily
6. Denture checks should be performed by treating dentists at least yearly to check for retention, fit, occlusion, and stability[17]

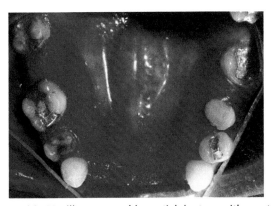

Fig. 1. Denture stomatitis. Maxillary removable partial denture with a noted deep red base. The lesions are typically outlined around the denture base. (*From* Muzyka BC, Epifanio RN. Update on oral fungal infections. Dent Clin North Am 2013;57(4):568; with permission.)

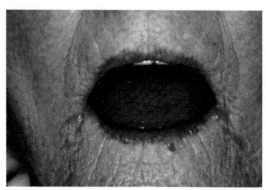

Fig. 2. Angular cheilitis (perleche). (*From* Scully C. Angular cheilitis (angular stomatitis). In: Oral and maxillofacial medicine—the basis of diagnosis and treatment. 3rd edition. Philadelphia: Elsevier; 2013. p. 223; with permission.)

Signs and Symptoms

The presentation of *Candida* infections and their associated signs and symptoms vary, depending on which type of infection the host is experiencing. **Table 3** includes a breakdown of several forms of *Candida* infections that can occur, with some being more superficial (such as thrush) and requiring less aggressive treatment compared with deeper infections such as candidemia or invasive candidiasis. Typical complaints of superficial infections include itching, burning, easy bleeding, discharge, soreness, and rash. A typical sign that could be picked up with a superficial infection would include a pseudomembrane that would be removable that shows underlying mucosal

Table 3	
Forms of candidiasis	
Various Presentations of Candida Infections in the Body	
Oral candidiasis (thrush/ pseudomembranous)	Osteoarticular
Oropharyngeal	Median rhomboid glossitis
Angular cheilitis	Denture stomatitis/erythematous (atrophic) oral candidiasis
Chronic mucocutaneous	Multifocal candidiasis
Esophageal	Urinary tract infection
Cutaneous	Vulvovaginitis
Severe forms	
Hyperplastic candidiasis/leukoplakic	Endocarditis
Candidemia	Endophthalmitis
Pneumonia	Invasive candidiasis
Disseminated (hepatosplenic)	

The infection by *Candida* can appear in several different forms from subtle superficial infections like pseudomembranous candidiasis to invasive endocarditis. Early identification is key for the treatment of more penetrating or deep infections involving *Candida*. For any presentation, a review of the patient's host defenses is necessary.
Courtesy of D.R. Telles, DDS, Huntington Beach, CA.

irritation with edema and erythema. With deeper infections, signs can vary based on the severity of infection, such as hemodynamic instability, shock, positive blood cultures, fever, and tachycardia; in compromised hosts, death can result if diagnosis is delayed.

Oropharyngeal

During the early evolvement of the HIV epidemic in the 1980s, oral thrush began appearing in otherwise young healthy men. As seen in **Fig. 3**, the presentation of oropharyngeal thrush typically presented as a pseudomembranous form. Clinically, the covering over the affected mucosa contains a white plaque, which can be wiped off with gauze to reveal red and at times bleeding mucosa underlying the plaque. In the 1980s, the initiation of thrush became highly suggestive of HIV infection. In contrast, there is an additional form known as atrophic candidiasis in which the mucosa of the tongue, palate, buccal mucosa, or lateral tongue can appear as red and erythematous and commonly presents with pain or a burning sensation.

Invariably, as treatment progressed and antiviral therapies improved, such as the introduction of HAART, oral thrush incidence decreased with the successful treatment of HIV infection. Specifically, Greenspan and colleagues[18] retrospectively studied 1280 HIV patients from 1990 to 1999. The study focused on determining the correlation between antiretroviral therapy (ART) or HAART therapies and the incidence of oral candidiasis, oral hairy leukoplakia, and oral warts (**Figs. 4** and **5**).

The study concluded that the incidence of oral candidiasis was found to decrease as the ART or HAART therapy advanced with the introduction of protease inhibitors.[18,19] After adjusting for CD4 count and viral load, the odds of having candidiasis were lower in patients on either ART therapy (odds ratio of 0.32) or HAART therapy (odds ratio of 0.28) compared with patients on neither of these therapies.[18] The mechanism behind the activity of protease inhibitors is activity against a major virulence factor of C albicans known as aspartyl proteinase (SAP) enzyme.[19] Cassone and colleagues[20,21] demonstrated that the use of protease therapy reduced SAP enzyme activity, resulting in decreased candidiasis incidence.

In an HIV individual, the highest-risk patients typically have a CD4 T-cell count of less than 200, which by definition is the onset of AIDS. Patients with CD4 counts between 350 and 500 rarely exhibit clinical findings of immunosuppression and those with CD4 counts between 200 and 350 typically present with illnesses such as candidiasis (oral thrush), mucosal infections, or herpes zoster.[19] In 2000, Patton[22] at the University of North Carolina at Chapel Hill studied 606 adults (455 men and 151

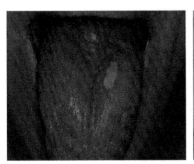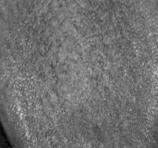

Fig. 3. Oral thrush (pseudomembranous candidiasis of the oral cavity). (*Courtesy of* M.W. Marshall, DDS, Huntington Beach, CA.)

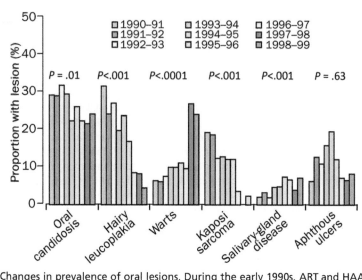

Fig. 4. Changes in prevalence of oral lesions. During the early 1990s, ART and HAART therapies did not include protease inhibitors. Notable was the decrease in oral candidiasis after the introduction of protease inhibitors from 1996 to 1999. (*From* Greenspan D, Canchola AJ, MacPhail LA, et al. Effect of highly active antiretroviral therapy on frequency of oral warts. Lancet 2001;357(9266):1411; with permission.)

women) infected with HIV who self-identified as HIV positive. The study concluded that certain common oral lesions, including pseudomembranous candidiasis, are strong indicators of immune suppression and thus serve as potential clinical markers of HIV. In an earlier study, Patton and colleagues[23] found in a sample of 250 individuals through a bivariate analysis, that HIV-infected individuals with oral lesions, including

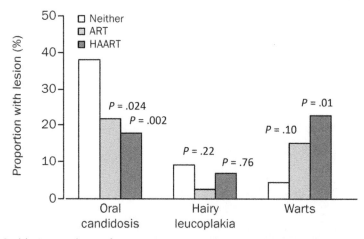

Fig. 5. Oral lesions and use of ART, 1996 to 1999. Decreases are noted in the incidence of oral candidosis (candidiasis) when taking either ART or HAART therapies versus not taking any treatment. (*From* Greenspan D, Canchola AJ, MacPhail LA, et al. Effect of highly active antiretroviral therapy on frequency of oral warts. Lancet 2001;357(9266):1411; with permission.)

hairy leukoplakia or oral candidiasis, were 1.8 times more likely to have a plasma HIV viral load of 20,000 copies/mL or higher than individuals without lesions.

Other typical causes of oral thrush can include the administration of broad-spectrum antibiotic, immunocompromised status, cancer, extremities of life (newborn or elderly), inhaled corticosteroids, and xerostomia. The intraoral locations of thrush can vary from patient to patient but typically involve the tongue, buccal mucosa, palate, and gingiva.

Median rhomboid glossitis (central papillary atrophy) is a variation in atrophic candidiasis that can present as a dorsal midline red lesion on the tongue (**Fig. 6**). The surface is typically de-papillated, but when biopsied with either brush or incisional, renders *Candida* infection. **Fig. 6** shows an example of the appearance of the lesion that typically affects men 3 times as often as women, according to Muzyka and Epifanio.[24]

Hyperplastic Candidiasis

With hyperplastic candidiasis, the provider is alerted that the patient has some form of leukoplakia/dysplasia or a verrucous variant of mucosal changes. As seen in the 3 photographs in **Fig. 7**, this patient has a white mottled-appearing lesion on the left buccal mucosa. Hyperplastic lesions have the tendency to extend into the lip commissure, similar to the lesions shown in the 3 photographs in **Fig. 7**. In addition, the lesions can appear nodular or speckled. Other areas that can present with this unique form of *Candida* include the lateral border of the tongue and palate.[25] This form of *Candida* has an increased risk for developing dysplasia or malignancies and therefore should be closely followed.[26] Fortunately, this form of oral pharyngeal candidiasis is rare.

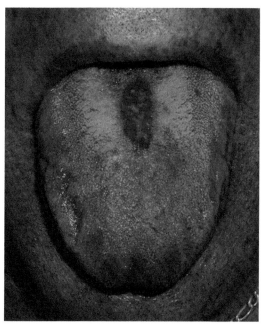

Fig. 6. Median rhomboid glossitis. (*From* Muzyka BC, Epifanio RN. Update on oral fungal infections. Dent Clin North Am 2013;57(4):568; with permission.)

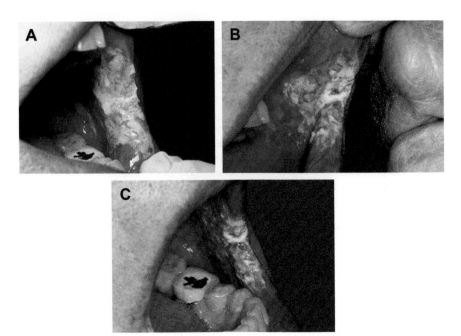

Fig. 7. Hyperplastic candidiasis. As shown in these 3 photographs (*A–C*), the presentation of nonwipeable plaques appear as white and red patches. When biopsied, this specimen rendered Candida infection with hyphae and pseudohyphae present on the H&E stain (hematoxylin-eosin, original magnification ×XX). The patient was treated with Ketoconazole successfully. (*Courtesy of* M.W. Marshall, DDS, Huntington Beach, CA.)

Esophagitis, Pneumonia, Bronchi

Esophageal candidiasis can result from swallowing *Candida* when a host already has an active oral fungal infection. When the passage of saliva includes infected tissues and food, the yeast can result in adherence to the esophageal lining. If esophageal candidiasis progresses, it can result in the following symptoms: scarring, obstructions, esophageal stricture, substernal discomfort or chest pain, nausea, and vomiting. Clearly, one of the first signs of *Candida* spreading presents as dysphagia or odynophagia.[27,28] In some cases, oral infection of candidiasis may not precede the development, and therefore, other causes must be explored. Esophagitis is associated with cancer, organ transplantation, proton pump inhibitors, progressive HIV infection to AIDs, or primary chronic mucocutaneous disorders. When symptoms of esophageal candidiasis are present, the gold standard is for direct endoscopy, and if patches or lesion are observed, then direct brush or incisional biopsy is indicated. Radiographic evaluation of the esophagus will also aid in the diagnosis of obstruction, fistula, bleeding, perforation, or stricture, which may require endoscopic dilation.[29] Medical management via antifungals, in conjunction with urgent referral to a gastrointestinal specialist, is indicated when suspicious of esophageal candidiasis. Respiratory infections can also develop, including involvement of the larynx, pharynx, bronchi, or pulmonary circuit. *Candida* has been well documented to have the ability to infect anywhere along the respiratory tract and has the potential to cause bronchitis or pneumonia. Typical presenting clinical manifestations include cough, tachypnea, dyspnea, tachycardia, and fever. In some cases, empyema and abscesses can result in lung damage and scarring. In addition to altered pulmonary functions tests, a clinical presentation of a patient with chronic pneumonia could include clubbing of the fingers due to chronic hypoxemia. Primary *Candida* pneumonia is a rare condition resulting from the aspiration of oropharyngeal contents into the respiratory tract. Secondary *Candida* pneumonia results from seeding of *Candida* in an individual with candidemia (blood infected with *Candida*). There is a small subset of patients in the pediatric population who are also at risk for developing *Candida* allergic reactions resulting in respiratory symptoms.[30] Treatment of all pneumonias is similar to the treatment of candidemia, which is discussed in the treatment section in later discussion.

Chronic Mucocutaneous

In contrast to isolated *Candida* infections, chronic mucocutaneous candidiasis can occur as a result of impaired immune function (acquired) or related primary T-cell immune deficiencies. Patients with either condition may have chronic recurrent *Candida* infections that can affect one or several areas of the body, including the skin, mouth, nails, eyes, and other mucous membranes. In primary immune deficiencies, patients with high susceptibility to chronic mucocutaneous candidiasis have deficiencies or impairment of the T-cell–mediated interleukin-17 (IL-17)–dependent T-cell immunity.[31,32]

This disorder is also seen in patients with endocrinopathies or autoimmune diseases, such as hypothyroidism and hypoparathyroidism, according to Coleman and Hay.[33] This condition is considered an autosomal-dominant disorder in which patients rarely develop disseminated or invasive candidiasis.[34]

Diagnosis

Typically, when *Candida* is seen in the superficial form, such as pseudomembranous, angular cheilitis, or other forms of mucocutaneous candidiasis, a presumptive diagnosis can be made with a trial of topical antifungal agents such as nystatin or clotrimazole. When superficial infections or lesions resolve, the proof is determined by the response of therapy. Laboratory testing for *Candida* infections can include incisional biopsy of a suspected lesion or brush biopsy (exfoliative cytology) followed by Gram staining or placement into a potassium hydroxide (KOH) preparation or periodic acid-Schiff. Histologically, the classic appearance of *Candida* hyphae will appear as clear tubes, whereas with Gram staining, the hyphae and yeast appear dark blue. In the PAS stain, the organism will appear red to purple.[24] It is important to remember, as stated previously, that *Candida* is a common organism found in the oral cavity, and therefore, the simple presence of *Candida* does not prove that the lesion is associated with a *Candida* infection. Therefore, quantitative culture counts have been recommended as guidelines to prove candidiasis in a respective culture taken.[11] In some cases, biopsy may be necessary, which includes variations in the presentation of *Candida* infections, such as leukoplakic candidiasis (hyperplastic candidiasis), invasive candidiasis, and mucocutaneous lesions, which are stored in 10% formalin in order to rule out dysplasia or other malignant conditions.

Treatment

Various systemic and nonsystemic (topical) agents are available for treating oropharyngeal candidiasis. Topical agents have served as the preferred therapy, particularly in uncomplicated cases. If possible, topical preparations should be used before systemic antifungal drugs. Topical agents are not absorbed systemically and thus lack the drug interactions and systemic adverse effects found with some systemic agents. Topical agents are commercially obtainable in a variety of formulations, including troches, oral rinses, vaginal tablets, powders, and creams. Systemic agents are preferred when topical agents are ineffective or not tolerated in cases such as immunocompromised HIV or patients with cancer.

Treatment of oral candidiasis available currently is summarized in **Table 4** for topical treatments and **Table 5** for systemic treatments of oral candidiasis (typical if refractory to topical treatment or recurrent).

Topical Therapy

Gentian Violet

Until the 1950s and the advent of the polyene-antifungals, Gentian Violet was classically used to treat oral candidiasis. To date, Gentian Violet is used in underserved or underdeveloped countries because of its cost-effectiveness and availability. This agent has particular side effects, including mucosa staining and mucosa irritation.[35] The dosage recommendations for this are 1.5 mL of a 0.5% solution administered twice daily until the lesions resolve, and the treatment typically is extended 5 to 7 days after the lesions have disappeared. This agent is not commonly used in the United States due to the increased efficacy of polyene alternatives.

Polyenes

Approximately 87 polyenes have been investigated; however, only 3 are commercially available, including nystatin, amphotericin B, and natamycin. Nystatin oral suspension remains the most commonly used polyene for the initial treatment of oral candidiasis. The drug is available as an oral suspension, lozenge, or cream. The typical formulation of a troche includes 100,000 units of nystatin, given 2 to 5 times daily for 7 to 14 days. It is important to ensure treatment extends several days after the lesions disappear in order to lower the rate or risk of recurrence of candidiasis. The general recommendation is to extend therapy 48 hours beyond resolution of perioral symptoms.[24] Nystatin is not absorbed systemically and therefore lacks serious toxicity. Adverse effects most often involve the gastrointestinal tract (ie, nausea, vomiting, and diarrhea). Although Nystatin is often used as prophylaxis for, or treatment of, oropharyngeal candidiasis in patients with cancer or patients with AIDS, several reports have cited disappointing findings, including frequent treatment failures and early relapses.[11]

Both Nystatin and amphotericin B are produced by *Streptomyces* species and act by binding to ergosterol and possibly to sterols in the cell membrane of fungi, altering cell membrane permeability by causing formation of aqueous pores or channels that leak cellular components and resulting in destruction of the *Candida* organism.

Azoles

The azoles are fungistatic, interfering with ergosterol synthesis, causing a change in the permeability of the cell membrane, leakage of cellular contents, and cell death.[11] Clotrimazole, an imidazole, was the first broad-spectrum antifungal of its class. Clotrimazole has been reported to be effective for prophylaxis and treatment of oropharyngeal candidiasis in patients with cancer, in whom it may prevent the development of esophagitis. However, it appears to be less effective than fluconazole in treating HIV-infected patients with oropharyngeal candidiasis.[11] Miconazole has also been shown to be effective in patients with oropharyngeal and esophageal candidiasis.[36]

When topical treatment does not effectively control oropharyngeal candidiasis, combining a topical agent with a systemic agent may successfully eradicate infection. In addition, combining topical and systemic agents may be beneficial by permitting the use of lower dosages and shorter courses compared with a single agent.

Table 4
Topical therapeutic options for the treatment of oral candidiasis

Agent	Vehicle or Form	Dose and Frequency	Side Effects and Special Features
Gentian Violet	• Solution	• 1.5 mL of 0.5% solution twice daily	• Skin irritation • Oral ulcers • Purple staining of clothes and skin
Nystatin	• Cream • Ointment • Suspension • Lozenge • Tablet (vaginal)	• Cream and ointment: Apply 3 to 4 times daily • Suspension: 100 U 4 times daily • Lozenge: 100,000 U a maximum of 5 times daily for 7–14 d • Tablet: 100,000 U 3 times daily	• Nausea and vomiting • Skin irritation
Amphotericin B	• Cream • Ointment • Lotion • Suspension	• Cream, ointment, lotion: 3 to 4 times daily for a maximum of 14 d • Suspension: 100 mg/mL	• Not absorbed from the gut
Miconazole	• Cream • Ointment • Gel • Lacquer	• 2% Cream and ointment: Twice daily for 2–3 wk • 2% Gel: 3 to 4 times daily for 2–3 wk • Lacquer: 1 g applied once weekly to dentures for 3 wk	• Skin irritation • Burning sensation • Maceration
Ketoconazole	• Cream	• 2% cream 2 to 3 times daily for 14–28 d	• Skin irritation • Headache
Clotrimazole	• Cream • Solution • Troche	• 1% cream twice daily to 3 times daily for 3–4 wk • 1% solution 3 to 4 times daily for 2–3 wk • 10 mg troche 5 times daily for 2 wk	• Skin irritation • Nausea and vomiting

From Millsop JW, Fazel N. Oral candidiasis. Clin Dermatol 2016;34(4):491; with permission.

Systemic therapy

Systemic therapy may be required in a patient with oropharyngeal candidiasis if the patient is refractory to topical treatment, cannot tolerate topical agents, and/or is at high risk for systemic infection. According to Pappas and colleagues,[37] for patients diagnosed with invasive forms of candidiasis or candidemia, the general recommendation is to extend drug treatment for a period of 14 days after the first negative culture. The invasive forms of candidiasis and their respective recommended treatment regimens are listed in **Table 6**.

Amphotericin B

Amphotericin B is another polyene antifungal, which is effective if given intravenously (IV) to patients having severe oropharyngeal candidiasis or patients with infections refractory to other agents. For invasive candidiasis, Amphotericin B is usually prescribed at 0.5 to 0.7 mg/kg daily and as high as 1 mg/kg for more resistant species.

Amphotericin B's principal use is in patients at risk for progressive and potentially fatal fungal infections. Its routine use is for oropharyngeal candidiasis, but it has been limited due to its toxic side effects. Notable toxic side effects include fever, chills, gastrointestinal effects, cardiovascular toxicity, pulmonary toxicity, and renal

Table 5
Systemic treatment options for the treatment of oral candidiasis

Agent	Vehicle or Form	Dose and Frequency	Side Effects and Special Features
Ketoconazole	• Tablet	• 200 mg daily or twice daily for 2 wk	• US Food and Drug Administration does not advise use of oral ketoconazole
Fluconazole	• Capsule	Initial loading dose of 250 mg; 50–200 mg daily thereafter for 7–14 d	• Nausea and emesis
Itraconazole	• Capsule • Oral solution	• 100–200 mg daily for 14 d • For severe recalcitrant cases, loading dose of 200 mg 3 times daily for 3 d	• Hepatotoxicity • Pregnancy risk category C • Interactions with other medications • Potential negative effects on male fertility
Posaconazole	• Suspension	• 100 mg twice daily on day 1, then 100 mg daily for 13 d • For refractory cases: 400 mg twice daily for 3 d, then 400 mg daily to twice daily for 25–28 d	• Hair loss • Adrenal insufficiency • Pregnancy risk category C • Gastrointestinal disturbance • Hepatotoxicity • Interactions with other medications • Take with food or acidic beverages • Pregnancy risk category C • Hepatic dysfunction • Gastrointestinal disturbance • Dizziness and headache • Pregnancy risk category C • Gastrointestinal upset • Neutropenia

From Millsop JW, Fazel N. Oral candidiasis. Clin Dermatol 2016;34(4):491; with permission.

toxicity.[11] However, despite such devastating side effects, amphotericin is considered a gold-standard treatment therapy for advanced *Candida* infections such as treatment of candidemia, meningitis, endocarditis, and so forth.

More recently, amphotericin is available as a nonsystemic oral rinse (topical treatment) for patients with oropharyngeal candidiasis. Amphotericin B lozenges are effective in patients susceptible to *Candida* infection. Lozenges provide delivery of a long-lasting concentration of the drug in the saliva. Unlike numerous other antifungal agents, resistance to Amphotericin B rarely occurs during therapy. In addition, the oral form of amphotericin lacks the ability to be absorbed; thus, toxic side effects are not evident.

Currently, there are 2 lipid forms of amphotericin B (LFAmB):

- Amphotericin B lipid complex
- Liposomal amphotericin B

When comparing LFAmB with Amphotericin B, LFAmB (typical dosage was 3–5 mg/kg per day), infusion-related reactions resulting in nephrotoxicity are diminished 6.6-fold compared with classic amphotericin B. Therefore, many clinicians have moved to using LFAmB for severe forms of *Candida* infections, especially in the intensive care unit setting.[38]

Azoles (imidazoles and triazoles)

Azoles are recommended to treat patients with either systemic or superficial fungal infections. Azoles are broken up into 2 categories: Imidazoles (Clotrimazole, Ketoconazole, Miconazole) and Triazoles (Fluconazole, Itraconazole, Posaconazole, Voriconazole). Oral azole drugs are effective against *C albicans*; however, they show limited use in resistant *C krusei* and *C glabrata*.[39]

Clotrimazole, when compared with historical treatment of oral candidiasis using nystatin rinses or troches, has shown superior efficacy in alleviating and preventing oral candidiasis. Clotrimazole is available in both creams and troches for treating all forms of oral candidiasis, including angular cheilitis. Based on the experience of the authors, it is their recommendation that first-line therapy start with 10 mg troches 5 times a day for a 14-day period. However, if patient compliance for this frequency of Clotrimazole presents a clinical dilemma, an effective alternative may include Miconazole 50 mg buccal tablet once daily placed daily for 14 days. Compliance with first-line therapy tends to present an inversely proportional variable in clinical efficacy based on the required amount of times an agent is to be taken per day.

Ketoconazole was the first imidazole found to have systemic activity. The typical dosage ranges from 200 to 400 mg orally daily. Although ketoconazole has been effective in treating oropharyngeal candidiasis, in patients with HIV infections and cancer, several studies have shown ketoconazole to be less effective than fluconazole in those patients with HIV infections. The most common adverse events reported for ketoconazole include nausea, vomiting, abdominal pain, and itching. However, the adverse event of greatest concern is hepatotoxicity; therefore, long prophylactic courses should be avoided. Asymptomatic increases in transaminase levels in serum have been reported in 2% to 10% of patients, with spontaneous resolution during therapy or resolution after discontinuation of therapy. When prescribing this medication, note that it must be taken with food and may not be adequately absorbed by patients having reduced gastric acidity.[39] For hepatitis with jaundice, although rare, hepatic failure has occurred in patients receiving systemic ketoconazole.

Two triazoles, fluconazole and itraconazole, are the newest azoles to become commercially available. Fluconazole is particularly useful for treating patients

Table 6
Treatment of candidemia and other forms of invasive candidiasis therapy

Condition	Primary	Alternative	Duration	Comments
Candidemia				
Nonneutropenic adults	Caspo 70 mg loading then 50 mg/d; Mica 100 mg/d; or Anid 200 mg loading, then 100 mg/d	Flu 800 mg/d loading, then 400 mg/d	14 d after last positive blood culture and resolution of signs and symptoms	Remove all intravascular catheters, if possible
Neonates	AmB 1.0 mg/kg/d IV; or Flu 12 mg/kg/d IV	LFAmB 3–5 mg/kg/d	14–21 d after resolution of signs and symptoms and negative repeat blood cultures	Occult central nervous system and other organ involvement must be ruled out; use LFAmB with caution if urinary involvement suspected
Neutropenia	Caspo 70 mg loading, then 50 mg/d; Mica 100 mg/d; or Anid 200 mg loading, then 100 mg/d	LFAmB 3–5 mg/kg/d or Flu 800 mg loading, then 400 mg/d	14 d after last positive blood culture and resolution of signs and symptoms and resolved neutropenia	Removal of all intravascular catheters is controversial in neutropenic patients; gastrointestinal source is common
Chronic disseminated candidiasis	LFAmB 3–5 mg/kg/d; or Caspo 70 mg loading, then 50 mg/d; or Mica 100 mg/d; or Anid 200 mg loading, then 100 mg/d	Flu, 6 mg/kg/d	3–6 mo and resolution or calcification of radiologic lesions	Flu may be given after 1–2 wk of LFAmB or an echinocandin if clinically stable or improved; steroids may be beneficial in those with persistent fever

Endocarditis	LFAmB 3–5 mg/kg/d ± 5-FC 25 mg/kg orally 4 times a day; or Caspo 150 mg/d; Mica 150 mg/d; Anid 200 mg/d	Flu 6–12 mg/kg/d IV/orally	At least 6 wk after valve replacement	Valve replacement is almost always necessary; long-term suppression with Flu has been successful among selected patients who cannot undergo valve replacement. Consider step down to Vori or Posa for susceptible, Flu-resistant isolates
Osteoarticular	Flu 400 mg/d or Caspo 50 mg/d; Mica 100 mg/d or Anid 100 md/d	LFAmB 3–5 mg/kg/d	6–12 mo ± surgery	Step down therapy to Flu after at least 2-wk induction with an echinocandin or LFAmB
Endophthalmitis	Flu 800 mg loading, then 400 mg/d; or Vori 400 mg × 2 loading, then 300 mg twice a day; or LFAmB 3–5 mg/kg/d	Intravitreal AmB 5–10 µg or Vori 100 µg	4–6 wk at least after surgery	Vitrectomy is usually performed when vitreitis is present
Cystitis	Flu 200 mg/d; or 5-FC 25 mg/kg 4 times a day for Flu-resistant isolates	AmB 0.3–0.6 mg/kg/d	1–2 wk	Echinocandins have minimal role in cystitis; for upper tract disease, treat as for candidemia

Abbreviations: 5-FC, 5-fluorocytosine; AmB, amphotericin B; Anid, anidulafungin; Caspo, caspofungin; Flu, fluconazole; Mica, micafungin; Posa, posaconazole; Vori, voriconazole.

From McCarty TP, Pappas PG. Invasive candidiasis. Infect Dis Clin N Am 2016;30(1):112–3; with permission.

requiring prolonged antifungal therapy because it is taken only once a day and is relatively well tolerated. Typical dosing of fluconazole varies (depending on specific infections) but ranges from 100 to 400 mg orally/IV. In one study comparing Fluconazole 100 mg daily dose orally with topically administered Clotrimazole troches (10 mg 5 times daily for 14 days), oral candidiasis was found to have a longer relapse time.[40] Both fluconazole and itraconazole have been shown to be effective in treating oropharyngeal candidiasis in patients with HIV infection and cancer. They are widely used in these patients. Further studies are needed to establish optimal doses in patients with HIV infection, different types of oropharyngeal candidiasis, and leukemia and bone marrow transplant patients.

ECHINOCANDINS (ANIDULAFUNGIN, CASPOFUNGIN, MICAFUNGIN)

The Echinocandins are antifungals with their own drug class. These agents act through the action against the β-(1,3)-D-glucan synthase enzyme complex, hence acting to inhibit the synthesis of fungal cell wall .[41] Caspofungin and micafungin are indicated in the treatment of refractory or invasive/disseminated candidiasis. Anidulafungin indications include candidemia, the treatment of esophageal candidiasis, as well as a prophylaxis for stem cell recipients. According to McCarty and colleagues,[42] echinocandins have been shown to be effective antifungal agents in 70% to 75% of *Candida* in randomized, comparative clinical trials. However, despite this drug class being available only as parenteral preparations, the few reported drug interactions, high clinical efficacy, and progressive concerns over fluconazole-resistant strains of *Candida*, more physicians have turned to echinocandins as a first-line therapy for patients with candidemia.[38] Typical dosing for these agents include the following:

- Caspofungin: loading dose of 70 mg followed by 50 mg daily;
- Anidulafungin: loading dose 200 mg and then 100 mg daily;
- Micafungin: 100 mg daily.

Seemingly, despite the high efficacy against candidemia, some *C glabrata* isolates have been shown to be resistant to echinocandins.

Pyrimidines (Flucytosine)

Flucystosine, a pyrimidine analogue, acts to disrupt RNA synthesis and hence protein and DNA syntheses and is a known fungicidal agent. When used as monotherapy, resistance to this agent develops quickly. Typically, flucytosine is used as a combination therapy with Amphotericin B, fluconazole, or itraconazole.[24] Dosing of Flucytosine comes in either an oral solution of 10 mg/mL or 250 mg oral capsule with a recommended dose of 50 to 150 mg/kg per day given every 6 hours.

Resistance to Treatment

Resistance of *Candida* to polyene agents is virtually unknown despite many years of clinical use. However, reports of resistance to azoles, particularly among patients with AIDS, are appearing with increasing frequency. In many situations, resistance appears to develop in those patients with advanced HIV disease or after repeated or long-term therapy.

It must be emphasized that all the azoles, particularly ketoconazole, can interact with many other agents, including antacids, histamine 2 antagonists, rifampin, omeprazole, phenytoin, astemizole, insulin, cyclosporine, oral anticoagulants, and corticosteroids. Such interaction may result in either decreased or increased blood levels of these antifungal agents, thus altering their potential efficacy or toxicity.

MUCORMYCOSIS

Zygomycosis is a term that was classically used to describe fungal infections that are caused by Zygomycetes, which consist of aseptate or septate irregular ribbonlike hyphae that have the capability of reproducing sexually through zygospores.[43] The main ways in which humans acquire mucormycosis is via inhalation of fungal spores or via direct penetration through the skin. The most common fungal organisms associated with mucormycosis are shown in **Fig. 8.**

Risk factors for the development mucormycosis include uncontrolled diabetes (especially with concurrent ketoacidosis), IV drug use, chelation therapy, high-dose glucocorticoids, penetrating trauma/burns, concurrent hemodialysis (especially when using the chelating agent desferrioxamine), use of occlusive dressings/boards, tongue blades, blast injury, malt/lumbar industrial workers, construction workers, malnutrition, and poor wound care. Other than direct penetration with Mucorales, the most common mode of transmission is through inhalation of fungal spores that can result in sinus, orbital, rhino, central nervous system, or pulmonary infections. Diabetics carry a particularly high risk of developing this infection, because when the disease is uncontrolled, this results in impairment of neutrophil function, phagocytosis, and oxidative reactions as well as increases free iron, which acts as a substrate, which enhances mucormycosis growth.[40,41]

In the oral and maxillofacial region, typical lesions that can be encountered include cutaneous (either primary or secondary to disseminated disease) or sinus mucormycosis. Primary penetration of fungal spores through breach of the skin barrier is the most common cause of cutaneous mucormycosis.

The presentation of oral and maxillofacial involvement including the face, nose, or palate is seen in 50% of cases but has been noted to be early diagnostic signs. An example of the eschar from mucormycosis is seen in **Fig. 9** extending from

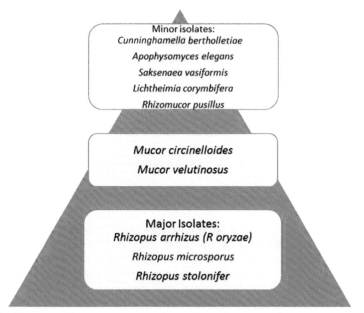

Fig. 8. The hierarchy of mucormycoses isolates. (*Data from* Farmakiotis D, Kontoyiannis D. Mucormycoses. Infectious Dis Clin N America 2016;30(1):143–63.)

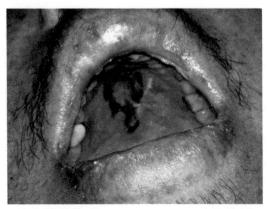

Fig. 9. Necrotic eschar of the palate as a result of extension of mucormycosis rhinosinusitis. (*From* Farmakiotis D, Kontoyiannis D. Mucormycoses. Infectious Dis Clin N America 2016;30(1):148; with permission.)

rhinosinusitis. If left untreated, extension into the orbit can lead to orbital cellulitis, corneal anesthesia, facial anhidrosis, proptosis, diplopia, loss of vision, ophthalmoplegia, or trigeminal/facial/orbital/optic nerve involvement.

Treatment of Mucormycosis

First-line treatment of mucormycosis is Amphotericin B. In a study by Chamilos and colleagues,[44] if initial Amphotericin B treatment is delayed, it is associated with significant increase in overall mortalities. Establishing an early diagnosis is essential and can be accomplished by doing a direct biopsy in conjunction with radiographic examination with either a computed tomographic scan or an MRI. As an alternative to Amphotericin B, posaconazole (an antifungal triazole) has shown a clinical efficacy in the treatment of refractory cases initially treated with Amphotericin B (known as salvage therapy). Currently, hyperbaric oxygen (HBO) therapy has been used by some clinicians in combination with traditional antifungal and surgical therapies. HBO therapy typically comprises pressured dives in an HBO chamber typically at 2 to 2.5 atm. HBO therapy has long been used as an adjunct to surgery when wound healing presents issues. The therapy provides reduction in tissue hypoxia and acidosis and provides high oxygen concentrations that are considered fungistatic, resulting in wound healing while enhancing neutrophilic action.[40,45] However, further studies are required in order to establish this as a standard adjunct for the treatment of mucormycosis.

HISTOPLASMOSIS

Histoplasmosis is an endemic fungal infection caused by the saprophytic and dimorphic fungus *Histoplasma capsulatum*. The spore form is found most commonly in moist, warm soil areas in the central and eastern United States, especially around the Mississippi and the Ohio River Valley and particularly in areas of exposure to excretions of bats and birds.[46] In the United States, incidence of histoplasmosis in adults 65 and older was found to be 3.4 cases per 100,000 population, with rates highest in the Midwest at 6.1 cases per 100,000.[47] There are approximately 500,000 cases of Histoplasmosis annually in the United States.[48,49]

Transmission

Transmission and infection is through aerosolization and inhalation of spores into the lungs.

Diagnosis

A new blood culture test is now available that uses a lysis-centrifugation blood culture technique that can rapidly detect organisms in patients with disseminated histoplasmosis. Biopsy and culture of tissue from biopsy, body fluids, and secretions are also used. Histoplasma antigen can also be detected in the urine.

Oral Manifestations

Oral manifestations of a histoplasma infection can present in all types of histoplasmosis (acute, chronic, and disseminated), but with variable occurrence. In one review of 78 patients with histoplasmosis, oral manifestations were found in 19% of acute cases, 31% of subacute cases, and 66% in disseminated cases.

The mucocutaneous presentation can be quite variable as well. These lesions can often appear similar in appearance to squamous cell carcinomas with a firm base, necrotic center, and rolled borders. **Fig. 10** shows that the most common locations intraorally are the tongue, buccal mucosa, and palate.[50] It is very rare for mucocutaneous lesions to be the only or primary finding, thus reinforcing the necessity of a complete and thorough health and travel history, clinical examination, and radiographic examination, if indicated. Biopsy of oral lesions is needed to confirm the diagnosis.[51]

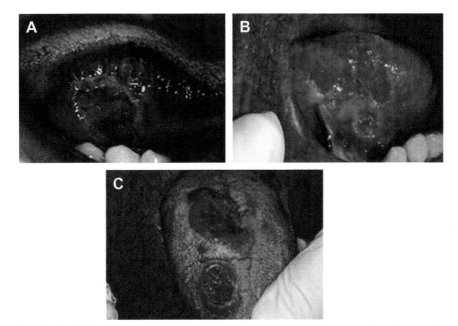

Fig. 10. (*A–C*) Histoplasma infections demonstrating ulcerated, granulomatous lesions with an inflamed base and firm rolled borders on the lateral and dorsal surface of the tongue. (*From* de Paulo LFB, Rosa RR, Durighetto AF. Primary localized histoplasmosis: oral manifestations in immunocompetent patients. Int J Infect Dis 2013;17(2):e139; with permission.)

Treatment

For most patients, a histoplasma infection is self-limiting and will resolve without treatment. However, if symptoms persist or worsen, antifungal therapy will be needed. Itraconazole is a commonly used antifungal agent and may be needed for 3 to 12 months.

BLASTOMYCOSIS

Blastomycosis infections are caused by the soil saprophyte *Blastomyces dermatitidis*, which flourishes in moist soils, or by decomposing matter such as dead leaves and wood. The endemic areas for *Blastomyces* in the United States include the Midwestern, south-central, and southeastern states with the highest concentration in the Ohio and Mississippi River valleys, the Great Lakes, and Saint Lawrence River. This rare fungal infection has a yearly incident rate of 1 to 2 cases per 100,000 in the United States. Wisconsin has the highest rate with 10 to 40 cases per 100,000.[52,53] Oral lesions are rare. Most oral lesions are ulcerative, but there may be verrucous lesions, granulomas, sessile-based projections, abscess in the mandible with radiographic bone loss, and mobile teeth.

CRYPTOCOCCOSIS

Cryptococcus is an encapsulated yeast that is often a cause of an invasive and opportunistic mycoses affecting different organ systems. More than 50 species of *Cryptococcus* have been identified, but only 2 species are known to cause human disease, namely, *Cryptococcus neoformans* and *Cryptococcus gattii*.[54]

C neoformans generally affects immunocompromised patients, with the highest-risk patients being patients with advanced AIDS. Only 11% to 14% of cases of disseminated infection occur in patients without AIDS.[55]

Oral lesions are encountered rarely, and there have only been a handful of reported cases, most being in the HIV population. Annie and colleagues[56] described a case of multiple facial Cryptococcal lesions in a patient with AIDS with disseminated disease. Oral Cryptococcosis can manifest as superficial ulcers, violaceous nodules, granuloma, cancerous looking lesions, or draining sinuses (**Fig. 11**).

Diagnosis of Cryptococcosis depends on isolation of the organism in culture from the involved site, including skin and oral lesions, blood, cerebrospinal fluid, and bronchoalveolar lavage.

Treatment

Management of Cryptococcosis depends on the site of involvement and the immune status of the patient. Clinical Practice Guidelines by the Infectious Diseases Society of America recommends treatment based on 3 risk groups: HIV-infected individuals, organ-transplant recipients, and non-HIV–infected and non-transplant patients.[57] The primary antifungal therapies used for management of Cryptococcosis include intravenous amphotericin B or its lipid formulation, oral flucytosine and oral fluconazole.

ASPERGILLOSIS

Aspergillosis is caused by *Aspergillus* species, which is a mold with hyaline hyphae. It is considered the second most common opportunistic fungal infection after the *Candida* species.[58] There are more than 800 species, out of which only a few can produce a spectrum of diseases, especially in immunocompromised patients, ranging

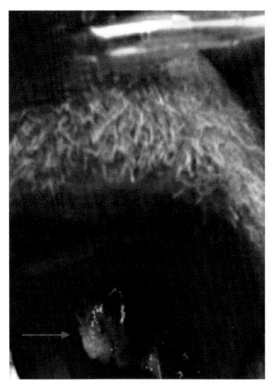

Fig. 11. A 1.5 × 1.5-cm ulceration with slightly heaped borders on the right lateral anterior oral tongue as shown by the arrow. (*From* Reinstadler DR, Dadwal S, Maghami E. Cryptococcal tongue lesion in a stem cell transplant patient: first reported case. Case Rep Otolaryngol 2012;2012:2; with permission.)

from noninvasive allergic forms to invasive disease.[59,60] *Aspergillus fumigatus* is the most frequently isolated species in invasive disease.[61] In recent years, mortality from invasive candidiasis has been on a decline, while an overall increase in deaths from invasive Aspergillosis and other molds has been noted.[62]

Aspergillus species are ubiquitous in the environment and are found in soil, water, air, and organic decaying vegetation. The most common portal of entry is by inhalation of fungal spores into the sinuses and the respiratory tract. Once inhaled, in the absence of appropriate host defenses, the spores enlarge, germinate, and disseminate hematogenously by vascular invasion.[63]

Individuals with a normal host defense rarely develop invasive disease. Defects in ciliary clearance in the airways, compromised innate and adaptive defense against *Aspergillus*, predispose an individual to develop disease.

In the oral and maxillary region, rhinosinusitis is the most common manifestation, either invasive, destructive invasive, or allergic form. Less commonly, the oral cavity, larynx, trachea, and ear are involved.[64–66]

Invasive rhinosinusitis often occurs in association with invasive pulmonary Aspergillosis. Spores occasionally get introduced to the antrum via an oroantral communication during a dental procedure, such as a root canal perforation or a dental extraction, and become pathogenic.[67,68] The maxillary sinus is the most common sinus to be affected. Invasive fungal sinusitis can have an acute and fulminant course with a high mortality occurring predominantly in the immunocompromised patient,[68] or a chronic indolent, granulomatous form with progression through the sinus mucosa, underlying bone and tissue. Clinically, *Aspergillus* rhinosinusitis can present with headache, fever, nasal congestion, facial swelling, purulent or bloody nasal discharge. It should be suspected in a patient with recurrent or refractory sinusitis not responding to antibiotic therapy.

Oral lesions associated with Aspergillosis and other systemic mycoses usually occur as a part of a disseminated disease from the lungs, but occasionally can reflect extension from a contiguous structure such as the maxillary sinus or a primary infection of the oral mucosa.[69] Perioral Aspergillosis can have a broad spectrum of clinical presentations. Necrotic ulcers are one of the most frequently encountered lesions, as shown in **Figs. 12** and **13**. Oral lesions show 3 distinctive clinicopathologic stages.[70] The early stages are characterized by isolated areas of violaceous marginal growth consisting of degenerated epithelium and fungal hyphae infiltrating connective tissue. In the advanced stage, these lesions transform into gray necrotic lesions extending into the attached gingiva with ulceration and pseudomembrane. Vascular invasion is found at the bases of the ulcers. In the late stage, progressive destruction of alveolar bone and surrounding facial muscles is noted, with histopathologic evidence of infiltration of fungal hyphae into the tissues. The presence of deep perioral ulceration in an immunocompromised patient should raise suspicion for fungal infection, including Aspergillosis.

Orofacial osteomyelitis, including of the paranasal sinuses, jaw, and skull base, has been reported. Gabrielli and colleagues[71] reviewed 310 cases of osteomyelitis caused by *Aspergillus* species and found 18% of the cases involved the maxillofacial area.

Diagnosis of aspergillosis requires a histopathologic examination and culture of affected tissue and fluid. The fungi appear with septate hyphae with dichotomous branching at acute angles. Angioinvasion is characteristic of *Aspergillus* along with tissue and bone necrosis.

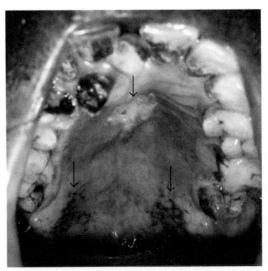

Fig. 12. Diffuse edematous swelling of the palatal mucosa (*bottom arrows*) with focal ulceration (*top arrow*). (*From* Syed A, Panta P, Shahid I, et al. Invasive aspergillosis associated with a foreign body. Case Rep Pathol 2015;2015:2; with permission.)

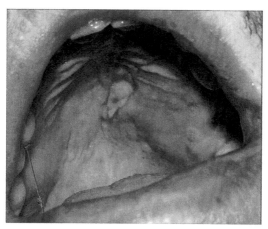

Fig. 13. Intraoral photograph showing the palatal ulceration. (*From* Rallis G, Gkinis G, Dais P, et al. Visual loss due to paranasal sinus invasive aspergillosis in a diabetic patient. Ann Maxillofac Surg 2014;4(2):248; with permission.)

The management of invasive Aspergillosis is usually multidisciplinary and involves using antifungal agents, with surgical debridement as indicated (local disease), and reduction of immunosuppression if feasible.[68]

COCCIDIOIDOMYCOSIS

Coccidioidomycosis or valley fever, commonly referred to as the "great imitator,"[72] is an endemic mycosis caused by the dimorphic fungi *Coccidioides immitis* and *Coccidioides posadasii*.[73] It was reclassified as a fungus in 1900 after being incorrectly identified as a protozoan in 1892.[74,75] It is endemic to the Southwestern United States such as Arizona and California, along with Central and South America. In Southern California, as much as 75% of the population is found to have immunity to the organism.[76] Patients from outside of these areas may acquire the disease by traveling to the endemic regions or by reactivation of latent disease during periods of immunosuppression.[77]

The usual acquisition of Coccidioidomycosis is via inhalation of soil dust containing infectious spores. Cutaneous involvement is the most frequent extrapulmonary manifestation, especially of the face and the extremities. On the face, it has a predilection for the nasolabial fold. Tongue and lip ulcers comprise almost 20% of the lesions.[78] Underlying skeletal and bone involvement can also occur.[79]

Diagnosis is based on histopathologic examination of tissue and fluid samples, culture, serology, polymerase chain reaction (not widely used), and imaging of the affected area. Serum antibodies immunoglobulin M (IgM) and IgG are the most frequently used diagnostic tests. IgM can be detected early in the disease (1–3 weeks), whereas IgG levels are raised after 8 to 10 weeks of symptom presentation.[80]

Because most of the patients who present with early infection will achieve resolution without treatment, specific antifungal therapy is not used in most cases. However, appropriate follow-up every 3 to 6 months should be performed in these patients until radiographic resolution is achieved.[77]

GEOTRICHOSIS

Geotrichosis is opportunistic mycoses most commonly caused by the yeast *Geotrichum candidum*. It is an infrequently encountered infection. However, many suggest that it may be underdiagnosed or misdiagnosed due to its close resemblance to diseases cause by *Candida* sp, particularly of the oral cavity.[81] *Geotrichum* species are ubiquitous yeasts and have been isolated in soil, plants, fruits, and vegetables. *G candidum* is considered a resident flora in humans and has been isolated from multiple sources, including the mouth, respiratory tract, gastrointestinal tract, skin, and vagina.[82]

Usually considered nonpathogenic in immunocompetent hosts, *G candidum* can cause invasive infection in the immunocompromised patient, especially patients with diabetes mellitus, HIV/AIDS, hematologic malignancies including leukemia and lymphoma, and patients on immunosuppressive agents (eg, steroids).[83,84] It has also been reported in patients on long-term antibiotic treatment.[85] Invasive disease has been associated with a high mortality, exceeding 50%.[86] Women and older patients are more susceptible.

Oral geotrichosis clinically resembles oral candidiasis. Bonifaz and colleagues[84] reported a total of 12 cases of oral geotrichosis and found 3 clinical varieties, with pseudomembranous being the most common type (75%), followed by hyperplastic and palatine ulcer. Pseudomembranous geotrichosis appears as white plaques on an erythematous background, which can be easily scraped off, and can be mistaken for candidiasis very easily. It mainly involves the tongue (glossitis) along with the buccal mucosa, soft palate, and rarely, the pharynx. It has also been associated with angular cheilitis.[84] Patients tend to present with burning and difficulty swallowing. Because treatment for oral geotrichosis is similar to treatment of candidiasis (ie, responds to typical anti-candidal drugs), it is thought that many cases are misdiagnosed. The villous manifestations of geotrichosis comparably resemble candidiasis as well as some viral infections. On the other hand, palatine ulcers are deeper and appear similar to other mold infections, such as mucormycosis or aspergillosis, which can be very aggressive with cerebral extension and carry a poor prognosis.

Diagnosis is based on microscopic examination of sample from lesions, prepared with 10% KOH and stained with methyl blue (cotton blue), showing hyphal septation with arthoconidia (**Fig. 14**). The hyphae may, however, be confused easily with pseudohyphae and blastoconidia of *Candida*. Cultures in Sabouraud glucose agar followed

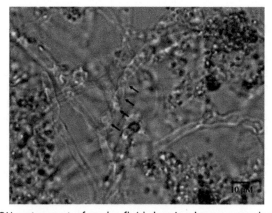

Fig. 14. Direct KOH wet mount of ocular fluid showing brown granular material and hyphae measuring 6 to 8 μM in width and chains of arthroconidia (*arrows*). (*From* Myint T, Dykhuizen MJ, McDonald CH, et al. Post operative fungal endopthalmitis due to Geotrichum candidum. Med Mycol Case Rep 2015;10:5; with permission.)

by biochemical tests are therefore needed for confirmation. Molecular biology is the most accurate technique and can identify different species.

Treatment of oral lesions consists of topical antifungals, such as nystatin or Gentian Violet 1%. Variable and limited data exist on *Geotrichum* species susceptibility for antifungals. Voriconazole has the lowest MIC (minimum inhibitory concentration) for azoles (Zaragoza),[87] whereas Amphotericin is the most widely used antifungal in deep seated and disseminated infections.[88,89] Duration of treatment is not clearly defined as it depends on site and extent of disease process.

SUMMARY

Oral and maxillofacial fungal infections are rare. When a host has an intact immune system, most fungal exposure should not progress into infection. When encountering fungal infections such as candidiasis, a thorough patient history is necessary, including any risk factors, partner history, familial history of diseases that can impact the immune system (eg, diabetes, immunosuppression, asthma, autoimmune disorders), smoking history, and hygiene regimens. It is imperative when encountering any oral fungal infections to explore the possibility of an underlying impairment; hence, it is warranted to involve the primary care physician early. An in-depth review of the patient may include a complete blood count, urine analysis, white blood cell count, sputum culture/Gram strain, glycosylated hemoglobin (HBA1c), HIV levels, CD4 count, albumin/prealbumin, brush biopsy/smear, incisional biopsy, and possibly fungal or blood cultures. In patients suspect for esophageal fungal infections, endoscopy or bronchoscopy with bronchial alveolar lavage may help to diagnose fungal infections. Molecular assays and DNA probes for identifying species that cause specific fungal infections still require additional research to validate use as a standard diagnostic tool. As a dental practitioner, early detection and diagnosis for most oral and maxillofacial fungal infections lead to decreased morbidity and mortality, especially with locally invasive infections such as Mucormycosis and Aspergillosis.

REFERENCES

1. Kauffman C. Chapter 346: Candidiaisis; Goldman's Cecil medicine. 24th edition, vol. 2. Philadelphia: Saunders; 2012. p. 1986–90.
2. Dignani M-C, Solomkin JS, Anaissie EJ. Chapter 8—candida clinical mycology. 2nd edition. Edinburgh (United Kingdom): Churchill Livingstone; 2009. p. 197–229.
3. Shoham S, Nucci M, Walsh, T. Mucocutaneous and deeply invasive candidiasis. Chapter 88, tropical infectious diseases: principles, pathogens and practice. 3rd edition. 2011. p. 589–96.
4. Colombo A, Guimarães T, Camargo LF, et al. Brazilian guidelines for the management of candidiasis—a joint meeting report of three medical societies. Braz J Infect Dis 2013;17(3):283–312.
5. Cannon RD, Holmes AR, Mason AB, et al. Oral Candida: clearance, colonization or Candidiasis? J Dent Res 1995;74:1152–61.
6. Odds FC, editor. Candida and candidosis. 2nd edition. London: Bailliere Tindall; 1998.
7. Elangovan S, Srinivasan S, Allareddy V. Hospital-based emergency department visits with oral candidiasis. Oral Surg Oral Med Oral Pathol Oral Radiol 2012; 114(2):e26–31.
8. Epstein JB, Polsky B. Oronpharyngeal candidiasis: a review of its clinical spectrum and current therapies. Clin Ther 1998;20(1):41–2.

9. Butz-Jorgensen E. Etiology, pathogenesis therapy and prophylaxis of oral yeast infections. Acta Odontol Scand 1990;48:61–9.
10. Scully C. Candidosis (candidiasis). In: Scully C, editor. Oral and Maxillofacial Medicine, The basis of diagnosis and treatment. 3rd edition. London: Churchill Livingstone; 2013. p. 254–63.
11. Epstein JB. Diagnosis and treatment of oropharyngeal candidiasis. Oral Maxillofacial Surg Clinic North America 2003;15:91–102.
12. Alsaeedi A, Sin DD, McAlister FA. The effects of inhaled corticosteroids on chronic obstructive pulmonary disease: a systematic review of randomized placebo-controlled trials. Am J Med 2002;113(1):59–65.
13. Nikawa H, Mikihira S, Egusa H, et al. Candida adherence and biofilm formation on oral surfaces. Nihon Ishinkin Gakkai Zasshi 2005;46(4):233–42.
14. Hoshi N, Mori H, Taguchi H, et al. Management of oral candidiasis in denture wearers. J Prosthodontic Res 2011;55:48–52.
15. Arendorf TM, Walker DM. Denture stomatitis: a review. J Oral Rehabil 1987;14: 217–27.
16. Scully C. Angular cheilitis (angular stomatitis). In: Scully C, editor. Oral and Maxillofacial Medicine, The basis of diagnosis and treatment. 3rd edition. China: Churchill Livingstone; 2013. p. 223–5.
17. Felton D, Cooper L, Duqum I, et al. Evidence-based guidelines for the care and maintenance of complete dentures: a publication of the American College of Prosthodontists. J Am Dent Assoc 2011;142:6s–7s.
18. Greenspan D, Canchola AJ, MacPhail LA, et al. Effect of highly active antiretroviral therapy on frequency of oral warts. Lancet 2001;357(9266):1411–2.
19. Smith J. HIV and AIDS in the adolescent and adult: an update for the oral and maxillofacial surgeon. Oral Maxillofacial Surg Clin North America 2008;20:535–65.
20. Cassone A, De Bernardis F, Tiisantucci A. In vitro and in vivo anticandidal activity of HIV virus protease inhibitors. J Infect Dis 1999;180(2):448–53.
21. Cassone A, Tacconelli E, De Bernardis F. Antiretroviral therapy with protease inhibitors has early, immune reconstitution-independent beneficial effect on Candida virulence and oral candidiasis in human immunodeficiency virus-infected subjects. J Infect Dis 2002;185(2):188–95.
22. Patton L. Sensitivity, specificity, positive predictive value of oral opportunistic infections in adults with HIV/AIDS as markers of immune suppression and viral burden. Oral Surg Oral Med Oral Pathol Oral Radiol Endod 2000;90:182–8.
23. Patton LL, McKaig RG, Eron JJ Jr, et al. Oral hairy leukoplakia, and oral candidiasis as predictors of HIV viral load. AIDS 1999;13:2174–6.
24. Muzyka B, Epifanio R. Update on oral fungal infections. Dent Clin North Am 2013; 57(4):561–81.
25. Millsop J, Nasim F. Oral candidiasis. Clin Dermatol 2016;34:487–94.
26. McCullough MJ, Savage NW. Oral candidiasis and the therapeutic use of antifungal agents in dentistry. Aust Dent J 2005;50:S36–9.
27. Edwards JE. Candida species. In: Mandell GL, Benette JE, editors. Mandell, Douglas, and Bennett's principles and practice of infectious diseases. 7th edition. Philadelphia: Churchill Livingstone Elsevier; 2010. p. 3225–40.
28. Nishimura S, Nagata N, Shimbo T, et al. Factors associated with esophageal candidiasis and its endoscopic severity in the era of antiretroviral therapy. PLos One 2013;8:e5821.
29. Marodi L, Cypowyj S, Tóth B, et al. Molecular mechanisms of mucocutaneous immunity against Candida and Staphylococcus species. J Allergy Clin Immunol 2012;130:101927.

30. Pasqualotto A. Candida and the paediatric lung. Paediatric Respir Rev 2009;10: 186–91.
31. Puel A, Cypowyj S, Marodi L, et al. Inborn errors of human IL-17 immunity under-lie chronic mucocutaneous candidiasis. Curr Opin Allergy Clin Immunol 2012;12: 61622.
32. Cypowyj S, Picard C, Marodi L, et al. Immunity to infection in IL-17-deficient mice and humans. Eur J Immunol 2012;42:224654.
33. Coleman R, Hay RJ. Chronic Mucocutaneous candidosis associated with hypo-thyroidism: a distinct syndrome? Br J Dermatol 1997;136:24–9.
34. Khosravi AR, Shokri H, Darvishi S. Altered immune responses in patients with chronic mucocutaneous candidiasis. J Med Mycol 2014;24(2):135–40.
35. Samaranayake LP, Kerguson MM. Delivery of anti-fungal agents to the oral cavity. Adv Drug Deliv Rev 1994;2(Suppl I):5–14.
36. Uchida K, Yamaguchi H. Susceptibility to miconazole (base) of isolates from the oral cavity and esophagus of patients with mycosis. Jpn J Antibiot 1991;44:109–16.
37. Pappas PG, Kauffman CA, Andes D, et al. Clinical practice guidelines for the management candidiasis: 2009 update by the Infectious Diseases Society of America. Clin Infect Dis 2009;48(5):503–35.
38. Bates DW, Su L, Yu DT. Mortality and cost of acute renal failure associated with Amphotercin B therapy. Clin Infec Dis 2001;32(5):686–93.
39. Greenspan D. Treatment of oral candidiasis in HIV infection. Oral Srgery Oral Med Oral Pathol 1994;78(2):211–5.
40. Walsh TJ, Roilides E, Rex JH, et al. Chapter 89-Mucormycosis. In: Guerrant RL, Walker DH, Weller PF, editors. Tropical infectious diseases: principles, pathogens and practice. 3rd edition. Edinburgh (United Kingdom): W.B. Saunders; 2011. p. 597–602.
41. Kontoyiannis DP, Lionakis MS, Lewis RE, et al. Zygomycosis in a tertiary-care cancer center in the era of Aspergillus-active antifungal therapy: a case control observational study of 27 recent cases. J Infect Dis 2005;191(8):1350–60.
42. McCarty TP, Pappas PG. Invasive candidiasis. Infect Dis Clin N Am 2016;30(1): 112–3.
43. Farmakiotis D, Kontoyiannis D. Mucormycoses. Infect Dis Clin N America 2016; 30:143–63.
44. Chamilos G, Lewis RE, Kontoyiannis DP. Delaying amphotericin B-based frontline therapy significantly increases mortality among patients with hematologic malig-nancy who have zygomycosis. Clin Infect Dis 2008;47:503.
45. Bentur Y, Shupak A, Ramon Y. Hyperbaric oxygen therapy for cutaneous/soft-tissue zygomycosis complicating diabetes mellitus. Plast Reconstr Surg 1998;102:822.
46. Akin L, Herford A, Cicciu M. Oral presentation of disseminated histoplasmosis: a case report and literature review. J Oral Maxillofacial Surg 2011;69(2):535–41.
47. Baddley JW, Winthrop KL, Patkar NM, et al. Geographic distribution of endemic fungal infections among older persons, United States. Emerg Infect Dis 2011; 17(9):1664–9.
48. Chu JH, Feudtner C, Heydon K, et al. Hospitalizations for endemic mycoses: a population-based national study. Clin Infect Dis 2006;42(6):822–5.
49. Wheat LJ, Slama TG, Eitzen HE, et al. A large urban outbreak of histoplasmosis—clinical-features. Ann Intern Med 1981;94(3):331–7.
50. Barbosa de Paulo LF, Rosa RR, Durighettojunior AF. Primary localized histoplas-mosis: oral manifestation in immunocompetent patients. Int J Infect Dis 2013;17: e139–40.

51. Latta R, Napoli C, Borghi E, et al. Rare mycoses of the oral cavity: a literature epidemiologic review. Oral Surg Oral Med Oral Pathol Oral Radiol Endod 2009; 108(5):647–55.

52. Klein BS, Vergeront JM, Weeks RJ, et al. Isolation of Blastomyces dermatitidis in soil associated with a large outbreak of blastomycosis in Wisconsin. N Engl J Med 1986;314(9):529–34.

53. Bradsher RW, Chapman SW, Pappas PG. Blastomycosis. Infect Dis Clin North Am 2003;17(1):21–40, vii.

54. Kwon-Chung KJ, Boekhout T, Fell JW, et al. Proposal to conserve the name Cryptococcus gattii against C. hondurianus and C. bacillisporus (Basidiomycota, Hymenomycetes, Tremellomycetidae). Taxon 2002;51:804–6.

55. DiNardo AR, Schmidt D, Mitchell A, et al. First description of oral cryptococcus neoformans causing osteomyelitis of the mandible, manubrium and third rib with associated soft tissue abscesses in an immunocompetent host. Clin Microbiol Case Rep 2015;1(3):17.

56. Yang A, Karki N, Henneberry J, et al. What is responsible for this cauliflower-like lesion? Consultant 2014;54(8):631.

57. Perfect JR, Dismukes WE, Dromer F, et al. Clinical practice guidelines for the management of cryptococcal disease: 2010 update by the Infectious Diseases Society of America. Clin Infect Dis 2010;50:291–322.

58. Hartwich RW, Batsakis JG. Sinus aspergillosis and allergic fungal sinusitis. Ann Otol Rhinol Laryngol 1991;100(5 Pt1):427–30.

59. Perfect JR, Cox GM, Lee JY, et al. The impact of culture isolation of Aspergillus species: a hospital based survey of Aspergillosis. Clin Infect Dis 2001;33(11):1824–33.

60. Hawksworth DL. Naming Aspergillus species: progress towards one name in each species. Med Mycol 2011;49(1):S70–6.

61. Cadena J, Thompson GR 3rd, Patterson TF, et al. Invasive Aspergillosis: current strategies for diagnosis and management. Infect Dis Clin N Am 2016;30:125–42.

62. Bhatt VR, Viola GM, Ferrajoli A. Invasive fungal infections in acute leukemia. Ther Adv Hematol 2011;2(4):231–47.

63. Kamai Y, Chiang LY, Lopes Bezerra LM, et al. Interactions of Aspergillus fumigatus with vascular endothelial cells. Med Mycol 2006;44(Suppl 1):S115–7.

64. Warman M, Lahav J, Feldberg E, et al. Invasive tracheal aspergillosis treated successfully with voriconazole: clinical report and review of literature. Ann Otol Rhinol Laryngol 2007;116(10):713–6.

65. Ganesh P, Nagarjuna M, Shetty S, et al. Invasive aspergillosis presenting as swelling of the buccal mucosa in an immunocompetent individual. Oral Surg Oral Med Oral Pathol Oral Radiol 2015;119(2):e60–4.

66. Rallis G, Gkinis G, Dais P, et al. Visual loss due to paranasal sinus invasive aspergillosis in a diabetic patient. Ann Maxillofac Surg 2014;4(2):247–50.

67. García-Reija MF, Crespo-Pinilla JI, Labayru-Echeverria C, et al. Invasive maxillary aspergillosis: report of a case and review of the literature. Med Oral 2002;7:200–5.

68. Peral-Cagigal B, Redondo-González LM, Verrier-Hernández A. Invasive maxillary sinus aspergillosis: a case report successfully treated with voriconazole and surgical debridement. J Clin Exp Dent 2014;6(4):e448–51.

69. Cho H, Lee KH, Colquhoun AN, et al. Invasive oral aspergillosis in a patient with acute myeloid leukemia. Aust Dent J 2010;55(2):214–8.

70. Myoken Y, Sugata T, Kyo TI, et al. Pathological features of invasive oral aspergillosis in patients with hematological malignancies. J Oral Maxillofac Surg 1996; 54(3):263–70.

71. Gabrielli E, Fothergill AW, Brescini L, et al. Osteomyelitis caused by Aspergillus species: a review of 310 cases. Clin Microb Infect 2014;20(6):559–65.
72. Huntington RW Jr. Coccidioidomycosis—a great imitator disease. Arch Pathol Lab Med 1986;110(3):182.
73. Fisher MC, Koenig GL, White TJ, et al. Molecular and phenotypic description of Coccidioides posadasii sp nov., previously recognized as the non-California population of Coccidioides immitis. Mycologia 2002;94:73–84.
74. Ophuls W, Moffitt HC. A new pathogenic mould (formerly described as a protozoan Coccidioides immitis pyogenes): preliminary report. Phila Med 1900;5: 1471–2.
75. Posada A. Un nuevo caso de micosis fungoidea con psorospermias. Ann Circulo Medico Argentino 1892;15:585–97.
76. Hicks MJ, Hagaman RM, Barbee RA, et al. The prevalence of cellular immunity to coccidioidomycosis in a highly endemic area. West J Med 1986;144(4):425–8.
77. Galgiani JN, et al. Treatment guidelines for coccidioidomycosis. Clin Infect Dis 2005;41:1217–23.
78. Filho D, Deus AC, Meneses Ade O, et al. Skin and mucous membrane manifestations of coccidioidomycosis: a study of thirty cases in the Brazilian states of Piauí and Maranhão. An Bras Dermatol 2010;85(1):45–51.
79. Gillespie R. Treatment of cranial osteomyelitis from disseminated coccidioidomycosis. West J Med 1986;145:694–7.
80. Laniado-Laborín R, Alcantar-Schramm JM, Cazares-Adame R. Coccidioidomycosis: an update. Curr Fungal Infect Rep 2012;6:113–20.
81. Kassamali H, Anaissie E, Ro J, et al. Disseminated Geotrichum candidum infection. J Clin Microbiol 1987;25:1782–3.
82. Peter M, Horváth G, Domokos L, et al. Data on the frequency of the genus Geotrichum in various human biological products. Med Intern (Bucur) 1967;19:875–8 [in Romanian].
83. Girmenia C, Pagano L, Martino B, et al. Invasive infections caused by Trichosporon species and Geotrichosis capitum in patients with hematological malignancies: a retrospective multicenter study from Italy and review of the literature. J Clin Microbiol 2005;43:1818–28.
84. Bonifaz A, Vázquez-González D, Macías B, et al. Oral Geotrichosis: report of 12 cases. J Oral Sci 2010;52(3):477–83.
85. Vázquez-González D, Perusquía-Ortiz AM, Hundeiker M, et al. Opportunistic yeast infections: candidiasis, cryptococcosis, trichosporonosis and geotrichosis. J Dtsch Dermatol Ges 2013;11:381–94.
86. Rolston K. Overview of systemic fungal infections. Oncology (Huntingt) 2001;15: 11–4.
87. Zaragoza O, Mesa-Arango AC, Gómez-López A, et al. Process analysis of variables for standardization of antifungal susceptibility testing of nonfermentative yeasts. Antimicrob Agents Chemother 2011;55:1563–70.
88. Sfakianakis A, Krasagakis K, Stefanidou M, et al. Invasive cutaneous infection with Geotrichum candidum: sequential treatment with amphotericin B and voriconazole. Med Mycol 2007;45:81–4.
89. Andre N, Coze C, Gentet JC, et al. Geotrichum candidum septicemia in a child with hepatoblastoma. Pediatr Infect Dis J 2004;23:86.

Oral Viral Infections
Diagnosis and Management

Earl Clarkson, DDS[a], Fatima Mashkoor, DDS[b],*, Saif Abdulateef, DMD[b]

KEYWORDS

- Herpes simplex • Varicella zoster • Mononucleosis • Cytomegalovirus
- Enteroviruses • Rubeola and rubella • Mumps and human papilloma virus
- Human herpes virus

KEY POINTS

- This article discusses common viral infections in the oral cavity that will be helpful to dental students, general dentists, and hygienists.
- This article includes common features seen clinically, as well as the histopathology, treatment, and prevention of viral diseases in the oral cavity.
- This helpful guide briefly discusses the main topics especially for the newly trained dentist and dental personnel.

INTRODUCTION

This article focuses on commonly seen viral infections in the oral cavity with associated systemic manifestations. The article discusses their clinical features, histopathology, diagnosis, treatment, and prevention. This will be a useful aid for general practitioners and other dental personnel wanting to expand their knowledge of oral pathology. This article encompasses the following viral infections: herpes simplex, varicella zoster, mononucleosis, cytomegalovirus (CMV), enteroviruses, rubeola, rubella, mumps, and human papillomavirus.

HUMAN HERPES VIRUSES

There are 8 types of human herpes viruses in the Herpetoviridae family. The most well-known, herpes simplex virus (HSV), exists in 2 types: HSV-1 and HSV-2. The remaining types in the Herpetoviridae family include varicella zoster virus (VZV), Epstein-Barr virus (EBV), CMV, HHV-6, HHV-7, and HHV-8.[1,2]

The authors have nothing to disclose.
[a] Department of Oral and Maxillofacial Surgery, Woodhull Medical Center, NYU Langone, 760 Broadway, Room 2C-320, Brooklyn, NY 11206, USA; [b] Department of Oral and Maxillofacial Surgery, Woodhull Medical Center, 760 Broadway, Room 2C-320, Brooklyn, NY 11206, USA
* Corresponding author.
E-mail address: fatima81@gmail.com

HERPES SIMPLEX VIRUS

According to the World Health Organization, in 2012 an estimated 3.7 billion people under 50 years of age (67%) tested positive for HSV-1 infection and approximately 417 million people aged 15 to 49 (11%) tested positive for HSV-2 infection.[3]

Herpes Simplex Virus Type 1

HSV type 1 is an enveloped, linear, double-stranded DNA virus that is usually acquired during childhood. Its primary mode of transmission is via infected saliva or direct contact of mucocutaneous lesions. Clinically they can be characterized in 2 forms:

1. Primary, which typically occurs in younger age groups and is often asymptomatic; or
2. Secondary, which occurs as a reactivation of the infection after a dormant phase.

In primary infection, the virus migrates to the sensory or autonomic ganglia (trigeminal ganglia) where it remains dormant until reactivation (secondary or recurrent form). Reactivation occurs during stress induced states (ie, fever, anxiety, immune compromised states). Incubation period ranges from several days to 2 weeks.[1,4,5]

Herpes Simplex Virus Type 2

HSV type 2 is structured the same as HSV-1, but has a predilection for genital mucosa lesions. Transmission occurs from oral to genital contact. Similar to HSV-1, HSV-2 becomes latent in the autonomic ganglia (lumbosacral region). However, HSV-2 is also capable of causing ocular lesions in newborns. Transmission occurs from infected mothers during the peripartum period owing to disrupted membranes and/or with direct contact with the infected mother's vaginal secretions.[1,4]

Clinical features

Primary herpetic gingivostomatitis Primary herpetic gingivostomatitis is an acute onset of the primary form of HSV-1 that occurs between the ages of 6 months and 5 years. Primary herpetic gingivostomatitis commonly presents with flulike symptoms (fever, chills, and cervical lymphadenopathy), intraoral mucosal lesions (usually 2–3 mm in size) and skin lesions. Lesions usually take about 7 to 10 days to resolve and heal without scar formation.[1]

Herpes labialis Herpes labialis is secondary or recrudescent herpes occurring around the perioral region, characterized by a burning and itching sensation before the appearance of vesicles. They can also appear in keratinized tissue of the hard palate and gingival tissues owing to the reactivation of the latent virus during conditions of stress or immunocompromised states[1] (**Fig. 1**).

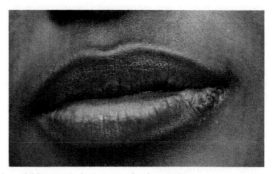

Fig. 1. A 3- to 4-day-old herpetic lesion on the lower lip.

Herpetic whitlow Herpetic whitlow occurs when the virulent orofacial lesions come in direct contact with fingers (**Fig. 2**). These lesions take about 4 to 6 weeks to resolve. Before the era of universal precaution, medical and dental providers were the most at risk to be infected.[1,5]

Histopathology
Microscopically, HSV contain intraepithelial cell balloonings, inflammatory cells, virus-infected epithelial cells, and acantholytic epithelial cells (Tzanck cells), although these findings are not specific for herpes.[1]

Diagnosis
Diagnosis is based on clinical presentation and virus cultures. Cultures usually require 2 to 4 days for positive identification and provide adjunctive confirmation along with clinical diagnosis. Immunologic assays using monoclonal antibodies or DNA in situ hybridization are also useful tools for positive testing.[1]

Treatment and prevention
Early treatment at the onset of prodromal symptoms are ideal. Acyclovir and its analogues show efficacy via viral DNA replication inhibition. Primary genital herpes can be treated by 200 to 400 mg acyclovir 5 times a day; with any primary lesion supportive therapy is indicated (analgesics, nonsteroidal antiinflammatory drugs, lavage, hydration). When symptoms arise, a 5% topical acyclovir ointment applied 5 times a day decreases the duration of herpes labialis. Prophylactic treatment with acyclovir 400 mg twice a day, valacyclovir 1 g daily, or famciclovir 250 mg twice daily reduces the prevalence and severity of recurrence. For dental and medical personnel, universal precaution and hygiene are of utmost importance to prevent self-inoculation or spreading the virus into the patient population.[1,2]

VARICELLA

The VZV is a highly contagious member of the herpes virus family, owing to similarities in its DNA core. Although its effects on children is more commonly known as chickenpox, it can reactivate in adults as shingles. Spreading in droplet form, it proliferates in macrophages, leading to viremia that overwhelms the body's defenses. Healthy individuals are able to limit replication and recover in a 2- to 3-week span. Children, older adults, and immunocompromised patients face a greater threat.[1,2]

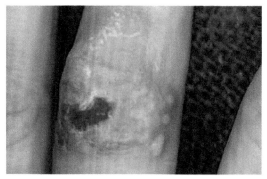

Fig. 2. Herpetic whitlow on the finger. (*From* Neville BW, Damm DD, Allen CM, et al. Oral and maxillofacial pathology. 4th edition. St Louis (MO): Elsevier; 2016. p. 221; with permission.)

Clinical Features

Varicella is common in children 6 to 11 years of age, commonly infecting siblings simultaneously. After the resolution of the condition, the virus remains latent at the dorsal root and trigeminal ganglia. Primary symptoms include low-grade fever, pruritis, malaise, and rash. Subsequently, vesicles develop. Initial lesions begins on the trunk and face and spread to the extremities.

Skin lesions are preceded typically by oral lesions, which tend to be painless. Further, immunocompromised patients risk involvement of the central nervous and pulmonary systems, resulting in a higher mortality rate.[1]

Histopathology

Microscopically, acantholysis of epithelial cells results in numerous free-floating Tzank cells, with margination of chromatin along the nuclear membrane and occasional multinucleation. In simple cases, the epithelium regenerates from ulcer margins with minimal scar formation.[1]

HERPES ZOSTER

Latent VZV is reactivated after many immunosuppressive states like human immunodeficiency virus (HIV) infection, radiation, or state of malignancy. Typically, it affects the sensory nerves of the trunk, head, and neck, resulting in symptoms of pain or paresthesia in those dermatomes. Vesicular primary lesions ulcerate and heal over in 1 to 2 weeks.[1,2]

Clinical Features

Vesicular development is distributed in a unilateral and linear distribution. The thoracic and lumbar dermatomes are the most typically involved, followed by craniofacial dermatomes. The second division of the trigeminal nerve is the most commonly affected, with corneal involvement leading to subsequent blindness. Lesions distribute on the forehead, upper eyelid, and upper and lower lips (**Fig. 3**). In 10% to 15% of these patients, postherpetic neuralgia later develops as a result of central and peripheral nerve injuries. The involvement of the geniculate ganglion is a rare but reported complication, also known as Ramsay Hunt syndrome.[1,2,5]

Histopathology

Vesicles of herpes zoster are indistinguishable microscopically from vesicles seen in primary varicella infection.[1]

Treatment for Varicella Zoster Virus and Herpes Zoster Infections

Since the advent of vaccinations, there has been a significant reduction in mortalities, hospitalizations, and complications related to varicella infections. In healthy patients, primary treatment includes supportive care with over-the-counter pain control, hydration, and a healthy lifestyle. Aspirin is avoided owing to reported incidences of Reye syndrome. However, in immunocompromised patients, an extensive regimen is indicated to prevent dissemination of the disease. Primary VZV infections are treated with a high dose of oral acyclovir, 800 mg 5 times daily for 7 days. Treatment should begin within hours of disease onset to reduce the risk of postherpetic neuralgia. Although commonly recommended, research has shown no long-term benefit when corticosteroids are added to an acyclovir regimen.[1,2,5]

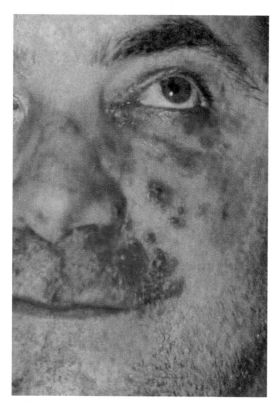

Fig. 3. Facial lesions from herpes zoster involving the second division of the trigeminal nerve. (*From* Regezi JA, Sciubba JJ, Jordan RCK. Oral pathology: clinical pathologic correlations. 6th edition. St Louis (MO): Elsevier; 2012; with permission.)

INFECTIOUS MONONUCLEOSIS (ALSO KNOWN AS "MONO" OR "KISSING DISEASE")

Mono is a disease of young adults, also known as kissing disease owing to its nature of transmission. It is primarily transmitted owing to close contact (sharing of straws, kissing, and other forms of saliva exchange). EBV and HHV-8 are the causal agents. EBV bind on the complement receptor on the B-cell and transform these cells. EBV is also associated with Burkitts lymphoma (B-cell lymphoma in children in central Africa).[1,2,4]

Clinical Features

Most children affected are asymptomatic; however, in young adults symptoms like fever, lymphadenopathy, pharyngitis, and tonsillitis are noted. Prodromal symptoms like malaise, fatigue precede 2 weeks before the development of fever, which can last 2 to 14 days in classic infectious mononucleosis cases. Some oral lesions are similar to petechiae on the soft and hard palates; necrotizing ulcerative gingivitis is also fairly common in infected patients.[1,4,5]

Diagnosis

Monospot test is a rapid screening test in which antibodies (hetrophile antibody) against EBV cross-react and agglutinates with sheep red blood cells. Complete blood count reveals elevated leukocytes and peripheral blood smears shows atypical lymphocytes.[1]

Treatment

Most cases resolves spontaneously within 4 to 6 weeks and only require treatment of clinical symptoms. Nonsteroidal antiinflammatory drugs are used for fever reduction and bed rest is advised for malaise and fatigue.[1,2]

CYTOMEGALOVIRUS

According to the Centers for Disease Control and Prevention, 50 to 80 adults in every 100 Americans are infected by 40 years of age. CMV establishes latency after initial infection in the salivary glandular cells, endothelium, macrophages, and lymphocytes. The virus can cross the placenta, causing congenital disease or infect newborns during delivery. Transmission can also occur by exchange of bodily fluids and blood transfusions.[1,2,6]

Clinical Features

Most infections are asymptomatic; less than 10% can present with flulike symptoms. In rare cases, other signs like hepatomegaly, splenomegaly, jaundice, and central nervous system involvement can occur. These symptoms should be taken seriously, especially in immunocompromised individuals. Oral lesions presenting with chronic mucosal ulcerations can present with coinfections of HSV, which is usually common in patients with AIDS (**Fig. 4**). CMV is the most common cause of mental retardation in viral infections causing multiple birth defects. Neonatal CMV infections can produce dental disorders exhibiting diffuse enamel hypoplasia, enamel hypomaturation, attrition, or discoloration of dentin.[1,2,5]

Diagnosis

Diagnosis is based on a combination of clinical features and other testing procedures, such as polymerase chain reaction or immunoassays serologic testing. Biopsy can be performed and should be done in chronic ulcers for immunocompromised patients that do not respond to conservative therapy.[1]

Treatment

Intravenous ganciclovir is recommended for treatment of CMV infections, although most resolve spontaneously. In patients with HIV/AIDS, the best treatment is improvement of their immune status such as treatment with highly active antiretroviral therapy.[1]

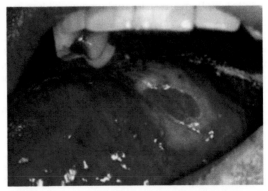

Fig. 4. Tongue ulceration from cytomegalovirus infection. (*From* Woo S. Oral pathology: a comprehensive atlas and text. Philadelphia: Elsevier; 2012; with permission.)

ENTEROVIRUSES

Enterovirus infections are classified into echoviruses, polioviruses, and coxsackieviruses A and B. In 1960, a new group of enteroviruses were discovered and designated as enterovirus 17. Some of these viruses have been linked to increased risk of type I diabetes mellitus and dilated cardiomyopathy. The annual incidence of symptomatic infections in the United States is 10 to 15 million. These infections affect any age group but are mostly seen in young children or infants. The most significant diseases among this group are herpangina; hand, foot, and mouth disease; and acute lymphonodular pharyngitis.[1,2]

HERPANGINA

The name, herpangina, is derived from herpes, which involves vesicular eruption and angina, which means inflammation. COXSACKIEVIRUS A (CVA) serotypes 1 to 10, 16, and 22 are the most common viruses isolated with this condition. Herpangina is transmitted by contaminated saliva or through contaminated feces. Outbreaks are very common in summer or early autumn.[1,2]

Clinical Features

Sore throat, fever, rhinorrhea, myalgia, and dysphagia are commonly seen with herpangina. Most cases are mild and symptoms last for 3 days. Clinically, oral lesions appear in the posterior areas of the mouth, usually the tonsillar pillars or soft palate. Small vesicles form but rapidly break down to 2- to 4-mm ulcers.[1,2,5]

Histopathology

Intracellular edema resulting in subepithelial vesicles with epithelial necrosis and ulceration are the final result.[1]

Treatment

Herpangina is mild, with minimal complications and a short duration. Therefore, supportive therapy is recommended. Contact with infected individual should be avoided to prevent spread of disease.[1,2]

ACUTE LYMPHONODULAR PHARYNGITIS

Acute lymphonodular pharyngitis is a variant of herpangina that is associated with CVA 10.

Clinical Features

Sore throat, headache, and a fever, which may last up to 10 days, are prominent features. Patients will develop diffuse small yellow to dark-pink nodules in the area of oropharynx.

Histopathology

Findings include lymphoid aggregate, which resolve without ulceration or vesiculation.

Treatment

No treatment is necessary; the condition is self-limiting.[1,2]

HAND, FOOT, AND MOUTH SYNDROME

This most common enterovirus condition mostly affects children younger than 5 years old, is highly contagious (seasonal mostly summer), and transmits through airborne spread or fecal–oral contamination. Coxsackie type A16 or enterovirus 71 viruses were linked to these infections. Hand, foot, and mouth syndrome tends to occur in epidemic clusters with high transmission rates.[1,2]

Clinical Features

Skin rash and oral lesions are associated with flulike symptoms, accompanied by cough, rhinorrhea, diarrhea, and headaches. Oral lesions precede skin lesions, first presenting as vesicles that rupture and become ulcers. Intraorally, these lesions tend to disseminate anywhere in the mouth although the palate, tongue, and buccal mucosa are favored sites. Cutaneous lesions primarily affect ventral surfaces and sides of the fingers and toes, borders of the palms, and soles of the feet. The legs and genitals are rarely affected. Skin lesions start as erythematous macules that develop central vesicles and heal without crusting.[1,2]

Histopathology

Distinguished histologic feature of skin lesions include reticular and ballooning degeneration of keratinocytes.[1]

Treatment

Management of hand, foot, and mouth disease is mainly supportive. Signs and symptoms usually clear up in 7 to 10 days. Over-the-counter pain medications such as acetaminophen (Tylenol, Johnson & Johnson, New Brunswick, NJ) or ibuprofen with topical oral anesthetics may help pain control.[1,2]

RUBEOLA (MEASLES)

Rubeola belongs to the family paramyxovirus, an RNA enveloped virus that is highly contagious. Rubeola is spread via airborne droplets through the nasopharyngeal respiratory epithelium.[4]

Clinical Features

Measles are uncommon in the 21st century owing to vaccination programs, but is commonly seen in unvaccinated individuals. The incubation period lasts from 10 to 12 days with the prodromal period lasting 1 to 7 days. There are 3 stages of measles, each typically lasting 3 days. The first stage includes the 3 Cs of coryza (runny nose), cough, and conjunctivitis. Oral manifestations, known as Koplik's spots, precede cutaneous lesions by 1 to 2 days. Koplik's spots are characterized as red macular lesions with a blue white center (**Fig. 5**). The second stage consists of erythematous maculopapular rashes that starts from the face and spreads down toward the extremities, along with a continuing fever. The third stage is when the fever resolves and the rashes began to subside. Complications are rare, but can include encephalitis and thrombocytopenic purpura. Otitis media and pneumonia can also occur as secondary infections.[1,2,4]

Diagnosis

Koplik's spots are a pathognomonic feature and histologically are seen as focal epithelial hyperparakeratosis. Diagnosis is clinically based with laboratory confirmation of rising serologic antibody titers.[1,2]

Treatment and Prevention

Supportive therapy includes adequate rest, fluids, and antipyretic and analgesics medications. The best therapy is prevention through vaccination. The Centers for

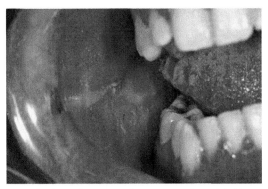

Fig. 5. Koplik's spot on the buccal mucosa. (*From* Regezi JA, Sciubba JJ, Jordan RCK. Oral pathology: clinical pathologic correlations. 6th edition. St Louis (MO): Elsevier; 2012; with permission.)

Disease Control and Prevention recommends childhood vaccination with the measles, mumps, and rubella (MMR) vaccine in 2 doses, first being around 12 to 15 months of age and the second around 4 to 6 years of age. Complete elimination of this disease is possible with a good vaccination program and requires global cooperation.[1,4,5]

GERMAN MEASLES (RUBELLA)

German measles are caused by the Togavirus family. It is a contagious disease with clinical features similar to measles. German measles are known to causes congenital birth defects in the developing fetus, especially if infections occur during the first trimester of pregnancy. The classic triad of rubella congenital syndrome includes heart disease, deafness, and cataracts. Prevention is through the MMR vaccines.[1,4]

MUMPS

Mumps are no longer common in the United States. Since the prevaccinated era there has been a reduction of 99% of cases in the United States. Belonging to the Paramyxoviridea virus family, the mumps virus primarily infects via salivary secretions or respiratory droplets.[1]

Clinical Features

One-third of mumps infections are subclinical and the rest have nonspecific symptoms such as fever, malaise, myalgia, and headache. The incubation period usually ranges from 2 to 4 weeks, with the patient at risk of spreading the virus 1 day before clinical symptoms to 2 weeks after resolution. Bilaterally, parotid gland involvement is the most commonly affected salivary gland; however, the sublingual and submandibular glands can also be involved. Swelling and pain begin from the ears and extend down to the mandible posteriorly and inferiorly, with pain during mastication.[1,2]

Diagnosis

Diagnosis is easily made clinically with serologic confirmation of rising titers of mumps, specifically immunoglobulin (Ig)G and IgM during the infectious stages.[1]

Treatment and Prevention

The recommended treatment is palliative care with nonsteroidal antiinflammatory drugs as analgesics, antipyretics, and bed rest. Hydration and diet precautions are recommended. Prevention is through prior MMR vaccinations.[1,5]

HUMAN PAPILLOMAVIRUS

Studies have shown that at least 25 strains of HPV have been associated with oral lesions. The most frequent lesions include: verruca vulgaris (common wart) and oral squamous papilloma. Owing to their immunocompromised state, HIV patients have an increased risk for papilloma related lesions. HPV-7, associated with butcher's warts, and HPV-32, often noted in multifocal epithelial hyperplasia, are most commonly seen in patients with HIV. Among the strains, the high-risk oncogenic HPV subtypes (primarily HPV 16, but also HPV 18, 31, 33, and 35) are commonly detected in oral squamous cell carcinomas.[1,2,5]

ORAL SQUAMOUS PAPILLOMA
Clinical Features

Intraorally, these lesions present as small, white, isolated, exophytic, and pedunculated growths. They are commonly found on the hard and soft palate, uvula, and vermillion of the lips. Lesions are prevalent in middle-aged male and females with a history of current sexual activity.[1]

Histopathology

Exaggerated growth of normal squamous epithelium. These lesions are exophytic with fingerlike extensions of the epithelium supported by connective tissue. This pattern resembles cutaneous warts.[1]

COMMON WART (VERRUCA VULGARIS)
Clinical Features

Common warts are found commonly on the skin and are caused by the cutaneous HPV subtypes 2 and 57. These warts are similar in appearance to squamous papillomas and tend to involve the lips, gingivae, and hard palate. Aerosolizing HPV particles should be suspected while locally excising these lesions with laser or electrocautery.[1,2]

CONDYLOMA ACUMINATUM
Clinical Features

Condyloma acuminatum is another condition resulting from a virus-induced proliferation of stratified squamous epithelium of the genitalia, perianal region, mouth, and larynx. HPV types 6 and 11 are usually detected in these lesions. Condyloma is regarded as a sexually transmitted disease with an incubation period of 1 to 2 months from the time of contact. These lesions might indicate sexual abuse when diagnosed in young children. Studies suggested vertical transmission from mothers with genital infections. Intraorally, these lesions commonly present as a group of multiple pink nodules on the labial mucosa, soft palate, and lingual frenum (**Fig. 6**). The average lesion size is 1.0 to 1.5 cm.[1,2]

Histopathology

Papillary projections are covered by stratified squamous epithelium, often parakeratotic but may be nonkeratinized. The epithelium is differentiated. However, prickle cells often demonstrate pyknotic nuclei surrounded by clear margin (Koilocytes).[1,2]

Treatment

Surgical excision with cryosurgery, scalpel excision, or laser ablation is the ultimate approach to manage these condition. Recurrences are common and perhaps are related to surrounding normal appearing tissue that may be harboring the infectious agent.[1,2]

HECK'S DISEASE (ALSO KNOWN AS FOCAL EPITHELIAL HYPERPLASIA/MULTIFOCAL EPITHELIAL HYPERPLASIA)
Clinical Features

Heck's disease is characterized by multiple asymptomatic well-circumscribed, smooth papules on the tongue and labial mucosa of children. These lesions are frequently seen in children but they can often be seen in older adults as well. HPV types 13 and 32 are detected in 75% to 100% of these lesions.[1]

Histopathology

Histopathologic evaluation reveals prominent acanthosis of the epithelium with elongated and wide rete ridges.[1]

METHODS OF COLLECTING SPECIMENS FOR VIRAL CULTURE AND DIAGNOSIS

As discussed, viral infections can be passed from host to host in several distinct modes (ie, airborne, contact, blood). To effectively isolate and diagnose virus specimens for testing purposes, they must be collected properly and transported in appropriate mediums for processing. Furthermore, because viral agents differ in genetic make up, composition, size, and structure, different testing modalities are used for diagnosis purposes. It should be noted, universal precautions should always be used when handling specimens. The purpose of this section is to review methods of collecting specimens for proper processing.[7]

To best identify the causative viral agents in a host, a physician should order the most specific and sensitive test for the expected agent based on clinical findings. As a treating physician, one must be aware of which agents can be isolated and identified based on the available testing modalities. Also, any relevant medical history should be provided to the laboratory to check for corresponding correlations. Diagnosis of viral infections rely on 4 primary modalities: antigen detection, culture, nucleic acid detection, and serology.[8,9]

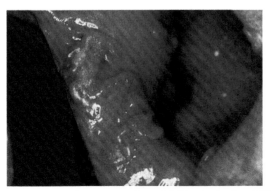

Fig. 6. Condyloma acuminatum. (*From* Regezi JA, Sciubba JJ, Jordan RCK. Oral pathology: clinical pathologic correlations. 6th edition. St Louis (MO): Elsevier; 2012; with permission.)

Viral agents can be identified readily from infected hosts by using specific antibody reagents. Direct fluorescent antibody testing (DFA) is the most common antigen test in use. It works by staining the collected specimen with a specific fluorescently labeled antibody and examining it under a microscopy. These tests are ordered commonly for skin and mucosal lesions, such as HSV and VZV. Other modified versions of DFA can help to identify viruses such as influenza A and adenovirus. A drawback to DFA testing is that it is labor intensive and technical expertise is needed for accurate diagnosis; however, test results are available much quicker and can be highly selective.[8,9]

Because viruses are intracellular pathogens, for diagnosis purposes, cultures require inoculation of viral agents into susceptible host cells. As these viral agents grow cell, cell staining with fluorescently labeled antibodies and characteristic cytopathic changes can be visualized for diagnosis purposes. Similar to DFA, this process is labor intensive; however, it takes a longer time and is less sensitive than other detection methods. One key advantage is this method may identify unsuspecting viral agents that was initially not clinically correlated.[8,9]

Nucleic acid detection is the most common method for testing many viral agents. Viral nucleic acids are amplified using polymerase chain reaction testing. Because nucleic acid testing does not rely on viable infectious viral agents, it allows for easier specimen collection and transport over other collection methods. Results are usually available within 24 hours.[8,9]

Serologic testing involves pathogen-specific antibodies produced by infected hosts. These tests can assist in diagnosis recent infections and determining immunity. Serologic testing is often used when other testing modalities are not available.[8]

ANTIVIRAL SUSCEPTIBILITY TESTING

With an increase of treating physicians to prescribe antimicrobial medications, it is well-documented that drug resistance is increasing. Antiviral susceptibility testing is available not widely and modalities are not standardized. Antiviral resistance develops as a result of mutations in viral genes. Currently, there are 2 main modalities to test resistance: genotypic antiviral resistance testing and phenotypic drug susceptibility testing. Genotypic antiviral resistance testing involve sequencing enzymatic genes to detect mutations that lead to drug resistance. Phenotypic drug susceptibility testing measures the ability of a virus to grow against different concentrations of antiretroviral drugs.[8,9]

SUMMARY

After reviewing the described lesions and viral infections, the general dentist and the dental hygienist will be able to diagnose these lesions based on clinical features. They will also be familiarized with details on basic histopathology, treatment, and prevention of commonly associated viral infections of the oral cavity.

REFERENCES

1. Neville BW. Oral and maxillofacial pathology. St Louis (MO): Saunders/Elsevier; 2009.
2. Regezi JA. Oral pathology: clinical pathologic correlations. 6th edition. St. Louis (MO): Elsevier; 2012.
3. Herpes simplex virus. World Health Organization. Available at: http://www.who.int/mediacentre/news/releases/2015/herpes/en/. Accessed July 17, 2016.
4. Gladwin M, Trattler B, Mahan CS. Clinical microbiology: made ridiculously simple. Miami (FL): Medmaster; 2014.

5. Woo SB. Oral pathology: a comprehensive atlas and Text. Philadelphia: Elsevier/ Saunders; 2012.
6. Centers for Disease Control and Prevention. Available at: https://www.cdc.gov/ cmv/overview.html. Accessed July 28, 2016.
7. Johnson FB. Transport of viral specimens. Clin Microbiol Rev 1990;3(2):120–31.
8. Hupp JR, Ferneini EM. Head, neck, and orofacial infections: an interdisciplinary approach. 1 edition. St Louis (MO): Elsevier; 2016.
9. Storch GA. Diagnostic virology. Clin Infect Dis 2000;31:739–51.

Recent Recommendations for Management of Human Immunodeficiency Virus–Positive Patients

Miriam R. Robbins, DDS, MS[a,b],*

KEYWORDS

- Human immunodeficiency virus • Acquired immune deficiency syndrome
- Dental management • Treatment planning considerations • Oral manifestations

KEY POINTS

- The delivery of oral health care is the same for the human immunodeficiency virus (HIV)-infected patient as for the non–HIV-infected one. HIV is not a valid reason to deny, delay, or alter treatment.
- There are no absolute contraindications and few complications associated with comprehensive oral health care treatment for asymptomatic HIV-infected patients and clinically stable patients with AIDS.
- Medical assessment of HIV-infected dental patients does not differ from that of any medically complex dental patient.
- The medical history of HIV-infected individuals most likely to impact the delivery of care is not related to HIV immunosuppression, but rather to non–HIV-associated conditions.
- Modifications in dental treatment may be necessary when treating patients with advanced HIV disease or other comorbid conditions that may be present in this population.

INTRODUCTION

Human immunodeficiency virus (HIV) is a retrovirus in the *Lentivirus* group that targets crucial immune cells called $CD4^+$ T cells. Two major types of HIV have been identified: HIV-1 (causes the majority of HIV infections globally) and HIV-2. The course of HIV infection is characterized by a long interval between initial infection and the gradual deterioration of immune function leading to AIDS.[1] Once considered a death

The author has nothing to disclose.
[a] Department of Dental Medicine, Winthrop University Hospital, 200 Old Country Road, Suite 460, Mineola, NY 11501, USA; [b] Department of Oral and Maxillofacial Pathology, Radiology and Medicine, New York University College of Dentistry, 345 E. 24th Street, New York, NY 10010, USA
* Department of Dental Medicine, Winthrop University Hospital, 200 Old Country Road, Suite 460, Mineola, NY 11501.
E-mail address: mrobbins@winthrop.org

Dent Clin N Am 61 (2017) 365–387
http://dx.doi.org/10.1016/j.cden.2016.12.006
0011-8532/17/© 2016 Elsevier Inc. All rights reserved.

dental.theclinics.com

sentence, treatment with current combination antiretroviral drugs (cART) can achieve viral suppression indefinitely, converting an HIV diagnosis to a chronic illness with people living with HIV for decades after diagnosis. In the absence of antiretroviral therapy, the average time between acquiring HIV and the development of AIDS is estimated to be between 10 and 15 years.[2] Over the past decade, the number of people living with HIV has increased, although the annual number of new HIV infections has remained relatively stable.

EPIDEMIOLOGY AND PREVALENCE

The first documented cases of AIDS were reported in 1981 by the Centers for Disease Control and Prevention (CDC), although the causative virus was not identified until 1983. Since the beginning of the epidemic, almost 71 million people have been infected with the HIV virus and about 34 million people have died of AIDS worldwide.[3] Currently, it is estimated that there are 36.9 million people living with HIV/AIDS worldwide, with 1.2 million adults in the United States.[4] There are about 50,000 new HIV infections per year, and 156,300 (12.8%) HIV-positive Americans do not know they are infected. Only 25% of patients being treated are considered to have controlled disease.[5] Currently, the CDC recommends that all individuals aged 13 to 64 years have an HIV test as part of routine medical care and that those with high-risk behavior receive annual testing. Specific separate consent for HIV antibody testing is no longer needed but different states have different requirements for pretest and posttest counseling.

PATHOGENESIS

HIV is present in bodily fluids including the blood, semen, vaginal fluid, breast milk, saliva, and tears as both free virus particles and infected immune cells. It is most commonly spread via sexual contact with an infected person or sharing needles contaminated with blood. Additionally, mother-to-child transmission can occur during birth or through breast feeding. HIV attaches to cells with CD4 surface molecule (primarily T lymphocytes, monocytes, tissue macrophages, and dendritic cells).[6] Once inside the cell, HIV replicates using the reverse transcriptase enzyme and the resulting DNA is imported into the cell nucleus and integrated. The infected cells then release new virus particles via surface budding. Cell death occurs either by direct cell killing via the budding virus, pyroptosis and apoptosis as a cellular reaction to the presence of the virus, or cell death by CD8 cytotoxic lymphocytes that recognize infected cells.[7,8] This resulting destruction of the cells of the immune systems progressively destroys the body's ability to fight opportunistic infections.

The laboratory criteria for defining a confirmed case were revised to incorporate a new multitest algorithm that expanded the number of tests that could be used and allowed for early detection of HIV infection (**Fig. 1**). Positive results from a fourth-generation combination HIV-1 p24 antigen/antibody enzyme-linked immunosorbent assay and a subsequent positive result from an orthogonal test are needed to determine HIV infection, such as:

- Qualitative HIV nucleic acid amplification testing (DNA or RNA)
- Quantitative HIV nucleic acid amplification testing (viral load assay)
- HIV p24 antigen test
- HIV isolation (viral culture)
- HIV nucleotide sequence (genotype)[9]

Point-of-care rapid tests (such as the OraQuick ADVANCE Rapid HIV-1/2 antibody test and OraQuick In-Home Test, Orasure Technologies, Inc, Bethlehem, PA) use an

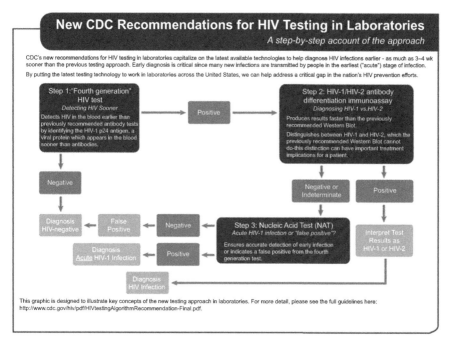

Fig. 1. Recommendations for human immunodeficiency virus (HIV) testing from the Centers for Disease Control and Prevention (CDC). (*From* Centers for Disease Control and Prevention and Association of Public Health Laboratories. Laboratory Testing for the Diagnosis of HIV Infection: Updated Recommendations. Available at: http://stacks.cdc.gov/view/cdc/23447. Published June 27, 2014. Accessed July 29, 2016.)

oral swab that detects HIV antibodies in mucosal exudate and can return results in as little as 20 minutes. They have a specificity of 99.98% (95% confidence interval, 99.90–100.0) and sensitivity of 93.0% (95% confidence interval, 86.6–96.9),[10] but are considered preliminary tests that must be followed by confirmatory blood tests.

The CDC defines 5 stages of HIV disease (0, 1, 2, 3, and unknown) based on the level of CD4+ lymphocytes and the presence of opportunistic diseases[9] (**Table 1**). Plasma HIV RNA load (the amount of virus present in the blood) is not used for staging HIV disease, but is used to estimate the level of viral replication and providing information about the rate of disease progression. The stage of HIV infection is based on the most advanced stage the person has ever experienced, regardless of their current CD4+ levels or state of health.

Table 1
Stages of HIV infection

Stage	CD4 Count (cells/mm³)	CD4%	Clinical Evidence
0	Early HIV infection		
1	≥500	≥26	No AIDS-defining conditions
2	200–499	14–26	No AIDS-defining conditions
3	<200	<15	Or documentation of AIDS-defining conditions
Unknown	No data	No data	No information

Abbreviation: HIV, human immunodeficiency virus.
Adapted from Centers for Disease Control and Prevention (CDC). Revised surveillance case definition for HIV infection—United States, 2014. MMWR Morb Mortal Wkly Rep 2014;63(3):7.

STAGE 0: VERY EARLY INFECTION

This stage indicates a very early infection that is diagnosed before standard antibody, antigen/antibody, or nucleic acid tests are positive. This stage is intended for patients with transiently low CD4 cell counts that are often seen right after infection but who do not have advanced disease.

STAGE 1: ACUTE HUMAN IMMUNODEFICIENCY VIRUS INFECTION

Among persons acutely infected with HIV, 40% to 90% will develop acute symptomatic illness within 28 days of infection.[11,12] Acute infection is associated with an acute flulike clinical syndrome with multiple nonspecific symptoms including fever, headache, malaise, lymphadenopathy, myalgias, and rash. The duration of the acute retroviral syndrome is usually 3 to 14 days and is frequently undiagnosed or misdiagnosed.[12,13] Very high plasma HIV RNA levels (viral load) and an initial decline in CD4+ T cells are seen during this period of initial infection. The immune system produces antibodies in response to HIV infections but it can take 6 to 8 weeks after exposure for detectable levels to be present through traditional testing. This "window" period represents a high risk for HIV transmission, because a person can receive a negative antibody test result and yet be highly infectious. A plasma HIV RNA assay used in conjunction with a p24 antigen/antibody combination screening test can detect HIV infection as short as 10 days[14] after infection (**Fig. 2**).

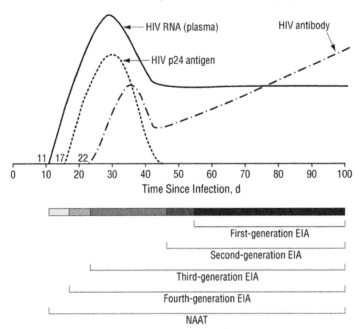

Fig. 2. Detection of human immunodeficiency virus (HIV) infection. EIA, enzyme immunoassay; NAAT, nucleic acid amplification. (*From* New York State Department of Health AIDS Institute. Johns Hopkins University Division of Infectious Diseases. HIV Clinical Guidelines Program. Diagnosis and Management of Acute HIV Infection. Available at: http://www.hivguidelines.org/clinical-guidelines/adults/diagnosis-and-management-of-acute-hiv-infection. This material was accessed on 2 June 2016 on the HIV Clinical Resource website (www.hivguidelines.org). The HIV Clinical Guidelines Program is a collaborative effort of the New York State Department of Health AIDS Institute and the Johns Hopkins University Division of Infectious Diseases. Copyright © Johns Hopkins University HIV Clinical Guidelines Program 2000–2016.)

STAGE 2: CLINICAL LATENCY

The production of antibodies and activation of CD8$^+$ T cells produce a period of clinical latency, also called asymptomatic or chronic HIV infection. Viral levels remain low although the virus continues to replicate at a low level. Infected persons usually have no HIV-related symptoms and CD4$^+$ cells can remain stable for a time. If there is no medical intervention, generally 10 to 15 years after primary infection, a slow decline in the immune function and HIV-related illnesses occur. The goal of all current HIV treatments is to prolong this period indefinitely by maintaining viral suppression.

STAGE 3: AIDS

According to the CDC definition, a person has AIDS if they are HIV-positive and have either:

- A CD4$^+$ T-cell count of less than 200 cells/mm^3
- A CD4$^+$ T-cell percentage of total lymphocytes of less than 14%
- Presence of AIDS-defining opportunistic infections (**Box 1**)

This is the stage where the immune system is badly damaged and opportunistic infections become common. People with AIDS survive an average of 3 years if medical care is not initiated or effective in reversing disease progression.

Box 1
AIDS-Defining Clinical Conditions

- Bacterial infections, multiple or recurrent (age ≤6 y)
- Candidiasis of bronchi, trachea, or lungs
- Candidiasis of esophagus
- Cervical cancer, invasive (age ≥6 y)
- Coccidioidomycosis, disseminated or extrapulmonary
- Cryptococcosis, extrapulmonary
- Cryptosporidiosis, chronic intestinal (>1 mo duration)
- Cytomegalovirus disease (other than liver, spleen, or nodes)
- Cytomegalovirus retinitis (with loss of vision)
- Encephalopathy attributed to HIV
- Herpes simplex: chronic ulcers (>1 mo duration) or bronchitis, pneumonitis, or esophagitis
- Histoplasmosis, disseminated or extrapulmonary
- Isosporiasis, chronic intestinal (>1 mo duration)
- Kaposi sarcoma

- Lymphoma
  - Burkitt
  - Immunoblastic
  - Primary, of brain
- *Mycobacterium avium* complex or *Mycobacterium kansasii*, disseminated or extrapulmonary
- *Mycobacterium tuberculosis* of any site
- Mycobacterium, other species or unidentified species, disseminated or extrapulmonary
- *Pneumocystis jirovecii* (previously known as *Pneumocystis carinii*) pneumonia
- Pneumonia, recurrent (age ≥6 y)
- Progressive multifocal leukoencephalopathy
- *Salmonella* septicemia, recurrent
- Toxoplasmosis of brain, onset at age >1 mo
- Wasting syndrome attributed to HIV

Abbreviation: HIV, human immunodeficiency virus.

Adapted from Centers for Disease Control and Prevention (CDC). Revised surveillance case definition for HIV infection—United States, 2014. MMWR Morb Mortal Wkly Rep 2014;63(3):1–10.

MEDICAL MANAGEMENT

Currently, the primary goal of HIV treatment is to reduce the active replication of the virus, thus preventing the immune system decline that leads to the development of opportunistic infections and cancers. A secondary goal is to reduce the risk of HIV transmission by reducing the level of viremia to undetectable levels, thereby decreasing infectivity.[15] This is achieved through the use of antiretroviral drugs that work at different stages of viral entry and replication. The 6 classes of drugs currently used for treatment are:

- Nucleoside and nucleotide reverse transcriptase inhibitors (NRTIs, NtRTIs)
  - Blocks the enzyme reverse transcriptase needed for HIV to copy itself
- Non-NRTIs (NNRTIs)
  - Alters reverse transcriptase
- Protease inhibitors (PIs)
  - Blocks the enzyme protease needed for replication
- Fusion inhibitors
  - Blocks HIV from entering $CD4^+$ cells
- Entry inhibitors
  - Blocks CCR5 coreceptor proteins on the $CD4^+$ cells needed for HIV entry
- Integrase strand transfer inhibitors
  - Blocks the enzyme integrase needed for HIV replication.

The Food and Drug Administration approved the NRTI zidovudine, the first anti-HIV drug approved for use in the United States, on March 20, 1987. Alone, it was unable to suppress the virus for long periods of time and patients would eventually develop one or more of the opportunistic infections and cancers seen in stage 3 disease, leading ultimately to death.[16] In 1995, highly active antiretroviral therapy was introduced, which combined 2 NRTIs with a PI with more promising results. The use of highly active antiretroviral therapy led to prolonged viral suppression and prevention of the immune system decline. Current antiretroviral treatments can achieve almost full suppression of viral replication, preventing HIV transmission, prolonging survival to almost normal life expectancies, and reducing HIV-related morbidity. However, even with no detectable viral load, latent reservoirs of HIV in resting T cells remain a major barrier to curing HIV infection.[17] Therefore, treatment of HIV infection requires lifelong adherence to combination therapy to maintain viral suppression.[18] A combination of 3 drugs from 2 or more classes is the current standard for chronic HIV treatment (cART) and it is now possible to achieve indefinite viral replication suppression on once-a-day single tablet regimens that combine multiple drugs with reduced side effects.[19] Currently, there are 25 Food and Drug Administration–approved HIV medicines and 14 combination medicines that contain 2 or more HIV medicines from different classes. Additionally, pharmacokinetic enhancers are used to increase the effectiveness of the HIV medications (**Fig. 3**).

Current treatment guidelines recommend initiation of cART at the time of HIV diagnosis, regardless of disease stage.[20] There is no standard cART regimen. For a treatment-naïve patient, an antiretroviral regimen generally consists of 2 NRTIs combined with an integrase strand transfer inhibitor, an NNRTI, or a pharmacologically boosted PI.[21] Which drugs are chosen depends on resistance testing, presenting viral load and $CD4^+$ at the time of diagnosis, and comorbid conditions. Treatment goals include long-term suppression of plasma HIV RNA to less than the level of detection by available assays, restoration and preservation of immune function to reduce the morbidity and mortality associated with infection, and prevention of HIV transmission.[22]

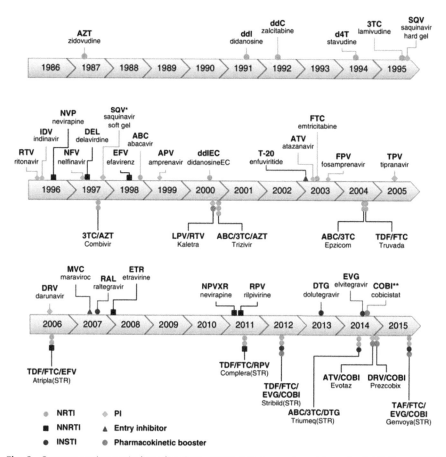

Fig. 3. Current antiretroviral medications. INSTI, integrase strand transfer inhibitor; NNRTI, nonnucleoside reverse transcriptase inhibitor; NRTI, nucleoside reverse transcriptase inhibitor; PI, protease inhibitor. **COBI has no antiretroviral activity. (*From* Cihlar T, Fordyce M. Current status and prospects of HIV treatment. Curr Opin Virol 2016;18:51; with permission.)

The success of cART has shifted the focus of medical care from the treatment and prevention of opportunistic infections to the surveillance of long-term toxicities and treatment of age-related conditions. By 2020, it is projected that 75% of the HIV-positive population in the United States will be 50 years or older.[23,24] People with durable viral suppression are living longer and dying from non–AIDS-related causes. However, compared with non–HIV-positive individuals, those with HIV have increased prevalence of premature age-associated diseases[25] and increased morbidity and mortality (**Box 2**).[26,27] Studies suggest that HIV is an independent risk factor for cardiovascular disease. HIV-positive patients are at a 2-fold increased risk of developing cardiovascular disease, including ischemic hearth disease, heart failure, and myocardial infarction[28–30] even after controlling for age and traditional cardiovascular risk factors, like tobacco use.[31] Rates of chronic and end-stage renal disease,[32,33] and liver disease (especially associated with alcohol abuse and coinfection with the hepatitis C virus) are also significantly higher. Significant hepatoxicity can also occur from cART medications. Use of some HIV medicines increase blood glucose levels and lead to the development of diabetes, especially in patients who are overweight,

---

Box 2
Age-related non-HIV complications more common in HIV-positive individuals

- Hypertension
- Cardiovascular disease
  - Ischemic heart disease
  - Myocardial infarction
  - Congestive heart failure
  - Stroke
- Hyperlipidemia
- Cancer
  - Lymphoma
  - Lung (independent of tobacco use)[86]
  - Colorectal
  - Skin
  - Anal
- Diabetes
- Liver disease
- Osteopenia and osteoporosis
- Neurologic
  - Peripheral neuropathy
  - Cognitive impairment
  - Dementia
- Pulmonary disease
  - COPD
  - Pulmonary hypertension
- Renal disease
  - Chronic
  - End stage

Abbreviations: COPD, chronic obstructive pulmonary disease; HIV, human immunodeficiency virus.

---

physically inactive, have a family history of diabetes, or have hepatitis C coinfection.[34] Osteopenia and osteoporosis are increased, especially in patients with renal disease. During the first 1 to 2 years after initiation of cART, patients may lose up to 6% of their bone mineral density at the hip and spine, resulting in an increased risk of fracture.[35] It is postulated that the premature development of these complications may be the result of a combination of natural aging, lifestyle factors (smoking, and drug and alcohol abuse), drug-specific toxicity, and persistent immune dysfunction and inflammation even in patients with nondetectable viral loads (**Fig. 4**).[36]

LABORATORY MONITORING

A number of routine laboratory tests are done to assess the patient's response to treatment and drug effectiveness, monitor the status of the immune system, and detect antiviral resistance and any possible toxicity or adverse reaction to medication. Possible toxicities include thrombocytopenia, anemia, neutropenia, peripheral neuropathy, hepatotoxicity, hyperglycemia, dyslipidemia, lipodystrophy, osteopenia, osteoporosis, and accelerated cardiovascular disease[37] (**Table 2**). Several factors may increase the incidence of adverse effects of cART, including the use of other medications with

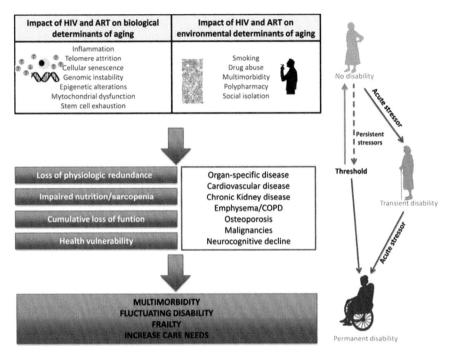

Impact of HIV and ART on biological determinants of aging	Impact of HIV and ART on environmental determinants of aging
Inflammation Telomere attrition Cellular senescence Genomic instability Epigenetic alterations Mytochondrial dysfunction Stem cell exhaustion	Smoking Drug abuse Multimorbidity Polypharmacy Social isolation

No disability

Acute stressor

Persistent stressors

Threshold

Transient disability

Loss of physiologic redundance

Impaired nutrition/sarcopenia

Cumulative loss of funtion

Health vulnerability

Organ-specific disease
Cardiovascular disease
Chronic Kidney disease
Emphysema/COPD
Osteoporosis
Malignancies
Neurocognitive decline

Acute stressor

MULTIMORBIDITY
FLUCTUATING DISABILITY
FRAILTY
INCREASE CARE NEEDS

Permanent disability

Fig. 4. Human immunodeficiency virus (HIV) infection as a chronic disease. ART, antiretroviral therapy; COPD, chronic obstructive pulmonary disease. (*From* Serrano-Villar S, Gutiérrez F, Miralles C, et al. Human immunodeficiency virus as a chronic disease: evaluation and management of nonacquired immune deficiency syndrome-defining conditions. Open Forum Infect Dis 2016;3(2):9; with permission.)

additive effects, comorbid conditions such as hepatitis or substance abuse, and low CD4$^+$ counts. Monitoring response to therapy is a long-term requirement, because more than 85% of HIV-infected individuals in the United States live more than 10 years from time of diagnosis.[38] CD4$^+$ cell counts in combination with levels of HIV replication (viral load) are the most reliable predictors of disease progression and prognosis.

CD4$^+$ Lymphocyte Counts

CD4$^+$ lymphocyte counts provide information on the overall immune function. The normal range is 500 to 1500 cells/μL. The CD4$^+$ count is a predictor of the risk of opportunistic infections as well as subsequent disease progression and survival. The CD4$^+$ count is used to determine the need for initiation and discontinuation of opportunistic infection prophylaxis. Systemic and oral opportunistic infections begin to appear when the CD4$^+$ count decreases to less than 500 cells/μL, and severe immunosuppression (CD4$^+$ <200 cells/μL) predisposes the patient to life-threatening infections. It is measured at entry to care and then every 4 to 6 months for the first 2 years. If the patient is virally suppressed and the CD4$^+$ counts are consistently greater than 500 cells/μL, then monitoring can be done annually.[39]

Human Immunodeficiency Virus RNA (Viral Load)

Viral load is used as a marker of viral replication. It measures the number of copies of HIV RNA that are present in the peripheral blood. The range is undetectable (<20–50 copies depending on the test used) to greater than 750,000 copies/mL. It is the most

Table 2
Adverse reactions to cART medications

Adverse Event	NRTIs	NNRTIs	PIs	INSTIs	EIs
Anemia/neutropenia	+	−	−	−	−
Bleeding events	−	−	+	−	−
Cardiovascular disease	+	−	+	−	−
Diabetes/insulin resistance	+	−	+	−	−
Dyslipidemia	+	+	+	+	−
Gastrointestinal effects	+	−	+	+	−
Hepatoxicity	+	+	+	−	+
Lipodystrophy	+	+	+	+	−
Nervous system/psychiatric	+	+	−	+	−
Osteopenia/osteoporosis	+	+	+	+	−
Renal effects	+	−	+	+	−
Steven-Johnson syndrome	+	+	+	+	−

Abbreviations: cART, combination antiretroviral drugs; EI, entry inhibitor; INSTI, integrase strand transfer inhibitor; NNRTI, nonnucleoside reverse transcriptase inhibitor; NRTI, nucleoside reverse transcriptase inhibitor; PI, protease inhibitor.

Adapted from Panel on Antiretroviral Guidelines for Adults and Adolescents. Guidelines for the use of antiretroviral agents in HIV-1-infected adults and adolescents. Department of Health and Human Services. Available at: http://aidsinfo.nih.gov/contentfiles/lvguidelines/AdultandAdolescent GL.pdf. Accessed February 15, 2016.

important indicator of response to highly active antiretroviral therapy, with viral loads of greater than 200 copies/mL in the presence of cART considered virologic failure.[40] It is measured at entry into care, at initiation of therapy, every 4 to 8 weeks until suppression is achieved, and then every 4 to 6 months in stable patients. Pretreatment viral load levels are also important in selecting the initial cART regimen because patients with high baseline viral loads may have poorer responses to some medications.

A complete blood count including a differential is important to monitor the level of neutrophils, red blood cells, hemoglobin and hematocrit, and platelets. Both HIV and cART medications can cause bone marrow suppression, leading to neutropenia, anemia, and thrombocytopenia, as well as increased susceptibility to infection and bleeding. These values are generally monitored every 6 months, although patients with more advanced HIV disease may require more frequent evaluations, especially before invasive procedures.

Other Tests

Blood chemistry tests including electrolytes, renal function, liver panel, glucose, and fasting lipids should be done at before beginning cART therapy and then monitored every 3 to 6 months to watch for medication-induced abnormalities. Comorbidities like coinfection with hepatitis C or substance abuse may necessitate more careful monitoring of liver function tests. Baseline testing for hepatitis B and C, tuberculosis, and sexually transmitted diseases should be performed at the time of initial diagnosis of HIV before initiation of cART.

PREVENTION OF NEW INFECTIONS

In pregnant and nursing women, cART can eliminate mother-to-child transmission.[41] Sexual transmission can be prevented in serodiscordant encounters if the

HIV-infected partner achieves and maintains viral suppression.[42] Additionally, in July of 2012, the Food and Drug Administration approved the use of emtricitabine/tenofovir (Truvada) as preexposure prophylaxis against HIV infection for HIV-negative individuals in conjunction with other risk reduction and safer sex strategies. Adherence is essential and preexposure prophylaxis only works as a preventive measure if it is taken daily.[43] Routine medical follow-up is needed, including HIV testing and sexually transmitted infection screening every 3 months. It is currently recommended for any HIV-seronegative person engaging in high-risk behavior, including[20,44,45]:

- Men who have unprotected sex with men or a diagnosis of a sexually transmitted disease within the last 6 months.
- Heterosexual men and women who have unprotected sex with partners of unknown HIV status with risk factors.
- A history of injection drug use in the last month with sharing of equipment.
- Discordant heterosexual and homosexual partners.

Postexposure prophylaxis is an emergency intervention in the event of an occupational (needle stick/sharp exposure or mucous membrane splash) or nonoccupational (sexual or injecting drugs) exposure to potentially infectious bodily fluids. Guidelines recommend postexposure prophylaxis initiation ideally within 2 hours of exposure. Efficacy begins to decrease within 24 to 36 hours and is not recommended if more than 72 hours has passed since exposure.[46] Treatment begins without waiting for confirmation of HIV serostatus of the source patient. Baseline assessment includes HIV testing with combination antibody/antigen test as well as hepatitis B and C serologies with follow-up testing of HIV serostatus at 4 weeks, 3 months, and 6 months after exposure. The recommended drug schedule is 28 days of daily emtricitabine/tenofovir plus twice-daily raltegravir (Isentress) or once-daily dolutegravir (Tivicay). An alternative regimen includes the use of daily tenofovir/emtricitabine/cobicistat/elvitegravir (Stribild).[47]

The risk of infection after an occupational exposure depends on a number of variables, including the quantity of blood or infectious fluid involved, exposure to the blood of an HIV-positive patient with a high viral load, injuries that occurred with a hollow-bore, blood-filled needle or sharp that was in the vein or artery of the source patient, a deep percutaneous injury, or contact with a mucous membrane or nonintact skin. The risk of infection varies for specific bloodborne pathogens from 0.09% to 30%[48] (**Box 3**).

Box 3	
Risk of infection for specific blood-borne pathogens	
Hepatitis B	
Hepatitis B surface antigen positive, hepatitis B e antigen negative	1%–6%
Hepatitis B surface antigen positive, hepatitis B e antigen positive	22%–30%
Hepatitis C	1.8%–3%
HIV	
Percutaneous exposure to blood	0.3%–0.5%
Mucous membrane exposure	0.09%
Abbreviation: HIV, human immunodeficiency virus.	
Data from Centers for Disease Control and Prevention (CDC). Oral health: infection control. Available at: http://www.cdc.gov/oralhealth/infectioncontrol/faq/bloodborne_exposures.htm. Accessed June 4, 2016.	

DENTAL MANAGEMENT

Because patients are living longer with HIV, more are seeking comprehensive dental care. Oral health care is an integral and important part of comprehensive health care for all patients with HIV/AIDS. Dental management of the asymptomatic HIV-infected patient is the same as treatment of the non–HIV-positive patient. Medical assessment of HIV-infected dental patients does not differ from that of any medically complex dental patient. The majority of HIV-infected patients are medically stable, requiring little to no modification in the delivery of dental care. The medical history of HIV-infected individuals that will most likely impact on the delivery of dental care will not be related to HIV immunosuppression, but rather will be related to non–HIV-associated conditions. Patients who report being HIV positive should be asked about any history of opportunistic diseases, knowledge of recent blood values, and any history of increased bleeding tendencies. Patients should be asked about comorbid conditions, especially cardiovascular disease, diabetes, or the presence of hepatitis-induced liver disease. Coinfection with hepatitis C occurs in up to 25% of all HIV-positive patients (>80% of HIV-infected injection drug users)[49] and can cause more rapid HIV progression as well as increasing hepatotoxicity from cART medications. Baseline vitals signs including blood pressure and pulse should be taken at the initial visit and before any invasive procedure. A social history including evaluation of prior or current use of tobacco, alcohol, or other illicit drugs should be obtained and patients should be counseled on modifiable risk factors, especially tobacco cessation. Medical consultation should be obtained based on detailed health history and physical findings. If the patient is on cART and is being monitored regularly by a medical provider and can verbally provide information about current blood values, there is no need to withhold noninvasive dental treatment (restorative, nonsurgical periodontal, or endodontic therapy) until medical consultation is obtained. For patients who are unable to provide information about their disease progression or current treatment regimens, patients with advanced disease (either HIV or comorbid conditions) and patients requiring surgical procedures, consultation with the medical provider and recent laboratory work including complete blood count with differential and platelets, should be obtained before initiating treatment.

Patients should be treated the same as any other patient, using standard universal precautions. The Americans with Disabilities Act of 1990 prohibits refusing to treat solely on the basis that a patient is HIV-infected.[50] Dentists may not:

- Plead ignorance as a reason for refusing to treat HIV-infected patients
- Refuse to treat HIV-infected patients because of the risk of transmission
- Inquire about a patient's HIV status unless the inquiry is asked of all patients
- Inquire how a patient obtain HIV unless in context of assessing other medical conditions
- Require HIV testing before treatment
- Increase the cost of service for additional precautions
- Limit the time of service unless procedure based

All new HIV-infected patients should have a comprehensive oral evaluation including appropriate radiographs, through extraoral and intraoral soft tissue examination and dental and periodontal examinations. Particular attention should be paid to identifying orofacial conditions that may be associated with reduced CD4$^+$ counts and HIV disease progression (**Box 4**). With the introduction of cART, the incidence of oral mucosal lesions associated with HIV has decreased with the exception of

---

Box 4
Orofacial conditions associated with immunosuppression

- Candidiasis
  - Psuedomembranous
  - Erythematous
  - Hyperplastic
  - Angular chelitis
- Hairy leukoplakia
- Kaposi's sarcoma
- Linear gingival erythema
- Necrotizing ulcerative gingivitis/periodontitis
- Necrotizing ulcerative stomatitis
- Major recurrent aphthous ulcers
- Oral warts
- Recurrent herpes simplex
- Salivary gland enlargement

---

human papillomavirus–associated oral lesions.[51,52] The appearance of oral lesions may be a sign of virologic failure and may indicate the need for the patient's cART regimen to be evaluated. Oral candidiasis is the most common oral lesion seen, especially in patients who smoke, wear removable prostheses, or have xerostomia.[53] Xerostomia may occur in up to 70% of HIV-positive patients as both a manifestation of HIV infection and as a side effect associated with medications used for the treatment of HIV and other medical comorbidities such as depression, hypertension, and diabetes.[54]

TREATMENT MODIFICATIONS

Treatment planning modifications for HIV-infected patients should be based on the patient's general medical health, not on the patient's HIV status. Modifications should occur if the patient has significant physical manifestations of HIV/AIDS or side effects from medications that impacts on their ability to withstand dental visits or compromises the outcome. Peripheral neuropathy as a side effect of some cART medications may impact on the patient's manual dexterity and may become a factor in terms of ability to perform adequate oral hygiene. Treatment planning should follow the same order as with other patients—alleviate pain, promote good oral health, control and prevent disease, restore function, and address functional and aesthetic concerns. The oral health care provider should recommend the preferred course of treatment, present alternative treatments (if any), and discuss the probable benefits, limitations, and risk associated with the proposed treatment.

Asymptomatic HIV-infected patients need no significant modifications in treatment planning or the delivery of care based solely on their HIV status. There are no contraindications for general dental procedures, including extractions, implant placement, and endodontic therapy. Baseline viral load and $CD4^+$ counts can be useful in determining where a patient is in terms of the stability of treatment and to alert the clinician to the need to monitor for opportunistic infections, but neither is necessary to deliver care. The viral load has no direct impact on the delivery of dental care, it does not give any information on current health status, does not predict how well a patient will tolerate a dental procedure, and is not used to determine the need for antibiotic prophylaxis before dental therapy. Likewise, the $CD4^+$ count has no direct impact on the delivery of dental care. A low $CD4^+$ count is not a valid reason to withhold or delay dental treatment and it should never be used to determine the need for antibiotic prophylaxis before dental therapy.

For patients with more advanced HIV/AIDS, patients need to be evaluated on a case-by-case basis. Laboratory tests become more important in helping to guide modifications in treatment. The HIV virus can have a direct myelosuppressive effect on the bone marrow, leading to anemia, neutropenia, and thrombocytopenia. Patients with coinfection with hepatitis B or C virus or those with medication induced hepatic changes may be at increased risk of bleeding owing to alteration in clotting factors. Bleeding abnormalities or increased susceptibility to bacterial infections should be managed the same as for the non–HIV-positive patient. Laboratory values for hemoglobin, white blood cells (particularly neutrophils, which are essential in preventing bacterial infections), platelets, and coagulation values should be checked to ensure they are above minimal levels needed to treat before undertaking invasive procedures (**Table 3**). If the patient has severe symptoms of AIDS that interfere with the provision of safe dental treatment or impair the patient's ability to endure treatment in a dental care setting, pain and infection should be managed, but elective treatment should be deferred until the patient's medical condition has improved.

There are no data to support routine antibiotic prophylaxis for patients with HIV disease based solely on $CD4^+$ counts before invasive procedures expected to produce transient bacteremias owing to mucosal manipulation. This is true even when the $CD4^+$ counts are less than 200 cell/mm^3. Susceptibility to infections may be determined by assessing the absolute neutrophil count, which provide defense against most bacterial infections. The absolute neutrophil count is usually provided as a part of a complete blood count with differential, but it can also be calculated by multiplying the total number of white blood cells by the percentage of neutrophils. Although there are no specific recommendations regarding the need for antibiotic prophylaxis, patients with severe neutropenia (<500 cells/mm^3) might benefit from a therapeutic antibiotic regimen starting with a loading dose at the time of the procedure and followed by 5 to 7 days of postoperative antibiotics.[55,56] Less than 1% of HIV-infected dental patients are likely to develop severe neutropenia[55] and it is generally only seen in patients with advanced disease. Antibiotic prophylaxis according to the 2007 American Heart Association guidelines are indicated for most dental procedures if the patient has a history of infectious endocarditis or cardiac valve replacement.[57]

DENTAL CARIES

Patients with HIV disease may be more prone to dental decay. Factors include HIV- and medication-induced xerostomia, medication related acid reflux, impaired ability to perform oral hygiene, cariogenic diet, and an increased rate of substance abuse. Caries management by risk assessment (CAMBRA)[58] should be used to formulate a therapeutic and preventive plan. Appropriate restorative procedures should be used for existing decay in conjunction with remineraliziation techniques such as fluoride varnishes and daily application of prescribed high-concentration fluoride toothpastes, rinses, or gels for those patients with identified risk factors to prevent future breakdown. The initiation of complex fixed restorations should be delayed until adequate caries control is achieved and the patient's ability to maintain good oral hygiene has been assessed. Patients at high risk should have more frequent periodic examinations

Table 3
Pertinent laboratory values

Cell Type	Normal (cells/mm³)		Minimum	Impact on Dental Care
Hemoglobin	14–18 g/dL (males); 12–16 g/dL (females)		<7 g/dL	Need to establish baseline value if excessive bleeding is anticipated. Medical consultation indicated for values <7 g/dL
White blood cells	4500–10,000 cells/μL (4.5–10.0)		2000 cells/μL	Neutrophil counts should be evaluated if total WBC <2000
Absolute neutrophil count	2,5000–7000 (2.5–7.0)		500 (0.5)	If <500 (0.5), antibiotic prophylaxis needed before invasive procedures
Platelets	150,000–450,000		50,000	Between 100,000 and 70,000: local hemostatic measures indicated. Between 70,000 and 50,000: case-by-case basis depending on other bleeding risk factors. <50,000: transfusion may be needed
CD4⁺/CD4%	544–1663	32–60		As CD4⁺/% decreases, OIs increases. No direct impact on dental care
	<500	<32		Primary immune suppression. No direct impact on dental care
	<400	<29		OIs including early oral lesions. Monitor oral cavity for candida. No direct impact of dental care
	200–400	14–28		Increased number and severity of OIs. Monitor oral cavity for oral OIs. Recent CBC/platelets before invasive procedures
	<200	<14		Severe immune suppression, major OIs, AIDS diagnosis. Patient should be closely monitored for presence of oral OIs; recare appointments every 3–4 mo. Recent CBC/platelets before invasive procedure
	<100			Fatal OIs, neoplasms, severe oral lesions. Patient should be monitored closely for the presence of oral OIs; recare appointments every 2–3 mo. Recent CBC/platelets before invasive procedure
Viral load	Range of detection <20–50 to >750,000 copies/mL			>200 copies/mL may indicate virologic failure. No direct impact on dental care
PT	11–14 s		<21 s	Medical consultation may be needed if procedure is expected to cause substantial bleeding. Good surgical technique with aggressive local hemostatic measures usually sufficient
PTT	25–35 s		<55 s	
INR	0.8–1.2		<3.5	

Abbreviations: CBC, complete blood count; OIs, opportunistic infections; INR, international normalized ratio; PT, prothrombin time; PTT, partial thromboplastin time.

to monitor for early signs of demineralization or decay and to reinforce preventive measures.

ENDODONTIC TREATMENT

Endodontic treatment offers many benefits and few drawbacks for HIV-infected patients. Although the DNA of the virus can be detected in periradicular lesions and in pulpal tissue,[59,60] there is no indication that HIV causes pulpal disease. Several retrospective and cohort studies have shown no increased incidence of postoperative complications and equal rates of healing of periapical lesions after endodontic therapy among HIV-positive patients, even in patients with $CD4^+$ cells of less than 200 cells/mm^3.[61–64] Postoperative infection rates were comparable with those among noninfected patients, even when no antibiotics were given.[65,66] The routine use of systemic antibiotics during endodontic therapy is not indicated.[67]

SURGICAL PROCEDURES AND IMPLANTS

The current platelet count and white blood cell count should be checked before any surgical intervention in patients with advanced HIV disease and any modification of treatment be based on abnormal results. Studies report no significant increase in postoperative surgical complications or infections in HIV-positive patients.[68] Complications, when they do occur, tend to be minor and easily treatable in an outpatient setting.[66,69] Prosthetic rehabilitation using dental implants is a viable and reasonable option regardless of $CD4^+$ cell count, viral load levels, or type of antiretroviral therapy.[70] Case selection is similar to any other population of patients, including bony anatomy and the presence of other medical contraindications such as poorly controlled diabetes, advanced renal or liver disease, or tobacco use.[71,72] Several studies and systematic reviews have shown no increased rate of infection and similar osseous integration in patients with well-controlled HIV as compared with a non-HIV cohort,[73–75] as well as similar healing from sinus lifts and bone augmentation surgeries.[76,77] Antibiotics should be used sparingly and should be based on clinical judgment rather than the patient's HIV status.

PERIODONTAL AND PREVENTIVE CARE

Among US adults, 46% have chronic periodontitis and the incidence increases with age.[78] Factors such as tobacco use and diabetes can contribute to the progression of periodontal disease. A risk assessment for periodontal disease should be done for each patient at their initial visit and include any history of HIV-related periodontal disease, such as linear gingival erythema or necrotizing gingivitis/periodontitis. A comprehensive gingival and periodontal examination with periodontal probing depths, plaque index, and assessment of oral hygiene performance should also be performed and include the evaluation of manual dexterity in the cases of medication-induced peripheral neuropathy. The importance of the maintenance of good daily oral hygiene should be stressed. Scaling and root planing are recommended for the nonsurgical treatment of periodontal disease. Surgical therapy, including open flap debridement, can be performed without postoperative complications as long as minimal hematologic levels are present. The modification of oral hygiene implements and adjunctive use of a daily antimicrobial mouth rinse such as 0.12% chlorhexidine may be considered for patients unable to maintain optimum oral health through routine preventive care.[79,80] Recare schedule should be individualized for each patient based on clinical findings with more frequent examinations and cleaning for those patients with a history of necrotizing gingivitis/periodontitis, diabetes, or chronic periodontitis.

MANAGEMENT OF ORAL CANDIDIASIS

Oral candidiasis remains the most common oral manifestations of HIV infection.[81] Risk factors include:

- Xerostomia
- Smoking
- Poor oral hygiene
- Removable prostheses
- CD4$^+$ counts of less than 300 cells[3]
- Uncontrolled diabetes
- Recent use of systemic antibiotics

A thorough soft tissue examination should be done at regular intervals to monitor for intraoral candida as well as angular chelitis. Patients with CD4$^+$ counts of less than 200 cells/mm^3 should be placed on a more frequent recare schedule to monitor for candida. Patients should be educated in ways to reduce predisposing factors such as improving oral and prosthetic hygiene, treatment of xerostomia with salivary substitutes and stimulants, smoking cessation, and decreasing dietary sugar intake.[82] Various topical and systemic antifungals are available for the treatment of oral candidiasis. Most topical rinses, creams, and ointments require multiple daily applications and have poor patient compliance. Oral troches and pastilles are ineffective in patients with xerostomia because they do not dissolve adequately. Fluconazole (either a 14-day regimen of 100 mg/d or a single-dose regimen of 750 mg)[83,84] or a 14-day course of once-daily 50 mg miconazole delivered in an adhesive buccal tab are effective treatments for most cases and have increased patient adherence. Patients should be instructed in daily denture care, including daily removal and cleaning of the prosthesis and soaking overnight in a commercially available denture cleaner. For patients who develop a candida infection, treatment of the prosthesis is necessary to prevent reinfection. This can be achieved by soaking the denture tissue side down in an antifungal nystatin solution or a dilute solution of water with bleach (patients should be instructed to thoroughly rinse the denture off before placing back in the oral cavity). Care should be taken to clean the denture cup daily with soap and water, as well as disinfecting toothbrushes (by soaking in commercially available antimicrobial mouth rinse or 0.12% chlorhexidine oral rinse)[85] after use. Older prosthesis, especially those in disrepair, might need to be refabricated to eliminate the presence of candida hyphae in the acrylic.

SUMMARY

With the advent of modern cART medications, HIV has become a chronic disease with patients living for decades after diagnosis (**Box 5**). HIV is not a valid reason to deny, delay, or withhold dental treatment. The delivery of oral health care is the same for the HIV-infected patient as for the non–HIV-infected patient. There are no absolute contraindications and few complications associated with comprehensive oral health care treatment delivered in an outpatient setting for asymptomatic HIV-infected patients and clinically stable patients with AIDS. Medical assessment of HIV-infected dental patients does not differ from that of any medically complex dental patient. The medical history of HIV-infected individuals that will most likely impact on the delivery of dental care will not be related to HIV immunosuppression but rather will be

> **Box 5**
> **Summary of dental considerations**
>
> - No contraindications to routine dental care in an outpatient setting
> - Get current laboratory values before any invasive procedure, especially if CD4$^+$ less than 200 cells/mm^3
>   - ANC and platelets most important values
> - Antibiotic prophylaxis based on ANC, not CD4$^+$/VL
> - Important to evaluate
>   - Ability to clot
>   - Ability to recover from bacteremia
>   - Ability to endure treatment in your dental care setting
>   - Comorbid conditions
>   - Cardiovascular
>   - Liver
>   - Diabetes
> - Awareness of potential drug side effects
> - May need more frequent recare appointments
>   - Decreased salivary flow and increased caries
>   - Increased frequency of periodontal disease
>   - Monitor oral cavity for signs of opportunistic infections
> - Rate of postoperative complications comparable to non-HIV population
>   - Most owing to non–HIV-related issues
>
> *Abbreviations:* ANC, absolute neutrophil count; HIV, human immunodeficiency virus; VL, viral load.

related to non–HIV-associated conditions. Consultation with the patient's medical provider and modifications in the delivery of dental treatment may be necessary when treating patients with advanced HIV disease or other comorbid conditions that may be present in this population especially cardiovascular disease, diabetes, and liver disease. Oral health care is an integral and important part of comprehensive health care for all patients with HIV/AIDS and the oral health care provider an essential part of the patient's primary health team.

REFERENCES

1. Weiss RA. How does HIV cause AIDS? Science 1993;260(5112):1273–9.
2. Moss AR, Bacchetti P. Natural history of HIV infection. AIDS 1989;3:55–61.
3. World Health Organization. Global Health Observatory (GHO) data. Available at: http://www.who.int/gho/hiv/en/. Accessed June 2, 2016.
4. HIV in the United States: At a glance. Available at: http://www.cdc.gov/hiv/statistics/overview/ataglance.html. Accessed June 2, 2016.
5. Centers for Disease Control and Prevention. HIV Surveillance Report, 2014. 2015. vol. 26. Available at: http://www.cdc.gov/hiv/library/reports/surveillance/. Accessed June 2, 2016.
6. Kumar V. Disease of the immune system. In: Aster JC, Abbas AK, Robbins SL, et al, editors. Robbins Basic Pathology. 9th edition. Philadelphia: Elsevier Saunders; 2013. p. 147.
7. Doitsh G, Galloway NL, Geng X, et al. Pyroptosis drives CD4 T-cell depletion in HIV-1 infection. Nature 2014;505(7484):509–14.

8. Douek DC, Roederer M, Koup RA. Emerging concepts in the immunopathogenesis of AIDS. Annu Rev Med 2009;60:471–84.
9. Centers for Disease Control and Prevention. Revised surveillance case definitions for HIV infection—United States, 2014. MMWR Recomm Rep 2014; 63(RR-03):1–10.
10. Pai NP, Balram B, Shivkumar S, et al. Head-to-head comparison of accuracy of a rapid point-of-care HIV test with oral versus whole-blood specimens: a systematic review and meta-analysis. Lancet Infect Dis 2012;12:373–80.
11. Kahn JO, Walker BD. Acute human immunodeficiency virus type 1 infection. N Engl J Med 1998;339:33–9.
12. Schacker T, Collier AC, Hughes J, et al. Clinical and epidemiologic features of primary HIV infection. Ann Intern Med 1996;125:257–64.
13. Hecht FM, Busch MP, Rawal B, et al. Use of laboratory tests and clinical symptoms for identification of primary HIV infection. AIDS 2002;16:1119–29.
14. Fiebig EW, Wright DJ, Rawal BD, et al. Dynamics of HIV viremia and antibody seroconversion in plasma donors: implications for diagnosis and staging of primary HIV infection. AIDS 2003;17:1871–9.
15. Cohen MS, Chen YQ, McCauley M, et al. Prevention of HIV-1 infection with early antiretroviral therapy. N Engl J Med 2011;365(6):493–505.
16. Moore RD, Chaisson RE. Natural history of opportunistic disease in an HIV-infected urban clinical cohort. Ann Intern Med 1996;124:633–42.
17. Siliciano JD, Siliciano RF. Recent developments in the effort to cure HIV infection: going beyond N= 1. J Clin Invest 2016;126(2):409.
18. Cihlar T, Fordyce M. Current status and prospects of HIV treatment. Curr Opin Virol 2016;18:50–6.
19. Gunthard HF, Saag MS, Benson CA, et al. Antiretroviral treatment of adult HIV infection: 2014 recommendations of the International antiviral society-USA panel. JAMA 2014;312(4):410–25.
20. Günthard HF, Saag MS, Benson CA, et al. Antiretroviral drugs for treatment and prevention of HIV infection in adults: 2016 recommendations of the international antiviral society-USA panel. JAMA 2016;316(2):191–210.
21. Recommendations Regarding Initial Combination Regimens for the Antiretroviral-Naïve Patient in Panel on Antiretroviral Guidelines for Adults and Adolescents. Guidelines for the use of antiretroviral agents in HIV-1-infected adults and adolescents. Department of Health and Human Services. Available at: http://aidsinfo.nih.gov/contentfiles/lvguidelines/AdultandAdolescentGL.pdf. Accessed June 2, 2016.
22. Panel on Antiretroviral Guidelines for Adults and Adolescents. Guidelines for the use of antiretroviral agents in HIV-1-infected adults and adolescents. Department of Health and Human Services. Available at: http://aidsinfo.nih.gov/contentfiles/lvguidelines/AdultandAdolescentGL.pdf. Accessed June 2, 2016.
23. Effros RB, Fletcher CV, Gebo K, et al. Aging and infectious diseases: workshop on HIV infection and aging: what is known and future research directions. Clin Infect Dis 2008;47:542–53.
24. Smith C, Sabin CA, Lundgren JD, et al. Factors associated with specific causes of death amongst HIV-positive individuals in the D.A.D Study. AIDS 2010;24:1537–48.
25. Serrano-Villar S, Gutierrez F, Miralles C, et al. HIV as a chronic disease: evaluation and management of non-AIDS defining conditions. Open Forum Infectious Disease 2016;3(2):ofw097.

26. Deeks SG, Phillips AN. HIV infection, antiretroviral treatment, ageing, and non-AIDS related morbidity. BMJ 2009;338:a3172.

27. Falutz J. Pathophysiology of HIV/AIDS. Managing the older adult patient with HIV. Switzerland: Springer International Publishing; 2016. p. 7–18.

28. Freiberg MS, Chang CC, Kuller LH, et al. HIV infection and the risk of acute myocardial infarction. JAMA Intern Med 2013;173:614–22.

29. Mary-Krause M, Cotte L, Simon A, et al. Increased risk of myocardial infarction with duration of protease inhibitor therapy in HIV-infected men. AIDS 2003;17: 2479–86.

30. Nou E, Lo J, Hadigan C, et al. Pathophysiology and management of cardiovascular disease in patients with HIV. Lancet Diabetes Endocrinol 2016;4(7): 598–610.

31. Triant VA, Lee H, Hadigan C, et al. Increased acute myocardial infarction rates and cardiovascular risk factors among patients with human immunodeficiency virus disease. J Clin Endocrinol Metab 2007;92:2506–12.

32. Kalayjian RC, Lau B, Mechekano RN, et al. Risk factors for chronic kidney disease in a large cohort of HIV-1 infected individuals initiating antiretroviral therapy in routine care. AIDS 2012;26:1907–15.

33. Mocroft A, Kirk O, Gatell J, et al. Chronic renal failure among HIV-1-infected patients. AIDS 2007;21:1119–27.

34. Side Effects of HIV Medicines: HIV and Diabetes. Available at: https://aidsinfo.nih.gov/education-materials/fact-sheets/22/59/hiv-and-diabetes#. Accessed July 29, 2016.

35. Alvarez E, Belloso WH, Boyd MA, et al. Which HIV patients should be screened for osteoporosis: an international perspective. Curr Opin HIV AIDS 2016;11(3): 268–76.

36. Goulet JL, Fultz SL, Rimland D, et al. Aging and infectious diseases: do patterns of comorbidity vary by HIV status, age, and HIV severity? Clin Infect Dis 2007;45: 1593–601.

37. Panel on Antiretroviral Guidelines for Adults and Adolescents. Guidelines for the use of antiretroviral agents in HIV-1-infected adults and adolescents. Department of Health and Human Services. Available at: http://www.aidsinfo.nih.gov/ContentFiles/AdultandAdolescentGL.pdf. Accessed June 4, 2016.

38. Centers for Disease Control and Prevention. HIV Surveillance Report, 2014. vol. 26. Available at: http://www.cdc.gov/hiv/library/reports/surveillance/. Accessed June 2, 2016.

39. Aberg JA, Gallant JE, Ghanem KG. Primary care guidelines for the management of persons infected with HIV: 2013 update by the HIV medicine Association of the Infectious Diseases Society of America. Clin Infect Dis 2014;58:e1–34.

40. Guidelines for the use of antiretroviral agents in HIV-1-infected adults and adolescents, January 20, 2011. Developed by the DHHS Panel on Antiretroviral Guidelines for Adults and Adolescents—A Working Group of the Office of AIDS Research Advisory Council (OARAC). Available at: http://www.aidsinfo.nih.gov/ContentFiles/AdultandAdolescentGL.pdf. Accessed February 16, 2016.

41. Townsend CL, Byrne L, Cortina-Borja M, et al. Earlier initiation of ART and further decline in mother-to-child HIV transmission rates, 2000-2011. AIDS 2014;28(7): 1049–57.

42. Donnell D, Baeten JM, Kiarie J, et al. Partners in Prevention HSV/HIV Transmission Study Team. Heterosexual HIV-1 transmission after initiation of antiretroviral therapy: a prospective cohort analysis. Lancet 2010;375(9731):2092–8.

43. Cottrell ML, Yang KH, Prince HM, et al. A translational pharmacology approach to predicting outcomes of preexposure prophylaxis against HIV in men and women using tenofovir disoproxil fumarate with or without emtricitabine. J Infect Dis 2016; 214(1):55–64.

44. Grant RM, Lama JR, Anderson PL, et al, iPrEx Study Team. Preexposure chemoprophylaxis for HIV prevention in men who have sex with men. N Engl J Med 2010;363(27):2587–99.

45. Volk JE, Marcus JL, Phengrasamy T, et al. No new HIV infections with increasing use of HIV preexposure prophylaxis in a clinical practice setting. Clin Infect Dis 2015;61(10):1601–3.

46. Centers for Disease Control and Prevention. Updated guidelines for antiretroviral postexposure prophylaxis after sexual, injection drug use, or other nonoccupational exposure to HIV—United States, 2016. Available at: http://www.cdc.gov/hiv/pdf/programresources/cdc-hiv-npep-guidelines.pdf. Accessed June 4, 2016.

47. Kuhar DT, Henderson DK, Struble KA, et al. Updated US Public Health Service guidelines for the management of occupational exposures to human immunodeficiency virus and recommendations for postexposure prophylaxis. Infect Control Hosp Epidemiol 2013;34(09):875–92.

48. Cleveland JL, Gray SK, Harte JA, et al. Transmission of blood-borne pathogens in US dental health care settings: 2016 Update. J Am Dental Assoc 2016;147(9): 729–38.

49. From: Viral Hepatitis-CDC Recommendations for Specific Populations: HIV/AIDS. Available at: www.cdc.gov/hepatitis/populations/hiv.htm. Accessed March 3, 2016.

50. Bragdon v. Abbott 524 US 624 (1998).

51. Patton LL, Ramirez-Amador V, Anaya-Saavedra G, et al. Urban legends series: oral manifestations of HIV infection. Oral Dis 2013;19:533–50.

52. Sanders AE, Slade GD, Patton LL. National prevalence of oral HPV infection and related risk factors in the U.S. adult population. Oral Dis 2012;18:430–41.

53. Baccaglini L, Atkinson JC, Patton LL, et al. Management of oral lesions in HIV-positive patients. Oral Surg Oral Med Oral Pathol Oral Radiol Endod 2007; 103(Suppl 1):S50–63.

54. Busato IM, Thomaz M, Toda AI, et al. Prevalence and impact of xerostomia on the quality of life of people living with HIV/AIDS from Brazil. Spec Care Dentist 2013; 33:128–32.

55. Patton LL. Hematologic abnormalities among HIV-infected patients: associations of significance for dentistry. Oral Surg Oral Med Oral Pathol Oral Radiol Endod 1999;88:561–7.

56. Campo J, Cano J, Del Romero J, et al. Oral complication risks after invasive and non-invasive dental procedures in HIV-positive patients. Oral Dis 2007;13:110–6.

57. Wilson W, Taubert KA, Gewitz M, et al. Prevention of Infective Endocarditis Guidelines From the American Heart Association: a guideline from the American Heart Association Rheumatic Fever, Endocarditis, and Kawasaki Disease Committee, Council on Cardiovascular Disease in the Young, and the Council on Clinical Cardiology, Council on Cardiovascular Surgery and Anesthesia, and the Quality of Care and Outcomes Research Interdisciplinary Working Group. Circulation 2007;116(15):1736–54.

58. Fontana M, Young DA, Wolff MS. Evidence-based caries, risk assessment, and treatment. Dent Clin North Am 2009;53(1):149–61.

59. Glick M, Trope M, Pliskin ME. Detection of HIV in the dental pulp of a patient with AIDS. J Am Dent Assoc 1989;119:649–50.

60. Elkins DA, Torabinejad M, Schmidt RE, et al. Polymerase chain reaction detection of immunodeficiency virus DNA in human periradicular lesions. J Endod 1994;20: 386–8.
61. Suchina JA, Levine D, Flaitz CM, et al. Retrospective clinical and radiologic evaluation of nonsurgical endodontic treatment in human immunodeficiency virus (HIV) infection. J Contemp Dent Pract 2006;7:1–8.
62. Quesnell BT, Alves M, Hawkinson RW Jr, et al. The effect of human immunodeficiency virus on endodontic treatment outcome. J Endod 2005;31:633–6.
63. Alley BS, Buchanan TH, Eleazer PD. Comparison of the success of root canal therapy in HIV/AIDS patients and non-infected controls. Gen Dent 2008;56: 155–7.
64. Fontes TV, Vidal F, Gonçalves LS. Endodontic infection in HIV-infected individuals: an overview. ENDO–Endodontic Pract Today 2015;9:15–23.
65. Cooper H. Root canal treatment on patients with HIV infection. Int Endod J 1993; 26:369–71.
66. Glick M, Abel SN, Muzyka BC, et al. Dental complications after treating patients with AIDS. J Am Dent Assoc 1994;125:296–301.
67. Aminoshariae A, Kulild JC. Evidence-based recommendations for antibiotic usage to treat endodontic infections and pain: a systematic review of randomized controlled trials. J Am Dental Assoc 2016;147(3):186–91.
68. Renton T, Woolcombe S, Taylor T, et al. Oral surgery: part 1. Introduction and the management of the medically compromised patient. Br Dent J 2013;215(5): 213–23.
69. Patton LL, Shugars DA, Bonito AJ. A systematic review of complication risks for HIV-positive patients receiving invasive dental treatments. J Am Dent Assoc 2002;133(2):195–203.
70. Oliveira MA, Gallottini M, Pallos D, et al. The success of endosseous implants in human immunodeficiency virus–positive patients receiving antiretroviral therapy: a pilot study. J Am Dental Assoc 2011;142(9):1010–6.
71. Gherlone EF, Capparé P, Tecco S, et al. A Prospective longitudinal study on implant prosthetic rehabilitation in controlled HIV-positive patients with 1-year follow-up: the role of CD4+ level, smoking habits, and oral hygiene. Clin Implant Dent Relat Res 2015;18(5):955–64.
72. Chambrone L, Preshaw PM, Ferreira JD, et al. Effects of tobacco smoking on the survival rate of dental implants placed in areas of maxillary sinus floor augmentation: a systematic review. Clin Oral Implants Res 2014;25(4):408–16.
73. Kolhatkar S, Khalid S, Rolecki A, et al. Immediate dental implant placement in HIV-positive patients receiving highly active antiretroviral therapy: a report of two cases and a review of the literature of implants placed in HIV-positive individuals. J Periodontol 2011;82(3):505–11.
74. Gay-Escoda C, Pérez-Álvarez D, Camps-Font O, et al. Long-term outcomes of oral rehabilitation with dental implants in HIV-positive patients: a retrospective case series. Med Oral Patol Oral Cir Bucal 2016;21(3):385–91.
75. Ata-Ali J, Ata-Ali F, Di-Benedetto N, et al. Does HIV infection have an impact upon dental implant osseointegration? A systematic review. Med Oral Patol Oral Cir Bucal 2015;20(3):347–56.
76. Stasko SB, Kolhatkar S, Bhola M. Sinus floor elevation and implant placement via the crestal and lateral approach in patients with human immunodeficiency virus/ acquired immunodeficiency syndrome: report of two cases. Clin Adv Periodontics 2014;4(4):217–25.

77. Diz P, Scully C, Sanz M. Dental implants in the medically compromised patient. J Dent 2013;41(3):195–206.
78. Eke PI, Dye BA, Wei L, et al. Update on prevalence of periodontitis in adults in the United States: NHANES 2009 to 2012. J Periodontol 2015;86(5):611–22.
79. Supranoto SC, Slot DE, Addy M, et al. The effect of chlorhexidine dentifrice or gel versus chlorhexidine mouthwash on plaque, gingivitis, bleeding and tooth discoloration: a systematic review. Int J Dent Hyg 2015;13(2):83–92.
80. Patton LL. Current strategies for prevention of oral manifestations of human immunodeficiency virus. Oral Surg Oral Med Oral Pathol Oral Radiol 2016;121(1): 29–38.
81. Shiboski CH, Webster-Cyriaque JY, Ghannoum M, et al. The Oral HIV/AIDS Research Alliance Program: lessons learned and future directions. Oral Dis 2016;22(S1):128–34.
82. Bajpai S, Pazare AR. Oral manifestations of HIV. Contemp Clin Dent 2010;1(1):1.
83. Hamza OJ, Matee MI, Breuggemann RJ, et al. Single-dose fluconazole versus standard 2-week therapy for oropharyngeal candidiasis in HIV-infected patients: a randomized, double blind, double-dummy trial. Clin Infect Dis 2008;47:1270–6.
84. Vazquez JA. Optimal management of oropharyngeal and esophageal candidiasis in patients living with HIV infection. HIV AIDS 2010;2:89–101.
85. Patel M, Shackleton JA, Coogan MM, et al. Antifungal effect of mouth rinses on oral Candida counts and salivary flow in HIV-infected patients. AIDS Patient Care STDS 2008;22:613–8.
86. Kirk GD, Merlo C, O'Driscoll P, et al. HIV infection is associated with an increased risk for lung cancer independent of smoking. Clin Infect Dis 2007;45:103–10.

Opportunistic Oral Infections

Parish P. Sedghizadeh, DDS, MS[a],*, Susan Mahabady, MS[a], Carl M. Allen, DDS, MS[b]

KEYWORDS

- Opportunistic infection • Oral • Pathogens • Microbiology • HIV

KEY POINTS

- An oral opportunistic infection (OI) is initiated by either exogenously acquired pathogens or resident host flora, and usually occurs in hosts with weakened immunity or known risk factors.
- Specific pathogens implicated in oral OIs include various species of bacteria, fungi, virus, and parasites, and infectious disease paradigms apply given the context of communicable disease.
- Microbiological diagnosis of oral OI can be achieved by biological, serologic, histologic, or molecular methods.
- Treatment of oral OIs is based on clinical presentation, causative pathogens, anatomic involvement, and also management of any underlying comorbidities.

INTRODUCTION

An opportunistic infection (OI) is a disease of microbial cause or pathogenesis generally thought to occur in hosts with weakened immunity, altered microbiota, or breached epithelium. As such, OIs can be associated with significant morbidity or mortality.[1] Local or systemic disease ensues during OIs, and, when affecting the oral cavity, disease can be primary or secondary. Oral OIs are initiated by either exogenously acquired pathogens or resident host flora. Indigenous microbes that cause oral OIs can consist of species native to the oral cavity, or arise from niches proximal or distal to the mouth; for example, microorganisms from the skin, gastrointestinal tract, or airway and sinuses.

Numerous pathogens have been associated with oral OIs, including biofilm (sessile) communities and planktonic (free-floating) microorganisms. The specific pathogens

Disclosures: The authors have nothing to disclose and no conflicts of interest related to this work.
[a] Division of Periodontology, Diagnostic Sciences and Dental Hygiene, Center for Biofilms, Ostrow School of Dentistry, University of Southern California, Los Angeles, 925 West 34th Street, Los Angeles, CA 90089, USA; [b] Division of Oral and Maxillofacial Pathology and Radiology, College of Dentistry, The Ohio State University, 305 West 12th Avenue, Columbus, OH 43210, USA
* Corresponding author. Center for Biofilms, Ostrow School of Dentistry, University of Southern California, Los Angeles, 925 West 34th Street #4110, Los Angeles, CA 90089.
E-mail address: sedghiza@usc.edu

Dent Clin N Am 61 (2017) 389–400
http://dx.doi.org/10.1016/j.cden.2016.12.007
0011-8532/17/© 2016 Elsevier Inc. All rights reserved.

dental.theclinics.com

implicated in oral OIs are extensive and include various species of bacteria, fungi, viruses, and parasites. Furthermore, parasitic diseases affecting the oral cavity can be caused by helminths, protozoa, or ectoparasites. Ectoparasites can also serve as vectors for prion-related diseases, although oral involvement is a rare finding in prion-mediated diseases and is not a stand-alone feature.[2,3] Most microbes associated with oral OIs do not cause disease in healthy hosts. Therefore, thorough medical history and knowledge of comorbidities in patients with suspected oral OI is essential for accurate diagnosis. Because treatment of oral OI should be individualized and predicated on a diagnosis and host-pathogen findings, identification of contributory pathogens is important. When indicated, culturing and antimicrobial susceptibility testing can aid in diagnosis and appropriate choice of antimicrobial therapy. In some cases of oral OI, empiric therapy is immediately instituted based on clinical judgment of microbial cause if culture is unavailable, or until culture and sensitivity results return from the laboratory. Biofilm-mediated infections may be culture negative and should not rule out the potential for infectious disease when clinical suspicion is high.[4] In addition, oral OIs can be polymicrobial, which may confound the cause, diagnosis, and treatment.

Oral health care providers should have basic knowledge of the pathogens implicated in oral OIs, how these pathogens are identified, and basic clinicopathologic features, all of which inform accurate clinical diagnosis, management, and prevention strategies. For reference, some of these pathogens and the diseases they cause have already been discussed in detail in other articles presented in this issue. The goal and scope of this article is to provide general practitioners with:

1. Basic knowledge of the pathogens and microbiology of oral OIs
2. The specific types of diseases seen with oral OIs
3. Risk factors for disease development and progression
4. Considerations relevant to diagnosis and patient care in this context

Clinical exemplars are used to clarify key points in the discussion to follow. Importantly, in some cases of oral OI (eg, atypical or challenging cases), a multidisciplinary approach to diagnosis and treatment is required and is beyond the scope of general dental practice, especially when systemic evaluation is necessary. Thus, appropriate specialty referral, such as infectious disease (ID) consultation, should be sought when applicable and on a case-by-case basis.

DISCUSSION
Microbiology

Oral OIs are associated with specific pathogens that include numerous bacteria, yeast, viruses, and parasites, as presented in **Table 1**. Each of these microorganisms have unique genotypic and phenotypic compositions and virulence factors. Common mechanisms for initiating or propagating disease, or evading host immunity, also exist. When an OI pathogen is acquired or not part of the host indigenous flora, possible modes of transmission, depending on the specific microbe, include sexual; zoonotic; or borne by vector, saliva, blood, food, water, soil, air, or droplets.[5,6] Moreover, infection via autoinoculation is possible with certain OI pathogens, and this should be taken into consideration for therapeutic decision making.[7] For example, cryotherapy may be favored rather than laser ablation for the treatment of oral condyloma to reduce the risk of acquiring or spreading human papilloma virus (HPV) in aerosolized plumes.[8]

Further, certain OI pathogens are endemic to specific geographic regions, as are various subtypes within a similar phylogenetic clade.[9,10] Also, not all microbial species within a similar clade are pathogenic to humans. Some are nonpathogenic, or only

Table 1
Representative pathogens by microbial category that can be encountered in patients with oral opportunistic infections

Bacteria	Fungi	Virus	Parasites
Actinomyces	Aspergillus	Bunyaviridae	Balantidium
Aggregatibacter	Candida	Cytomegalovirus	Calliphora
Bacteroides	Cryptococcus	Coxsackievirus	Cestodes
Bartonella	Geotrichum	Echovirus	Chrysomya
Brucella	Histoplasma	Epstein-Barr virus	Ciliophora
Campylobacter	Mucoraceae	Herpes simplex virus	Cochliomyia
Capnocytophaga	Paracoccidioides	Human papillomavirus	Cordylobia
Corynebacterium	Penicillium	Kaposi sarcoma virus	Cryptosporidium
Coxiella	Sporothrix	Paramyxovirus	Demodex
Dialister	Trichophyton	Poxvirus	Dermatobia
Eikenella		Roseolovirus	Entamoeba
Enterobacter		Togavirus	Giardia
Escherichia		Varicella zoster virus	Hypoderma
Francisella			Larvae forms
Fusobacterium			Lucilia
Haemophilus			Musca
Klebsiella			Nematodes
Micrococcus			Oestrus
Micromonas			Plasmodium
Mycobacteria			Rhinosporidium
Peptostreptococcus			Trematodes
Porphyromonas			Trichomonas
Prevotella			Trypanosomes
Propionibacterium			Wohlfahrtia
Pseudomonas			
Salmonella			
Serratia			
Staphylococci			
Streptococcus			
Tannerella			
Treponema			
Veillonella			
Yersinia			

pathogenic to nonprimates and seen in veterinary medicine. Therefore, clinicians in different regions should be familiar with the epidemiology of pathogenic strains endemic to their region. However, with widespread travel throughout the world, OI cases not usually endemic to a region can also be observed, stressing the importance of travel history in such cases.[11]

Microbiological diagnosis of OI can be achieved by biological, serologic, histologic, or molecular methods.[12,13] All have advantages and disadvantages, but sensitivity and specificity are generally high for these modalities and vary based on the specific test, sample, and organism.[14] False-negatives and cross reactivity are possible confounders in any methodology. Therefore, correlation of results with clinical findings, and a combination of tests, usually provides higher accuracy for definitive diagnosis. Parasites can be especially difficult to culture in vitro and time consuming because of the complex life cycle of these organisms and the many variables involved.[15]

Contemporary diagnostic microbiology is progressively adopting molecular methods (eg, DNA/RNA-based assays) as first-line tests for a variety of samples.[14] Serologic assessments for circulating antigens or antibodies can be useful for many infections.

Molecular methodology includes assays based on polymerase chain reaction, in situ hybridization, immunosorbent techniques, direct and indirect immunofluorescence, next-generation sequencing, and spectroscopy. For dentists in private practice or not in a hospital setting, one challenge in clinical diagnostic microbiology of oral OIs is limited knowledge of commercial laboratories able to perform all needed tests or specific tests, particularly for rare conditions or organisms not routinely investigated in many laboratories, such as certain viral or parasitic pathogens. Additional challenges in diagnostic microbiology include heterogeneity in laboratory methodology, lack of universal standardization or harmonization, and microbial heterogeneity.[16,17]

Risk Factors

Patients most susceptible to OIs in general are those with compromised immunity.[18] Accordingly, comorbidities such as human immunodeficiency virus (HIV)/acquired immunodeficiency syndrome (AIDS), diabetes, cancer, or neutropenia can play a significant role in susceptibility to oral OI and the course of disease. For example, it has been shown that in transplant patients and hemodialyzed patients (diabetic and nondiabetic), multiorgan disturbances influence both the occurrence of secondary clinical oral manifestations and prevalence and species composition of oral pathogens.[19] **Box 1** lists

---

Box 1
Risk factors for oral opportunistic infections

Age

Chemotherapy

Chronic steroid therapy (local or systemic)

Diabetes (uncontrolled)

Drugs/medications

Genotype

Geography

Head and neck radiotherapy

HIV/AIDS

Hospitalization/nosocomial

Leukopenia/lymphopenia/neutropenia

Poor oral hygiene

Pregnancy

Sexual exposure

Smoking

Surgery

Syndromes

Transplant-associated immunosuppression

Trauma

Vector transmission

Xerostomia

Zoonosis

some of the at-risk populations or risk factors associated with oral OIs that have been reported in the literature.[20–24] Familiarity with comorbidities and factors linked to the development of oral OI proves useful for clinical risk assessment, diagnosis, treatment planning, and prevention. In certain cases of oral OI, treatment of the underlying comorbidity and elimination of risk factors is necessary to achieve clinical resolution of secondary infection.

Diseases

Table 2 lists the various opportunistic IDs that can be encountered clinically in the oral cavity and oropharynx by microbial category. Many of the conditions listed in **Table 2** can affect regions other than the oral cavity, and can also be seen in immunocompetent individuals. In contrast, some conditions almost exclusively affect the oral cavity, such as secondary infection or osteomyelitis in medication-related osteonecrosis of the jaw (MRONJ), as shown in **Fig. 1**.[25] MRONJ is more prevalent and severe in patients with comorbidities such as cancer or immunosuppression, and clinical suppuration and oral trauma have been shown to be independent risk factors for disease onset.[26] MRONJ is also known to be associated with bacterial biofilms, making treatment more challenging.[27,28] In this case, ID consultation was sought, and culture and antibiotic susceptibility testing (AST) was performed from exudate swabs and tissue samples. Gram-staining results were nonspecific and positive for gram-negative pleomorphic rods and white blood cells. Molecular results specifically identified *Serratia marcescens* as the predominant pathogen and AST using Kirby-Bauer methodology revealed sensitivity to ceftriaxone, gentamicin, moxifloxacin, and trimethoprim/sulfamethoxazole (antibiotics not routinely used in dentistry), and resistance to ampicillin, cefazolin, and amoxicillin, which are more commonly used in dentistry. This case of MRONJ shows the importance of familiarity with risk factors for specific oral OIs, such as cancer, chemotherapy, suppuration, and tooth extraction with MRONJ. It also shows how a resident pathogen can become opportunistic in a susceptible patient. It further shows the relevance of sampling and culture for

Table 2			
Opportunistic infections that can affect the oral cavity by microbial category			
Bacterial	**Fungal**	**Viral**	**Parasitic**
Actinomycosis	Aspergillosis	Aggressive periodontitis	Amebiasis
Bacillary angiomatosis	Blastomycosis	Condyloma acuminatum	Chagas disease
Cat-scratch disease	Candidiasis	Hand-foot-and-mouth	Cysticercosis
Cellulitis	Coccidioidomycosis	disease	Dirofilariasis
Leprosy	Cryptococcosis	Heck disease	Filariasis
Linear gingival	Histoplasmosis	Herpes zoster	Leishmaniasis
erythema	Mucormycosis	Infectious mononucleosis	Mesomycetozoea
Mucositis	Paracoccidioidomycosis	Kaposi sarcoma	Myiasis
Necrotizing ulcerative	Penicilliosis	Mucocutaneous ulcers	Toxoplasmosis
gingivitis	Phycomycosis	Molluscum contagiosum	
Necrotizing ulcerative	Sporotrichosis	Oral hairy leukoplakia	
periodontitis		Papillomas	
Necrotizing ulcerative		Papillomatosis	
stomatitis		Parotitis	
Oral syphilis		Recurrent herpes	
Oral tuberculosis			
Osteomyelitis			
Osteonecrosis			
Parotitis			

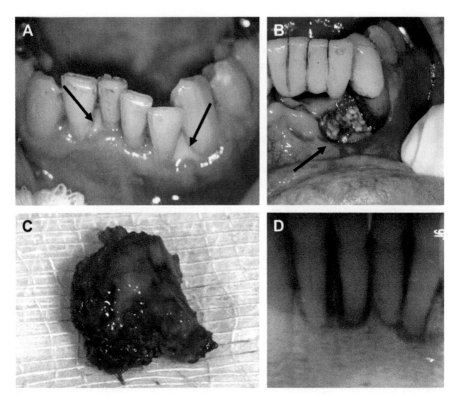

Fig. 1. A 71-year-old man with advanced-stage prostate cancer who was undergoing active chemotherapy (monthly intravenous zoledronate) and developed an oral OI of MRONJ. (*A*) Copious purulence is seen (*arrows*) extruding from the interdental space of the jaw, which was painful, and teeth tested nonvital. (*B*) A large area of exposed sequestrum is observed (*arrow*) at the nonhealing site following tooth extractions. (*C*) Gross specimen debrided from the infection for culture and histopathologic evaluation. (*D*) Radiograph of the jawbone showing ill-defined osteolysis around the anterior mandibular teeth with loss of lamina dura. (*Courtesy of* Allan C. Jones DDS, MS, Torrance, CA.)

pathogen identification and more targeted therapeutics, and the utility of radiographs to assess hard tissue involvement given the anatomic location of disease. Further, in cases like this, tissue samples for culture may be just as important as, or more relevant than, swab cultures for molecular diagnosis. Microscopic evaluation of tissue in MRONJ cases can also be useful to rule out metastatic cancer to the jaws or other differentials in the clinical diagnosis, and the histopathology in this case was consistent with an osteomyelitis of the jaw, although not specific enough for accurate microbiological diagnosis.

When dealing with potential OI, ID paradigms apply given the context of communicable disease, and infection control measures and universal precautions should be used. In some cases, the presence and identification of an oral OI, or multiple lesions of oral OI in the same patient, may raise clinical suspicion for undiagnosed immunosuppression. In such cases, systemic evaluation and ID consultation should be sought because further laboratory and medical investigations may be warranted to assess systemic health and immune status, as shown in **Fig. 2**. In the context of HIV, early diagnosis of infection and immunosuppression, along with access to medical care

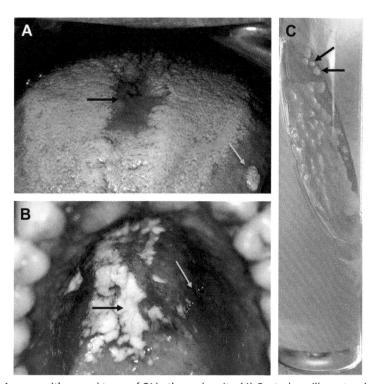

Fig. 2. An man with several types of OI in the oral cavity. (*A*) Central papillary atrophy (*black arrow*) of the tongue and a wart or papilloma (*green arrow*) of the lateral tongue is seen. (*B*) The palate shows evidence of pseudomembranous (*black arrow*) and erythematous (*green arrow*) candidiasis. (*C*) A Sabouraud dextrose agar slant from clinical swab for fungal culture is strongly positive and fungal colony-forming units (*black arrows*) can be seen. These combined findings should raise suspicion for immunosuppression and HIV, which was subsequently confirmed with additional testing and serology.

and antiretroviral therapy, plays an important role in HIV-related oral disease prevention.[29] Vaccination for HIV-related IDs is also a consideration in patients with HIV to prevent specific OIs.[30] This case also shows that not just rare pathogens but common organisms, such as *Candida* spp, can be opportunistic or more virulent in immunocompromised patients. Furthermore, less common *Candida* species may be seen in immunocompromised hosts, such as *Candida tropicalis*, *Candida glabrata*, *Candida parapsilosis*, *Candida krusei*, *Candida dubliniensis*, or *Candida geotrichum*. This finding reinforces the need in some cases for culture and molecular diagnostics for more definitive subtyping. Overall, there has been a reduction in HIV-related oral OIs, except for an increase in HPV-related lesions in the era since highly active and combined antiretroviral therapy.[31,32]

Clinicopathologic Considerations

The clinical presentation of oral OIs is diverse. Tissue damage can occur as a direct result of invading pathogens, or secondary to host immune responses. Systemic findings, if present, may include fever, malaise, fatigue, malnutrition, or lesions analogous to or different from those found in the oral cavity. Lymphadenopathy may or may not be a feature with oral OIs. In some cases of oral OI, serologic studies may reveal increased levels of nonspecific inflammatory markers such as C-reactive protein, or an increased erythrocyte sedimentation rate. Determining microbial etiopathogenesis (ie, bacterial, fungal, viral, or parasitic) based on clinical features, history, and signs and symptoms can be helpful for informing initial empiric pharmacotherapy until further testing and results.

Oral lesions associated with OIs can present with a broad range of morphologies, including ulcer, plaque, cyst, wart, erosion, granuloma, nodule, sequestrum, or abscess. None of these are pathognomonic for a specific disease, but can aid in identifying causes and guide further testing for a more definitive diagnosis, such as culture or biopsy. For example, an oral abscess would be more appropriate for swab culture, as opposed to solid warts (**Fig. 3**) or nodules, which would be more suitable to biopsy and histopathologic evaluation for definitive diagnosis. Molecular confirmation with in situ hybridization is useful for diagnosis in oral condyloma acuminatum, as in this case.

When a nonhealing oral lesion is available for biopsy, results can be informative for diagnosis or further testing. For example, **Fig. 4** shows histopathologic findings for a patient with a nonhealing area of necrotizing ulcerative gingivitis clinically that was nonresponsive to local therapy and antibiotics. Biopsy was performed and suggestive of histoplasmosis fungal infection with associated inflammatory response. Without biopsy these organisms and diagnosis could easily have been missed, and even with biopsy the diagnosis is challenging. Parasitic protozoa that cause diseases like

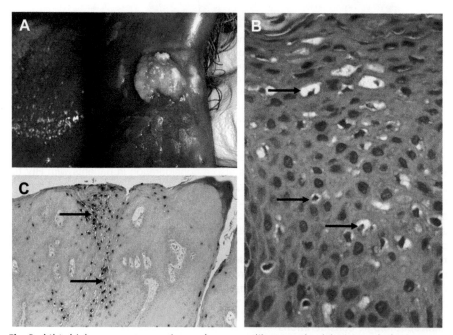

Fig. 3. (*A*) Labial mucosa at commissure shows wartlike growths. (*B*) Histopathologic examination of biopsy reveals koilocytosis (*black arrows*), which represents squamous cells with large and irregular, well-defined perinuclear halos and cytoplasmic thickening; nuclear irregularity and variation in size is also observed (hematoxylin-eosin 100, original magnification ×40). (*C*) Digoxigenin-labeled probe counterstained with nuclear red (original magnification × 10).

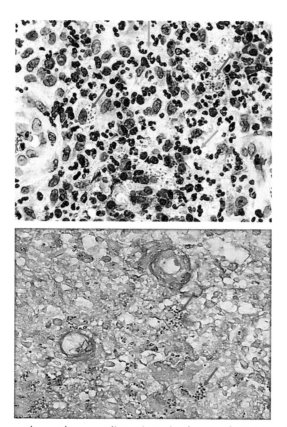

Fig. 4. The top image shows a hematoxylin-eosin–stained section from a necrotizing ulcerative gingivitis biopsy. Histopathologic evidence of acute inflammation or neutrophils (*blue arrows*) is seen in a background of chronic inflammation comprising macrophages and histiocytes. Vague granulomas (*top left*) were also observed. Intracellular microbes consistent with histo-plasmosis could be seen (*red arrows*) in a granular cytoplasm within phagocytic cells. The bot-tom image shows a periodic acid–Schiff stain, which highlights fungal cell walls and more readily shows tissue pathogens (*red arrows*). Top-(20 × original magnification), Bottom-(10 × original magnification). (*Courtesy of* Audrey Boros, MSc, DDS, Los Angeles, CA.)

leishmania and Chagas disease have similar histopathologic findings to histoplasmo-sis because all are intracellular parasites. *Histoplasma* organisms are uniform in size and morphology, with a characteristic clear halo encompassing the cell wall, whereas protozoa may be of various sizes and morphologies without a clear halo. However, diagnosis can be difficult on histopathology alone, especially when organisms are not readily identifiable on hematoxylin-eosin sections, requiring further testing or special stains. Periodic acid–Schiff or silver-based stains are useful for identifying structures with high carbohydrate content, such as the cell wall of fungi, aiding in discrimination from protozoa. Other fungi and fungal diseases in the differential diag-nosis of histoplasmosis, such as *Cryptococcus*, blastomycosis, coccidioidomycosis, paracoccidioidomycosis, and mucormycosis have different histomorphologic features (eg, hyphae or sporulation) from histoplasmosis and are usually geographically spe-cific. This case also shows how clinical and epidemiologic correlation and additional testing or stains are warranted for definitive diagnosis, and ID specialty referral is essential after oral diagnosis to rule out pulmonary, pericardial, meningeal/cerebrospinal fluid, or other systemic involvement that can be seen with histoplasmosis, and also to assess immune status and provide appropriate systemic antifungal therapy. ID consultation can also be useful when intravenous antimicrobials are indicated for treatment.

Histopathology is also useful for identifying infections associated with granulomatous inflammation, but is limited for definitive diagnosis. In granulomatous cases, additional stains include Gomori methenamine silver, Giemsa, periodic acid–Schiff, and Ziehl-Neelson.[33] In addition, the histopathology of an oral OI caused by a parasitic helminth is shown in **Fig. 5** from a patient with an enlarging oral submucosal mass. A larval form of a parasite was identified in the biopsy specimen, warranting ID consultation for blood, urine, and fecal testing for systemic molecular diagnosis. Advanced imaging studies such as computed tomography scans or MRI can also be useful in such cases for systemic evaluation.

In general, treatment of oral OIs is based on clinical presentation, causative pathogens, anatomic involvement, and also management of any underlying comorbidities. Current reference materials can provide up-to-date approaches to treatment of most oral OIs and specific causative pathogens (eg, antibiotic, antifungal, antiviral, or antiparasitic drugs), but again this first requires an accurate diagnosis and knowledge of causal pathogens.

The information and cases presented herein show the heterogeneity in clinical presentations and manifestations of oral OIs. Case exemplars from each causal category (bacterial, fungal, viral, and parasitic) are presented in this article to highlight microbiological and clinicopathologic considerations relevant to practice. Importantly, some oral OIs may be associated with an increased risk for cancer development in affected patients and require long-term follow-up and surveillance. Examples include Kaposi sarcoma in patients with HIV/AIDS, or the increase in oropharyngeal cancers in younger patients caused by high-risk HPV subtypes.[34] Therefore, clinical risk assessment and history with review of systems, and again accurate diagnosis, treatment, and follow-up, are essential in cases of oral OI for improved patient outcomes. Because many of the pathogens associated with oral OIs are transmissible or communicable, infectious disease paradigms apply and ID consultation may be appropriate in some cases as this article has shown. Further, the oral cavity with its robust microbiota can act as a source of pathogens to induce clinically significant OIs, particularly in immunosuppressed individuals. Thus, evaluation of the oral cavity in patient populations susceptible to OIs in general is highly recommended.

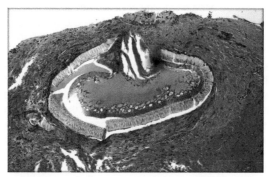

Fig. 5. Oral submucosal mass consistent with helminth larvae (*red arrows*) at a cross section of the parasite's digestive tract. (*Courtesy of* Yeshwant Rawal, BDS, MDS, MS, Seattle, WA.)

REFERENCES

1. Masur H, Read SW. Opportunistic infections and mortality: still room for improvement. J Infect Dis 2015;212(9):1348–50.
2. Jayanthi P, Thomas P, Bindhu P, et al. Prion diseases in humans: oral and dental implications. North Am J Med Sci 2013;5(7):399–403.
3. Lupi O. Could ectoparasites act as vectors for prion diseases? Int J Dermatol 2003;42(6):425–9.
4. Costerton JW, Post JC, Ehrlich GD, et al. New methods for the detection of orthopedic and other biofilm infections. FEMS Immunol Med Microbiol 2011;61(2): 133–40.
5. Galletti B, Mannella VK, Santoro R, et al. Ear, nose and throat (ENT) involvement in zoonotic diseases: a systematic review. J Infect Dev Ctries 2014;8(1):17–23.
6. Coffield DJ Jr, Spagnuolo AM, Shillor M, et al. A model for Chagas disease with oral and congenital transmission. PLoS One 2013;8(6):e67267.
7. Stojanov IJ, Woo SB. Human papillomavirus and Epstein-Barr virus associated conditions of the oral mucosa. Semin Diagn Pathol 2015;32(1):3–11.
8. Gloster HM Jr, Roenigk RK. Risk of acquiring human papillomavirus from the plume produced by the carbon dioxide laser in the treatment of warts. J Am Acad Dermatol 1995;32(3):436–41.
9. Norman FF, Monge-Maillo B, Martínez-Pérez Á, et al. Parasitic infections in travelers and immigrants: part II helminths and ectoparasites. Future Microbiol 2015;10(1):87–99.
10. Hassona Y, Scully C, Aguida M, et al. Flies and the mouth. J Investig Clin Dent 2014;5(2):98–103.
11. Chen LH, Blair BM. Infectious risks of traveling abroad. Microbiol Spectr 2015; 3(4). http://dx.doi.org/10.1128/microbiolspec.IOL5-0005-2015.
12. Ndao M. Diagnosis of parasitic diseases: old and new approaches. Interdiscip Perspect Infect Dis 2009;2009:278246.
13. Guarner J, Brandt ME. Histopathologic diagnosis of fungal infections in the 21st century. Clin Microbiol Rev 2011;24(2):247–80.
14. Bloomfield MG, Balm MN, Blackmore TK. Molecular testing for viral and bacterial enteric pathogens: gold standard for viruses, but don't let culture go just yet? Pathology 2015;47(3):227–33.
15. Visvesvara GS, Garcia LS. Culture of protozoan parasites. Clin Microbiol Rev 2002;15(3):327–8.
16. Abass E, Kang C, Martinkovic F, et al. Heterogeneity of *Leishmania donovani* parasites complicates diagnosis of visceral leishmaniasis: comparison of different serological tests in three endemic regions. PLoS One 2015;10(3):e0116408.
17. He Q, Barkoff AM, Mertsola J, et al. European *Bordetella* expert group (EUpertstrain); European Surveillance Network for Vaccine-preventable Diseases (EU-VAC.NET). High heterogeneity in methods used for the laboratory confirmation of pertussis diagnosis among European countries, 2010: integration of epidemiological and laboratory surveillance must include standardisation of methodologies and quality assurance. Euro Surveill 2012;17(32) [pii:20239].
18. George MP, Masur H, Norris KA, et al. Infections in the immunosuppressed host. Ann Am Thorac Soc 2014;11(Suppl 4):S211–20.
19. Piekarczyk J, Fiedor P, Chomicz L, et al. Oral cavity as a potential source of infections in recipients with diabetes mellitus. Transplant Proc 2003;35(6):2207–8.
20. Youssef J, Novosad SA, Winthrop KL. Infection risk and safety of corticosteroid use. Rheum Dis Clin North Am 2016;42(1):157–76.

21. Ghidini M, Hahne JC, Trevisani F, et al. New developments in the treatment of chemotherapy-induced neutropenia: focus on balugrastim. Ther Clin Risk Manag 2016;12:1009–15.

22. Schuurhuis JM, Stokman MA, Witjes MJ, et al. Head and neck intensity modulated radiation therapy leads to an increase of opportunistic oral pathogens. Oral Oncol 2016;58:32–40.

23. Pana ZD, Farmaki E, Roilides E. Host genetics and opportunistic fungal infections. Clin Microbiol Infect 2014;20(12):1254–64.

24. Patton LL, Phelan JA, Ramos-Gomez FJ, et al. Prevalence and classification of HIV-associated oral lesions. Oral Dis 2002;8(Suppl 2):98–109.

25. Katsarelis H, Shah NP, Dhariwal DK, et al. Infection and medication-related osteonecrosis of the jaw. J Dent Res 2015;94(4):534–9.

26. Barasch A, Cunha-Cruz J, Curro FA, et al. Risk factors for osteonecrosis of the jaws: a case-control study from the CONDOR Dental PBRN. Tex Dent J 2013; 130(4):299–307.

27. Kumar SK, Gorur A, Schaudinn C, et al. The role of microbial biofilms in osteonecrosis of the jaw associated with bisphosphonate therapy. Curr Osteoporos Rep 2010;8(1):40–8.

28. Sedghizadeh PP, Kumar SK, Gorur A, et al. Microbial biofilms in osteomyelitis of the jaw and osteonecrosis of the jaw secondary to bisphosphonate therapy. J Am Dent Assoc 2009;140(10):1259–65.

29. Patton LL. Current strategies for prevention of oral manifestations of human immunodeficiency virus. Oral Surg Oral Med Oral Pathol Oral Radiol 2016;121(1): 29–38.

30. Nicolini LA, Giacobbe DR, Di Biagio A, et al. Insights on common vaccinations in HIV-infection: efficacy and safety. J Prev Med Hyg 2015;56(1):E28–32.

31. Patton LL, Ramirez-Amador V, Anaya-Saavedra G, et al. Urban legends series: oral manifestations of HIV infection. Oral Dis 2013;19(6):533–50.

32. Patton LL. Oral lesions associated with human immunodeficiency virus disease. Dent Clin North Am 2013;57(4):673–98.

33. Majeed MM, Bukhari MH. Evaluation for granulomatous inflammation on fine needle aspiration cytology using special stains. Patholog Res Int 2011;2011:851524.

34. Young D, Xiao CC, Murphy B, et al. Increase in head and neck cancer in younger patients due to human papillomavirus (HPV). Oral Oncol 2015;51(8):727–30.

Immunizations

An Evolving Paradigm for Oral Health Care Providers

Leslie R. Halpern, DDS, MD, PhD, MPH[a],*, Charles Mouton, MD, MS[b]

KEYWORDS

- Vaccine-preventable diseases • Vaccine effectiveness • Active
- Passive immunization • Vaccine Adverse Event Reporting System (VAERS)
- CDC Standard precautions

KEY POINTS

- The pervasive increase in transmissible vectors of infectious diseases has created great concern in the health of populations globally.
- Oral health care professionals are especially at risk for the transmission of significant microorganisms, both bacterial and viral.
- The provider needs to be knowledgeable about the exposure/transmission of life-threatening infections in their daily practice, as well as options for prevention.
- This article is designed to increase the oral health care provider's awareness of vaccine-preventable diseases that pose a high risk in the dental health care setting.
- Specific dosing strategies are suggested for the prevention of infections caused by several bacterial and viral microorganisms based on available evidence and the epidemiologic changes described recently.

INTRODUCTION

The pervasive increase in transmissible vectors of infectious diseases has created great concern in the health of populations globally. The World Health Organization has approximately 36 million health care workers worldwide with more than 3 million who have not received vaccinations/immunizations.[1,2] These health care providers are exposed to a cornucopia of infectious agents as they perform their professional duties, including being at high risk for injuries and transmission from exposure to blood borne pathogens (BBPs).[1,2] Of occupational exposures, 75% are percutaneous; the remaining 25% are mucosal–cutaneous.[1–4] Infection transmission in the oral health arena has

[a] Residency Program, Oral and Maxillofacial Surgery, Meharry Medical College, 1005 DB Todd Junior Boulevard, Nashville, TN 37208, USA; [b] Department of Family and Community Medicine, Meharry Medical College, School of Medicine, Nashville, TN 37208, USA
* Corresponding author.
E-mail address: lhalpern@mmc.edu

Dent Clin N Am 61 (2017) 401–424
http://dx.doi.org/10.1016/j.cden.2016.12.010
0011-8532/17/© 2016 Elsevier Inc. All rights reserved.

been a global public health concern since the 1980s, when the human immunodeficiency virus (HIV) epidemic came to light. Risk factor identification revealed the high risk of contact between dentists and their patients serving as a vector for transmission.[5,6] Furthermore, dentists experience puncture wounds by needles more than any other health care specialist.[4–7] As such, oral health care professionals are especially at greatest risk for the transmission of significant microorganisms, both bacterial and viral (**Table 1**). There are numerous reports across the globe that document significant cases where dentists still do not engage in safe practices with regard to barrier protection; that is, gloves, eye glasses, facemasks, and other protective shields.[3,4,6]

In the 1980s, viral hepatitis, that is, hepatitis B virus (HBV) infection, was 4 times greater among oral health care workers, which has declined significantly owing to high compliance with HBV immunizations of the dental staff, as well as infection control practices referred to as universal precautions.[8,9] The Centers for Disease Control and Prevention (CDC) in 1996 expanded the "concept" of universal precautions to

Table 1 Representative infectious diseases in dentistry		
Disease Name	**Etiologic Agent**	**Incubation Time**
Bacterial		
Staphylococcal infections	*Staphylococcus aureus*	4–10 d
Streptococcal infections	*Streptococcus pyogenic*	2–3 d
Tuberculosis infections	*Mycobacterium tuberculosis*	Up to 6 mo
Diphtheria	*Corynebacterium* diphtherias	—
Pertussis	*Bordetella pertussis*	—
Viral		
Recurrent herpetic	Herpes simplex type 1 and type 2	2 wk
Rubella	Rubella togavirus	9–11 d
Measles	Paramyxovirus	10–12 d
Mumps	Paramyxovirus	16–18 d
Influenza	Live attenuated vaccine/H1N1	—
Hepatitis A	Hepatitis A virus	14–28 d
Hepatitis B	Hepatitis B virus	6 wk–6 mo
Hepatitis C	Hepatitis C virus (non-A non-B hepatitis)	Weeks–months
Hepatitis D (delta)	Hepatitis D virus (delta)	Weeks–months
Varicella virus	Varicella zoster	—
Infectious mononucleosis	Epstein–Barr virus	4–7 wk
Hand–foot–mouth disease	Cocksackie virus A, B	2 d–3 wk
Herpangina	Cocksackie virus A	5 d
AIDS	Human immunodeficiency virus	Weeks–months
Fungal		
Dermatomycosis	*Trichophyton microorganism*	Days–weeks
Superficial skin infections	*Epidermophyton/Candida*	—
Candidiasis miscellaneous	*Candida albicans*/esophagitis	Days–weeks
Superficial infections from hands and eyes	Numerous organisms	2–3 d

Adapted from Molinari JA. Infection control: its evolution to the current standard precautions. J Am Dent Assoc 2003;134(5):570; with permission.

standard precautions and in 2003 updated Guidelines for Infection Control in the Dental Health-care Setting.[8,9] In 2016, the CDC reissued a "Summary of Infection Prevention Practices in Dental Settings: Basic Expectations for Safe Care."[8–10] Because of the significant risk of exposure to BBPs, such as HBV, the oral health care provider continues to be at high risk for not only viral infections, but also numerous bacterial infections that are now increasing nationally and globally.

Although the immunization protocols for HBV are well-followed in the dental profession, few infection control guidelines have applied immunization paradigms against other bacterial and viral diseases that pose a true risk for infection in dental health personnel and their patients, including measles, rubella, tuberculosis (TB), and diphtheria.[3,4,11,12] Another caveat to this dilemma is assessing the state of vaccine confidence in the United States based on the incidence and risk for these diseases. Vaccine confidence defines the trust that health care providers and patients have with respect to vaccine administration and recommended immunization schedules.[11–13] There is judicious monitoring of adverse effects of vaccine administration by the Vaccine Adverse Event Reporting system, who are in turn monitored by the US Food and Drug Administration and the CDC.[13] This is further discussed elsewhere in this article.

This article is designed to increase the oral health care provider's awareness of the latest assessment of vaccine and immunization prevention for vaccine-preventable diseases that pose a high risk in the dental health care setting. Basic principles of immunology and immunization and vaccination are described, followed by recommendations for the prevention and control of infectious diseases that can affect dental health care personnel and their patients. Specific dosing strategies are suggested for the prevention of infections caused by several bacterial and viral microorganisms based on available evidence and the epidemiologic changes in diseases described in recent years to provide a clear understanding of risks and benefits of vaccine-preventable diseases that pose a public health consequence in the oral health care setting.

IMMUNOGENESIS, IMMUNIZATION, AND VACCINATION
Immunogenesis

The normal response of the immune system is predicated on a series of cellular events and inflammatory cascades. The building blocks for immune mechanisms have their origin within the reticuloendothelial system. The cells of the bone marrow, when exposed to an antigenic agent, undergo a cascade of cellular differentiation to form either lymphoid or myeloid cell lines.

Lymphoid cell line

This pleuripotential cell line can give rise to B, T, non-B, or non-T lymphocytes that when exposed to the periphery mature and act on the allergen. Specifically, the B lymphocytes are the catalyst for antibody production by interacting with an antigen on the cell surface. B cells that mature into plasma cells can secret immunoglobulins, as well as become memory cells that, when reexposed to an antigen, exert a secondary immunologic response. This interaction between B cells and antigen causes a cascade of signals that act within the cytoplasm and cause the events of an allergic reaction. T lymphocytes orchestrate a series of immunologic events at the level of the B lymphocyte, macrophage, and natural killer cells. These lymphocytes also activate acute phase reactants such as cytokines, and surface membrane molecules of the CD series and major histocompatibility complex pathways. Major histocompatibility complex pathways allow for the T lymphocyte to interact with an antigen to protect the host.

Myeloid cell line

The myeloid cell line can mature into several types of blood cells. This cell lines' pleuripotency allows for a stem cell–like action, the differential capacity of cellular elements that will form either mononuclear phagocytes or granulocytes. The mononuclear cells enter the bloodstream and populate the endothelial environment as macrophages that can phagocytize bacteria or initiate inflammatory cascades by their production of acute phase reactants. In addition, they can interact with B lymphocytes to promote the processing of antigen. Neutrophils that arise from this cell line are the catalysts for the acute inflammatory response. The two main other cell lines from myeloid precursors are eosinophils and basophils. It is these two cells that are most important in the early and late phases of the allergic reaction.

Immunoglobulins, complements, and acute phase reactants

There are five classes of immunoglobulins (Ig): IgA, IgD, IgE, IgG, and IgM. These proteins are secreted by B cells. The immunoglobulin IgE is the most important in the immediate hypersensitivity reaction seen in anaphylaxis. The complement system is the most important in host resistance to infection. This group of proteins activates mast cells, and modulates vascular permeability, the release of inflammatory mediators, and the initiation of polymorphonuclear leukocytic infiltration during antigen or bacterial invasion. The acute phase reactants, cytokines, act as stimulators of inflammatory cascades and mediators of immune cell maturation.

Immunizations and Vaccinations

The terms immunization and vaccination are often considered synonymous and involve the use of any pathogen or immune biologic as a preventive strategy against a disease caused by a specific antigen.[14] Immunization is considered a broader term or less specific because vaccines were originally derived from a specific vaccine developed from cowpox to treat smallpox, that is, a "vaccination an example of an immunization."[4]

Knowledge of the immune response is essential to understand the significant value of immunization and vaccinations in infectious diseases because vaccines are considered an effective public health tool for disease prevention. Their mechanisms of action reside within the immune responses that are either active or passive (**Box 1**).

Active immunization

Active immunization is acquired through an induction of immunity after exposure to an antigen. The antibody response is elicited by a vaccine or toxoid and the humoral immunity of the host is relative to the specific pathogen of interest. The response can take several days to weeks and can last a lifetime. An example is the hepatitis A vaccine (see elsewhere in this article for specific immunization).

Passive immunization

Passive immunization, often thought of as acquired, is a process of providing IgG antibodies to protect against infections; it is immediate and can be short lived. An example is the transfer of maternal tetanus antibodies across the placenta to the unborn child. Acquired passive immunity is through serum from immune individuals to a susceptible donor.[15]

Vaccines

Vaccines are biologic preparations that provide active acquired immunity against a specific infectious disease. Vaccinations can be separated into 2 types: inactivated or attenuated. Inactivated forms are derived from previously virulent microbes that

> **Box 1**
> **Building blocks for immunization and vaccination**
>
> *Immunobiologic*
> Antigenic substance or antibody containing preparation used to induce immunity and prevent infectious diseases.
>
> Active immunization
> Use of an antigenic substance to induce immunity by stimulating an immune response.
>
> Vaccine
> A suspension of live (usually attenuated) or inactivated microorganisms, or fractions thereof.
> 1. Monovalent
>   A vaccine consisting of a single strain or type of organism.
> 2. Trivalent
>   A vaccine consisting of 3 types of strains of a single organism (influenza vaccine), or 3 different organisms (diphtheria, pertussis, tetanus vaccine).
> 3. Polyvalent
>   Multiple strains or types of organisms in the vaccine (23-valent pneumococcal vaccine).
>
> Toxoid
> A modified (nontoxic) bacterial toxin that is capable of stimulating antitoxin formation.
>
> Passive immunization
> Use of an antibody containing preparation to enhance or restore immunity. Immune globulin: A sterile solution containing antibodies from human blood.
>
> Antitoxin
> A solution of antibodies derived from the serum of animals immunized with specific antigens.
>
> *From* Quaranta P. Immunizations and oral health care providers. Dent Clin North Am 2003;47(4):644; with permission.

are killed by biologic agents, heat, or radiation. Examples are the influenza, polio, and hepatitis A vaccines.[4,12] Attenuated forms contain live microbes, most which are viruses that are cultured to become disabled. Examples are measles, yellow fever, rubella, and mumps. Bacteria such as *Mycobacterium tuberculin* and typhoid are made noncontagious and used as an antigen to provide active immunity. An example is the Bacillus of Calmette and Guerin (BCG) vaccine. It must be remembered that these strains must not be administered to medically compromised and immunocompromised patients because they can mutate and cause disease.[16]

Toxoid vaccines are produced from inactivated toxic compounds of the microbes such as tetanus and diphtheria that serve as a modified (nontoxic) bacterial toxin capable of stimulating antitoxin antibody formation (the reader is referred to Quaranta[4] for further examples of vaccines types).

IMMUNIZATIONS DESIGNATED FOR ORAL HEALTH CARE PROVIDERS

The CDC estimates that 40 to 50,000 vaccine-preventable deaths occur every year in the United States and estimates the health care burden of vaccine-preventable diseases are at $10 billion.[8–10] As such, maintenance of immunity is an important part of disease prevention and the use of vaccines safeguard the health of various types of oral health care providers, their staff, and their patients. Within the last 2 decades the Advisory Committee on Immunization Practices (ACIP) advocated for infection control guidelines with respect to immunoprophylaxis of dentists against the BBP HBV and standard precautions against hepatitis C virus (HCV), for which there is no vaccine (reviewed elsewhere in this article).[10] All healthy adults within the United States are encouraged to be vaccinated for measles, mumps, rubella (MMR) and pneumococcal diseases. Recommendations for all health care workers including dentists according to the CDC are described in **Box 2**. Despite these recommendations, many practices have not implemented these precautions.

Dentists are at greater risk for infections caused by bacteria and viruses owing to numerous encounters with the use of sharps and must be judicious with respect to his/her awareness of preventive measures against vaccine-preventable diseases within their clinical practice.[2–4,9] Studies have shown a low level of awareness toward vaccine-preventable diseases within the oral health care setting. Petti and colleagues[3] applied a survey questionnaire to 379 dental practitioners to evaluate their awareness toward vaccine-preventable diseases. The results concluded that practitioners had a low awareness of vaccine-preventable diseases, and the authors suggested a need for greater attention to immunization focusing on vaccine-preventable diseases that poses a significant risk to both the clinician and patients they serve. The survey evidence obtained with this dental population can be used as a foundation for designing immunization programs tailored specifically for the oral health care setting.[3,16]

Box 2
Health care personnel vaccination recommendations

Vaccines and Recommendations
Hepatitis B

In unvaccinated HCPs give a 3-dose series (dose 1 now, dose 2 in 1 month and dose 3 approximately 5–6 months after dose 2). IM dosing may be given to HCPs who perform tasks that may involve exposure to blood or body fluids. Testing of anti-Hbs titers occur 1 to 2 months after dose 1. Anti-Hbs of 10 mLU/mL or greater signifies positive immunity and no other titers are needed. Anti-Hbs of less than 10 mLU/mL is not protective of infection and therefore, 3 doses of vaccine are needed over the routine schedule stated, with additional titer testing 1 to 2 months after.

If the anti-Hbs titer remains less than 10 mLU/mL after 6 doses, the person is considered a nonresponder and is counseled of precautions of exposure. Nonresponses may also be HBsAg positive and therefore HBsAg testing is needed. HCP that are in this group must be counseled and medically evaluated.

Influenza

Vaccination is by 1 dose of influenza annually. The inactivated formula is given IM, except when using the intradermal influenza vaccine. LAIV is administered intranasally. All HCP must receive vaccinations annually and LAIV administered only to nonpregnant HCP ages 49 or younger. Inactivated injectable vaccines are preferred when HCPs are caring for immunocompromised patients, especially those in isolation.

MMR

HCPs born in 1957 or after without titer measurements or prior vaccination should receive 2 doses of MMR, 4 weeks apart. HCPs born before 1957 should have been exposed but if not then should be administered 2 doses of MMR or subcutaneously. One dose of MMR is considered for an HCP with no evidence of disease of immunity to rubella. In this group 2 doses of MMR are required if there is an outbreak of measles or mumps; 1 dose for an outbreak of rubella.

Meningococcal

Vaccinations are required for HCPs exposed on a routine basis to isolates of *Neisseria meningitis*. MenACWY and MenB strains are used with a booster every 5 years if risk of exposure continues. Each vaccination is given at a separate site on the body. Subcutaneous can be used in the form of MPSV4 if necessary.

Tetanus, Diphtheria, Pertussis

HCPs should receive a dose of Tdap vaccine if they are either unsure of a previous dose or received a dose regardless of the past interval between last dose HCPs who are pregnant should receive a dose of Tdap for each pregnancy and all HCPs require a booster every 10 years. All vaccines are given IM.

Varicella (Chickenpox)

All HCPs are strongly recommended to receive immunity against varicella zoster, whether or not they were exposed either to Chickenpox or Shingles. Two doses of vaccines are given 28 days apart and tested for degree of immunity.

Abbreviations: Hbs, hepatitis B surface; HBSAg, hepatitis B surface antigen; HCP, health care provider; IM, intramuscularly; LAIV, live attenuated influenza vaccine; MenACWY, meningococcal A, C, and Y diseases; MenB, meningococcal B disease; MMR, measles, mumps, rubella; MPSV4, meningococcal vaccine; Tdap, tetanus toxoid, acellular pertussis and reduced diphtheria toxoid.

Adapted from Immunization action coalition, healthcare personnel vaccination recommendations. 2016. Available at: www.immunize.org/catg.d/p2017.pdf. Accessed December 2, 2016.

VACCINE-PREVENTABLE DISEASES OF IMPORTANCE FOR ORAL HEALTH CARE PROVIDERS

The following vaccine-preventable diseases that require awareness by the oral health care provider to avoid transmission within their practice setting and patient population are presented in this section.

Hepatitis A Virus

Hepatitis A virus (HAV) infection arises from an RNA virus and transmitted through a fecal–oral route. It can elicit symptoms or may be asymptomatic. Although self-limiting, this virus can cause significant morbidity.[11,12,16] HAV exposure has been under control since 1995, when two forms of inactivated vaccine were developed: Havrix, given to ages 18 or greater in two doses 6 to 12 months apart and Vaqta given to patients 17 or older in two doses; 6 months apart.[12,16–18] Since 2006, the ACIP has recommended vaccination of children 1 year and older. It is also available in combination with the HBV vaccine (Twinrix). Immunogenicity studies indicate a 95% to 100% seroconversion when the vaccine is given and immunogenicity can remain active for 20 to 30 years.[4,11,12] The ACIP recommends HAV vaccination in travelers and at-risk populations, namely, intravenous drug users, men who have sex with men, those who are previously exposed to HAV, patients receiving clotting factors, and those who travel to areas that are endemic to the viral infection.[11,12,16] Adverse effects include anorexia, headaches, and malaise. HAV exposure without vaccination can be treated with either immunoglobulin or a single dose of the vaccine. The CDC recommends vaccinations to people exposed to anyone who they are in personal contact with, such as adoptee children from other countries.[11,12] HAV is recommended for oral health care providers that work in special needs facilities as well as penal institutions.[4]

Hepatitis B Virus

HBV infection is a global public health problem and is 1 of 2 forms of chronic hepatitis worldwide.[1] More than 240 million people are chronically infected, with more than 300,000 fatalities owing to cirrhosis and more than 340,000 owing to hepatocellular carcinoma.[1,3,4] There are at least 10 separate genotypes that are geographically separated, with genotype A in Europe and North America, genotypes B and C in Asia, genotype D in the Mediterranean, genotype E in Africa, genotype F in Central America, and so on.[6,19] Age of infection varies and will determine the chronicity of infection; that is, 90% of babies born to hepatitis B e antigen–positive mothers may be at risk and regions that are highly endemic for HBV have acquired the infection at birth or early childhood.[1] Infectivity within Western Europe is markedly lower with HBs-Ag positive individuals who have acquired HBV via sexual contact, intravenous drug use, or parenteral exposure of the BBPs by splashing or spillage.[1,4,10,12] With respect to spillage, HBV can survive at room temperature on surfaces for 1 week.[1] Within the United States, unprotected sexual contact as well as intravenous drug use is the major risk factors. Blood donor screening has been successful in reducing exposure of HBV to 1 to 4 cases per 1,000,000 in areas of low prevalence and 1 per 20,000 in areas of high prevalence.[1,3,12]

Studies on HBV infection in health care workers vary throughout the globe and range from 0.1% (in the United States) up to 73% (in Africa), depending on country of origin.[1,3,6,12] Vectors of transmission include blood via stick or aerosol, saliva, and nasopharyngeal secretions transmitted through male sex, older age, dental treatment, blood transfusion, and working in a health care setting.[1,9,10] Serum HBV has an incubation period of 50 to 100 days. A recent 2016 update examined the transmission of BBPs in the US dental health care setting (Cleveland and colleagues[9]) indicated that transmission of BBPs in the dental setting was rare since 2003, that is, 3 events reported. Failure to adhere to CDC guidelines resulted in these adverse events.[10]

HBV infection is the most significant occupational hazard in the oral health care arena, with a significantly higher incidence in dental staff, as well as oral surgeons, periodontists, and endodontists.[3,4,10] Patients with periodontal disease demonstrate increased HBV surface antigens, anti–hepatitis B core, and anti-HCV in saliva than comparable control patients.[6,19] To decrease the burden of HBV in the dental care setting, all doctors and staff should receive vaccinations (discussed elsewhere in this article) as well as using other standard procedures; that is, gloves, gowns, protective equipment. It is mandatory within the United States to be vaccinated against HBV before admission into dental schools and colleges.[9,10] In a literature review by Cleveland and colleagues,[9] from 2010 to 2015 there have been only 3 reports of transmission of HBV and HCV in the dental care setting. The rare occurrence of transmission was owing to failure of sterilization of instruments, a lack of training of staff on BBPs, and the use of multidose vials inappropriately. The 2016 CDC prevention recommendations are in place to be implemented as standard precautions to be applied by all oral health care providers in their practice settings (**Table 2**).[9,10] The 2016 update by the CDC's guidelines for infection control in dental health care settings emphasizes the elements of standard precautions and basic prevention of infection in the dental clinic setting in the form of a checklist that can be designed based on the specific needs of the practice. Dental staff can apply their checklist to daily procedures and how well they adhere to the guidelines that provide a safe environment from HBV transmission.[10] **Table 2** depicts examples of methods and their evaluation.

Hepatitis B virus vaccine

The hepatitis vaccine has been available in the United States since 1986.[20] Any health care worker performing procedures that expose them to BBP should be

Table 2
Guidelines for providing a safe environment for infection prevention

Program Risk Predictor	Outcome Assessment
Immunization of DHCP	Annual review of personnel records for Immune status
Education/CE training	Score CE credit and conduct audit when there is a cross-training of new skills that affect the employee exposure
Assess occupational exposure	Report exposures with an incident report on time, place, and prevention for future events
Postexposure/medical management	Postexposure protocols are expected and all staff understands the protocols including access for further Questions/concerns; that is, toll free numbers to CDC
Hand hygiene protocol	Observe/document hand washing before/after patient contact
Personal protective equipment	Observe/document barrier precaution use/review with staff
Sterilization protocol monitor	Monitor records/logs/temperature of autoclave/spore Check, on a weekly basis and correct if critical deficiency
Evaluate safety devices	Annual review of medical devices and repairs
Compliance of water EPA	Monitor dental water quality using test kits that are self-maintained or use commercial laboratories for testing
Disposal of medical waste	Safe disposal protocol and measures if hazardous waste
Health care infection	Assess patient treatment follow-up for any undue infectious process

Abbreviations: CDC, Centers for Disease Control and Prevention; CE, continuing education; DHCP, dental health care provider; EPA, Environmental Protection Agency.
Adapted from Centers for Disease Control and Prevention (CDC). Guidelines for infection control in dental health-care settings — 2003. MMWR Morb Mortal Wkly Rep 2003;52:1–61.

vaccinated.[3,10,20] There are 2 recombinant preparations of HBV vaccines. There is no need for serologic testing before vaccinations; however, if exposure of HBV is a possibility before HBV vaccination then hepatitis B immunoglobulin should be administered.[4,12] The immunization protocol involves 3 doses.[4,12] The first dose is administered followed 1 month by the second dose and the third dose is administered 2 months after the second dose and at least 4 months after the first dose. The first 2 doses are primers to enhance the immune response so that the third dose acts as a booster. Immunogenicity from HBV vaccine can last for greater than 15 years in hosts who are not immunosuppressed.[4] Nondetectable circulating anti–hepatitis B surface antigen is not indicative of loss of immunity and boosters are not normally recommended; however, antibodies should be detectable 30 to 60 days after the last dosing schedule.[4,11,12] If there is no detectable antibody titer, another dose can be administered. If there is still no response or a titer of 10 mLU/ml, then this group of patients and providers needs to be counseled appropriately about their susceptibility to HBV infectivity.

Adverse effects of HBV include soreness at site of injection, myalgia, and fevers. Several studies have associated exposure to HBV vaccine and predisposition to demyelinating neurologic diseases such as Guillain-Barre syndrome and multiple sclerosis, although no epidemiologic data indicate this risk.[4,21] The ACIP recommends that diabetics greater than 60 years of age be vaccinated against HBV when the diabetes is diagnosed.[11] Studies have shown an increased risk for HBV infection in diabetics that are in facilities where their blood glucose is being monitored constantly.[11] Testing for circulating antibodies is also recommended for clinicians older than age 30 because advancing age is correlated with lower seroconversion rates; 42% seroconversion for those older than age 60 compared with 83.3% of those younger than age 50.[4,22] Oral health care workers who suffer from immunocompromised diseases should not be exposed to live vaccines if they are receiving chemotherapy and/or radiation. The time between ending therapy and getting vaccinated is 3 months and the CDC has outlined specifics for HIV-infected health care providers.[4,9,10]

Hepatitis C Virus

HCV was first identified as the causative vector in 95% of cases of non-A non-B hepatitis during the 1980s.[6] The incubation period can vary from 3 to 20 weeks and can present in an asymptomatic fashion, because exposure is associated with a transient increase in liver alanine transferase of up to 10-fold before symptoms present.[6,23] HCV infection progresses to chronicity and is a major health problem that leads to cirrhosis and hepatocellular carcinoma.[4,6,23] The World Health Organization reports that 130 to 150 million people are infected and HCV exposure is regionally variable, with high prevalence rates in the Middle East and Northern Africa and low rates in North American and Western Europe.[24] Seven strains of HCV have been recorded and HVC genotype 1 is the most prevalent worldwide followed by HCV 3. The transmission of infection was through infected blood products until 1989, and routine screening for antibodies to HCV occurred in the 1990s, which has reduced transmission significantly. More recent risk for HCV exposure has been through acupuncture, body piercing, tattooing, nail scissors, hair clippers, and needle stick injury to health care workers.[25] HCV and HBV have never been infectious with exposure to vomit, urine, sweat, or tears.[6] HCV transmission occurs in 10% of health care workers after parenteral exposure from percutaneous and mucosal blood of an HCV RNA-positive patient.[1,6]

Cleveland and colleagues[10] reported a study within the oral health care setting of an oral surgery office that a patient became infected with HCV from another patient owing to multiple lapses of infection prevention and control. Dental assistants in this setting were administering medications without appropriate training and exposed a patient to HCV. The use of multidose vials for more than 1 patient and a lack of autoclave monitoring resulted in transmission of HCV.[10] Other studies related to infectivity have identified that HCV can survive in the environment for up to 6 weeks on a dry surface.[10] Whether or not this can act as a route remains to be determined because only a percutaneous path has been identified as the source of contact. The prevalence of HCV antibodies in US dentists who participated in the American Dental Association health screens are well below that of the population at large (0.5% vs 1.6%) suggesting a very low risk for occupational exposure as compared with studies worldwide that show greater anti-HCV positivity in health care providers.[9,10]

HCV vaccine

A report by the Committee on a National Strategy for the Elimination of Hepatitis B and C, Board on Population Health and Public Health Practice (Health and Medicine Division; National Academies of Sciences, Engineering, and Medicine; Buckley GJ, Strom BL, editors) is examining the feasibility of hepatitis B and C elimination in the United States. Although there is no vaccine for HCV, new direct-acting antivirals may cure 95% of chronic infections, although these drugs are unlikely to reach all chronically infected people anytime soon. As such, per the CDC guidelines, all oral health care workers should follow standard procedures by meticulously applying infection control checklists, as well as vaccinations specific to risk of exposure.

Measles, Mumps, and Rubella Vaccine

Measles is a paramyxovirus spread by respiratory transmission to the nasopharynx with an incubation period of 10 to 12 days.[12] It spreads to the lymphatic system and respiratory tract with resultant coughing, conjunctivitis, and coryza followed by Koplick spots or a rash. It can lead to encephalitis and pneumonia. Successful immunization with vaccine has eliminated its endemic spread and so it is one of the major vaccine-preventable diseases.[11–14] Most adults born before 1956 should have antibody immunity; however, history alone is no longer considered to be presumptive for antibody immunity.[11,12] Laboratory confirmation of antibody immunity is required for health care personnel for measles, mumps, and rubella. (see vaccine protocol).

Mumps is a paramyxovirus also spread to the nasopharynx and can spread to the meninges and glands such as the testes and parotids, and can lead to orchitis in men.[12] The incubation is 16 to 18 days and can be either symptomatic or asymptomatic. Aseptic meningitis can also occur as well as loss of hearing in 1 in 20,000 infections.[26] Introduction of the live vaccine (MMR; see below) has reduced cases in the United States and supports the premise of vaccine-preventable diseases.[12,26]

Rubella is a togavirus and spread through respiratory transmission with an incubation period of 14 days followed by a maculopapular rash and arthralgias and arthritis. There are rare complications of thrombocytopenia and encephalitis. The devastating complication, however, is congenital rubella syndrome that results in deafness, cataracts, cardiac defects, mental retardation, and fetal demise.[12,27] These sequelae stress the importance of the rubella vaccine (part of the MMR compound). Nonimmune women should be immunized to avoid the risk of congenital rubella in their offspring.[12,27]

Measles, mumps, and rubella vaccine

The MMR vaccine is highly effective in eliciting an antibody response and immunity to each component of the virus.[12,26,27] Measles antibodies develop after 1 dose and up to 99% after the second dose. One dose of the MMR is effective in eliciting antibodies to mumps and rubella and gives lifelong immunity. The CDC recommends that, if appropriate, vaccination is not documented a serologic test is done and if the health care provider is not protected 2 doses of MMR vaccine is administered 4 weeks apart.[6,12] Because MMR is a live vaccine, female providers are recommended to avoid getting pregnant for 3 months after receiving the MMR vaccine.[11,12,28] Adverse reactions include fever and a transient rash. Egg allergies should be documented and vaccines should not be administered because MMR vaccine components are extracted from chick embryos.[11,12]

Varicella zoster virus

The varicella zoster virus is a member of the herpes virus family of DNA viruses. It is a common vector for illness in the United States with the majority of exposure presenting as Chickenpox initially. It has the propensity to reactivate later in life within the dorsal root ganglia of the nervous system; herpes zoster virus commonly known as "shingles." The latter is more common with advancing age and in patients with immunosuppression owing to other diseases.[29] The varicella zoster virus is transmitted by direct exposure via inhalation of aerosols from vesicular fluid or respiratory tract secretions. The illness starts with a mild prodromal phase followed by a rash that progresses to a macular/papule lesion before crusting. The infectious period is 1 to 2 days before the rash and continues until all lesions become crusted.

The varicella virus was endemic to the United States at significant levels before the introduction of a vaccine in 1995.[12,29] Two vaccines are available for prevention of the primary infection: Varivax and a combination of MMR and varicella called ProQuad.[12] The dosing schedule is over 4 to 8 weeks, with 78% of adults mounting an antibody response after the first dose and 99% after second dose with full immugenicity 4 to 8 weeks later, which lasts a lifetime in the majority of cases.[12] Routine vaccination is recommended for all nonpregnant patients/staff because vaccination with varicella virus during pregnancy poses a risk for the unborn child. Pregnant women should be tested for immunity. If nonimmune, they are given a choice. Because the vaccine is attenuated, women should not become pregnant for 4 weeks after immuniza-tion.[12,29,30] For oral health care providers who are nonimmune, 2 doses should be given 4 weeks apart.

Herpes zoster (shingles) is a localized painful cutaneous eruption seen in older and immunocompromised adults. It usually has a dermatome distribution and is caused by a reactivation of the herpes virus within the dorsal root ganglia supplying area of the eruption. A complication of shingles is postherpetic neuralgia, a painful condition that can last over months to years. It occurs in 10% to 18% of individuals with shin-gles.[11,12,29] Another complication is the Ramsay-Hunt syndrome that results from a peripheral facial nerve paralysis owing to herpes zoster involving the geniculate gan-glion of the facial nerve. The herpes zoster vaccine (Zostavax) was approved in 2006 by the US Food and Drug Administration for use in 60 years of age or older, but also condones its use in those 50 to 59 years of age.[11,12] The ACIP has not commented on this age range, but does agree with the use in patients 60 year of age and older. A history of zoster is not a contraindication for vaccination and it may potentiate the anti-body response form the initial exposure by acting like a booster.[11,12] Randomized, controlled trials have suggested that protection can last at least 4 years. Efficacy seems to decrease with age.[29]

Influenza

Over the past 5 years, the CDC and the ACIP have strongly recommended that all health care workers, as well as all patients including children be immunized against influenza.[4,11,12] The epidemiology, morbidity, and mortality of influenza have described and the rates of serious illness and death among patients age 65 and older is approximately 36,000 deaths in the 1990s.[31] Influenza is a strongly infectious path-ogen causing a severe respiratory illness with concomitant fever, headaches, coryza, vomiting, and diarrhea. Transmission is via respiratory droplets. Influenza A and B cause epidemic disease outbreaks worldwide.[12,31] Type A is broken down further into subtypes based on surface antigens (neuraminidase and hemagglutinin). Anti-genic shifts can result in serious pandemics based on mutational changes within the antigen structure.[11,12,31]

Influenza vaccines

Randomized clinical trials have looked at the efficacy of vaccine-preventable disease and health care worker absenteeism.[12] Results suggest an increased cost effective-ness in the immunization of all health care workers during the flu season.[32] There are 2 types of influenza vaccine for adults: the trivalent inactivated form (TIV) and the attenuated form influenza vaccine (live attenuated influenza vaccine).[12,31] The latter is administered nasally.[33] The attenuated form is sensitive to temperature and cannot replicate within the human core range. These are adapted to cold and require coolness for activation of immunity protection. The live attenuated influenza vaccine is more effective in children and is not approved in ages for those 50 years of age and older, in pregnant women, in immunocompromised patients (ie, HIV), chronic obstructive pulmonary disease, renal disease, hepatic dysfunction, or metabolic sequelae of diabetes. There is a new trivalent vaccine (TIVI) given intradermally to ages those 18 to 64 in the deltoid muscle. Adverse reactions include pain erythema, induration, and pruritus. The TIVHD is an alternative to TIV if the patient is older than 65 years of age. Both the live attenuated influenza vaccine and TIV are equivalent to influenza A subtype H3N2, H1N1, and 1 influenza B virus.[12,32] With reference to allergic reactions, the ACIP recommended in 2011 to revise the egg allergy contraindication to a precaution strategy if there is no history to anaphylaxis and egg exposure. The issue of the older patient relates to their immune system undergoing an "immunosenescence" and, therefore, higher doses of vaccine may be warranted. This hypothesis is still under investigation.[33]

Streptococcus pneumoniae
S pneumoniae is a gram-positive anaerobic bacteria inhabiting the respiratory tract and seen in 70% of healthy subjects. The vector is via respiratory droplets and results in serious exacerbations of pneumonia, meningitis, and septic bacteremia. Epidemiologic evidence indicates up to 40,000 cases in the United States and 1.6 million deaths of pneumococcal disease worldwide in the elderly and children.[12,34] As such, there has been a global public health effort to decrease the death rate from septicemia through the use of immunization against pneumococcal disease.

Pneumococcal Polysaccharide Vaccine
Pneumococcal polysaccharide vaccine is a purified pneumococcal polysaccharide preparation originally made in the late 1970s and now available as Pneumovax, a 23-valent vaccine (pneumococcal polysaccharide vaccine 23).[12,34] It is recommended for persons 65 or older. Both the ACIP and CDC in 2008 added smokers and asthmatics as high risk in need of the pneumococcal vaccine to reduce the severity of pneumonia.[35] Recent studies also suggest that this vaccine can prevent myocardial infarctions owing to its effects on inflammation from thrombotic events.[12,34] At least 80% of adults who receive the vaccine develop antibody protection for at least for 5 years, although those who are immunocompromised have less of the efficacy of protection (ie, HIV and cancer patients undergoing chemotherapy and radiation).[12,34] Health care workers should be judicious in recommending that patients who are newly diagnosed with malignancies get vaccinated with the pneumococcal polysaccharide vaccine 23 and wait at least 2 weeks before initiating therapeutic interventions.[12,34] Patient who are more than 65 years old and had a vaccination should get a second after 5 years to act as a booster.[36]

Tetanus, diphtheria, and pertussis
Tetanus, diphtheria, and pertussis, although not seen quite frequently in the United States, remain a concern for certain populations that have either never been previously vaccinated or have a new onset exposure.[11]

Tetanus
Clostridium tetani is a gram-positive anaerobic organism whose exotoxins prevent the release of neurotransmitters leading to uncontrolled muscle spasms and trismus. They enter via an open wound and can exacerbate/prevent swallowing and breathing leading to death. During the 1940s, tetanus toxoid was introduced as part of the routine immunization package in children consisting of 3 spaced doses with a recurrent

booster every 10 years except if there is an exposure such as stepping on a rusty nail or open wounds in soil.[11,12] C tetani produces a toxin that destroys tissue on any mucous membrane but most often on the tonsils and pharyngeal tissue. These locations of injury can cause respiratory obstruction and death.

Pertussis

Among the 3 diseases, pertussis remains an endemic health problem with between 800,000 and 3.3 million cases in the United States annually.[12] Bordetella pertussis is a gram-negative coccobacillus that attacks the respiratory epithelium. There are 3 phases of the disease process:

1. Catarrhal consisting of coryza, coughing, and sneezing;
2. Paroxysmal stage with continued coughing, followed by a long inspiration and a whooping for 4 to 6 weeks; and
3. A convalescent stage, where the coughing decreases.

Older individuals are often vectors for transmission to young children. The latter is on the rise owing to the debate about vaccine effectiveness (discussed elsewhere in this article).[13,37]

Diphtheria

Corynebacterium diphtheria is an aerobic gram-positive bacteria producing a toxin that acts to destroy tissue within the mucous membranes. Diphtheria was a significant cause of mortality in children during the 1940s, but with toxoid immunization this disease has been eradicated with only 5 cases reported within the last 15 years.[12]

Tetanus-Diphtheria-Pertussis Vaccine

Within the United States, there are 2 preparations of vaccines—Adacel and Boostrix—each containing tetanus toxoid, acellular pertussis and reduced diphtheria toxoid (Tdap).[11,12,38] One dose of Tdap is as efficacious as 3 doses of diphtheria toxoid, acellular pertussis, and tetanus toxoid with respect to the antibody response. Boostrix is available for those ages 10 to 64 years and Adacel is approved for those ages 11 to 64 years.[11,12] The ACIP suggest that Tdap can be administered to those greater than 65 years of age if the patients are in contact with young children because morbidity and mortality are greatest in children.[12,38] Furthermore, if parents are immunized their young children are protected more than 50% of the time they are exposed. The ACIP has structured a vaccination protocol for Tdap (see **Box 2**).[38]

Human Papillomavirus

HPV is a double-stranded DNA virus that infects basal epithelium. HPV type 16 and 18 are responsible for the majority of cervical dysplasia seen, as well as 40% of penile cancers seen in the United States and worldwide.[11,12,39,40] It is the most common sexually transmitted disease and out of 80% of females who are sexually active, 41% can be exposed to HPV type 16 by age 50.[41] HPV can cause skin warts and cervical dysplasia that can mature into squamous cell carcinoma in the vagina, anus, vulva, and oral cavity.[40,41] Pregnant women can transmit the virus to their newborn at the time of birth. Other risk factors are numerous sex partners and a partner's sex history. HPV 16 is especially responsible for more than 85% of head and neck squamous cell cancers.[12,39,40] The progression of HPV infection from precancerous to cancer can occur over a period of 10 years. Most HPV infections, however, can clear over 8 months to 2 years.[11,12,40]

Human papillomavirus vaccine

There are 2 vaccines available to prevent human papillomavirus (HPV) infections, and as of 2011, both are licensed in the United States; Cervarix is protective against HPV 16 and 18 and Gardasil is protective against HPV 6, 11, 16, and 18. Both are composed of viruslike particles from recombinant capsid proteins of HPV, neither are live, and both have an efficacy greater than 90% in preventing precancerous cervical lesions.[12,41,42] Gardasil is used for girls and young women 9 to 26 years of age for the prevention of vulva, vaginal, anal, and cervical precancerous lesions, as well as vaginal warts. The ACIP recommends Gardasil for all unvaccinated men ages 22 to 26, as well as those who are immunocompromised, test positive for HIV, and/or who have sex with men. Cervarix is recommended for women ages 10 to 25 for the prevention of cervical cancer and precancerous lesions.[41,42]

The dosing schedule for both vaccines is based on ACIP recommendations of 3 inoculations.[42] Each dose is 0.5 mL administered intramuscularly. The first dose is followed by a second dose 1 to 2 months after, followed by a third dose 6 months after the first dose. With respect to oropharyngeal cancer protection, there are no studies to support the use of these vaccines. Studies do not support the vaccination of pregnant women, but there are no conclusive data that show morbidity.[11,41,42] Further studies are underway, as well as studies that examine the decrease in disease in women given the vaccine up to age 45.[12] HPV vaccines should be administered before sexual contact; however, the vaccine is still recommended even after contact. Studies are now in progress to determine the duration of antibody efficacy and as such there is no recommendation for booster vaccinations.[11,12,42]

Typhoid and tuberculosis

Typhoid and TB vaccinations are not routinely recommended for health care providers in the United States. TB, however, is still quite common in certain parts of the world such as Africa.[16,43] The World Health Organization reports the highest incidence rate to be Southern Africa.[43] The overall risk of acquiring infection from *Mycobacterium tuberculosis* is very low in the United States; however, there are numerous cases of children emigrating from other parts of the world to the United States who are given the attenuated BCG vaccine to prevent TB. This results in false positive findings when the standard tuberculin test is given.[44] The CDC recommends stringent criteria for health care workers to receive BCG coverage:

1. The workers are treating have a high percentage of TB-active individuals who are resistant to rifampin and isoniazid; and
2. Transmission of active infection is likely owing to inadequate infection control measures.[4,16,45]

Two new blood tests are now being used to increase the specificity of exposure to TB, an enzyme-linked immunosorbent assay and an immunosorbent assay that measures T-cell activity and latent TB infection.[44] The oral health care provider must be judicious in his or her decision to take the BCG vaccine because it may interfere with the ability to detect newly acquired infection and so only those who are in regular contact with infected patients should weigh the risks and benefits of vaccination.[3,4,11]

Although the incidence within the United States of acquired typhoid fever is declining, the proportion of cases resulting from foreign travel has continued to increase.[16,46] A major advance in the control of typhoid fever was the development of an oral live, attenuated vaccine (Ty21a). Ty21a in a formulation given over 1 week provides 69% efficacy for at least 4 years. A series of 4 doses confers maximum protection.[46,47] Travelers to areas of high risk should be vaccinated as well as being vigilant for careful selection of food and water; the protection of the vaccine can be overcome by large inoculates of *S typhi*. With respect to oral health care, this vector of infection is not routinely listed as one that necessitates a vaccine-preventable disease strategy.[46,47]

VACCINE-PREVENTABLE DISEASES IN THE IMMUNOSUPPRESSED ORAL HEALTH CARE WORKER

The advances in health science, technology, and vaccine-preventable disease strategies have afforded opportunities for health care workers who have debilitating illnesses to continue practicing their specialties. Immunocompromised patients with primary immune deficiency, secondary immune deficiency, and immune-regulated abnormalities can be vaccinated with a protective effect (**Box 3** describes each immunocompromised condition).[47,48] Examples of immune conditions that oral health care providers are infected with include HIV, HCV, acquired malignancies, and autoimmune diseases being treated with corticosteroid therapy regimens. Vaccines that contain killed virus components do not pose a problem to this population of health care providers if protocols are followed that mimic the dosing of patients who are in a similar situation. Specific vaccines that are recommended include the polysaccharide vaccines such as *Haemophilus influenza* type B, pneumococcal, and meningococcal vaccines (discussed elsewhere in this article). There should be no administration of an attenuated form of vaccine if one is undergoing chemotherapy and/or radiation until 3 months after the final treatment is given because the ability to mount an antibody reservoir can be impeded. Those who are under corticosteroid regimens need to be scrutinized carefully. The CDC recommends no contraindication to live vaccine administration if steroid therapy was less than 2 weeks but supports no vaccinations

---

Box 3
Characteristics and strategies for vaccine-preventable disease in primary, secondary and immune regulatory abnormalities

PID
  Increase susceptibility to infection, autoimmune and inflammatory sequelae
  Diagnosis requires thorough evaluation of T-cell, B-cell, and innate immunity
  Antibody deficiency often cause of PID
  Inactivated vaccines recommended
  Attenuated vaccines; that is, MMR, VAR, rotavirus, live influenza, oral polio contraindicated

SID/IRA
  Usually owing to consequences of immunosuppression and/or modulatory treatment
  Human immunodeficiency virus infection, hematologic malignancies, tumors, solid organ transplant recipients, multiple sclerosis, inflammatory bowel disease, autoimmune/ inflammatory diseases, chronic diabetes, heart, lung disease and complement deficiencies.
  Immune impairment may be may be a combination of B- and T-cell deficiencies.
  Yearly vaccination of inactivated PCV and pneumococcal polysaccharide vaccine 23 highly recommended, as well as quadrivalent meningococcal vaccines and hepatitis B.
  Live vaccines administration is predicated upon severity of immune state with need for risk to benefit decisions by an immunologist.
  SID/IRA patients require higher dosing and more frequent immunizations.

Abbreviations: IRA, immune-regulatory abnormalities; MMR, measles, mumps, rubella; PID, primary immune deficiency; SID, secondary immune deficiency; VAR, varicella.
Adapted from Eibl MM, Wolf HM. Vaccination in patients with primary immune deficiency, secondary immune deficiency and autoimmunity with immune regulatory abnormalities. Immunotherapy 2015;7(12):1286.

until 3 months after steroid therapy that exceeds 2 week duration. It is most important to weigh the risk to benefit ratio with the provider's physician of record. Evaluation and monitoring within this population would define and improve treatment decisions for greater cost effectiveness, reduction of complications owing to their disease state, and a better health-related quality of life.

ASSESSMENT OF VACCINE CONFIDENCE

The US population generally has great confidence in the efficacy and reliability of the vaccine program and the latest measles cases provided yet another reminder of the importance of vaccines and timely vaccination.[13] Although the source case traced to the tourist destination is not known, the first identified case of measles stemmed from an individual who had not been vaccinated against the disease and most of the subsequent infections involved people who were unvaccinated. Unfortunately, in many cases, the unvaccinated children were likely unvaccinated by choice.[13] The recommended measles vaccination must have been delayed or declined, a choice that left them vulnerable and the rest of the unvaccinated population susceptible to measles. These cases are a lesson to health providers who chose not to be vaccinated and lack immunity to vaccine-preventable infectious diseases.[49]

Immunity is often silent or invisible until it is tested—and measles is one of the most sensitive "stress tests" we have. The need to maintain the high immunization rates, particularly in health workers, along with evidence that more parents are hesitating or delaying when it comes to following vaccination recommendations, prompted the Assistant Secretary for Health of the Department of Health and Human Services to ask the National Vaccine Advisory Committee to assess how confidence in vaccines affects vaccination in the United States.[13,49,50]

Vaccines are one of the most effective and successful public health tools to prevent disease, illness, and premature death from preventable infectious diseases. and there is much good news in the United States when it comes to recommended vaccines and vaccinations.[13,51] When there are high levels of immunity in a community induced by vaccination, a transmitting case is unlikely to encounter a susceptible host, thus terminating transmission and preventing exposure of others in the community who are either not protected by vaccination (no vaccine is 100% effective[5]), cannot be vaccinated (ie, have a legitimate contraindication to vaccination), or who are not eligible for vaccination (eg, children too young for some recommended vaccines).[50,51] Thus, what makes vaccines unique is that with high levels of vaccination both the individual and the community are protected, a phenomenon, characterized often as "herd immunity." However, high vaccination coverage rates are required for community protection. In the United States, high vaccination rates have been reached for many recommended vaccines, leading to the near elimination of the corresponding vaccine-preventable diseases and 99% to 100% reductions in mortality from vaccine-preventable diseases, leading to thousands of lives saved each year.[13,51] Not all recommended vaccinations have reached high coverage rates and there are places in the country where coverage is not high enough to achieve population protection, leaving the people, including young children and health professionals, vulnerable to vaccine-preventable diseases, especially in the event of a disease outbreak. Vaccination rates among children are high and, for most parents, following the recommended schedule is the norm. Health care providers are highly supportive of vaccines and immunization recommendations and, for most parents, are a trusted source of information and guidance. When it comes to vaccine confidence, trust in health care providers, health care provider communication and endorsement, social norms, and communication play central roles in instilling, maintaining, and fostering vaccine confidence. Health care providers can also demonstrate this trust by being fully immunized against vaccine-preventable disease.[13,49,50]

The Working Group recognized several challenges that threaten successful utilization of recommended vaccines. There are communities and places (eg, schools) where vaccination levels are below and sometimes far below the levels needed to protect those who are unvaccinated. There are also parents whose reluctance, hesitation, concerns, or lack of confidence has caused them to question or forego recommended vaccines. In some cases, the children are vaccinated, but vaccinations are delayed beyond recommended ages, alternative schedules are used, or vaccines are totally declined, health workers are declining vaccination, and others fail to recognize their lack of immunogenicity. In these cases, the individual is left susceptible to the disease and, if infected, can transmit it to others.[13,49–51]

PUBLIC CONFIDENCE

As the World Health Organization's Strategic Advisory Group of Experts' vaccine hesitancy efforts illustrate, building and fostering vaccine confidence and acceptance is not just a problem in the United States, but an issue of urgent importance in global health.[52] More efforts are needed to identify, develop, and evaluate strategies and approaches to find the ones that facilitate or instill confidence, and the resources and systems need to be in place to share lessons learned and effective practices. Along these lines, it is also the case that vaccine confidence and acceptance efforts need to encompass health care providers.[13,52] Not only is it imperative that they have high confidence in recommended vaccines and vaccinations, they must have the resources, capacities and capabilities needed to effectively educate and address individuals' questions and concerns. In most cases, it is health care providers who directly affect workers' confidence and acceptance of recommended vaccines and vaccinations.

Vaccination in accordance with the CDC's ACIP recommended immunization schedule continues to be the social norm in the United States and high vaccination coverage has been achieved for most recommended vaccines on the recommended childhood immunization schedule.[13,51] For infant and early childhood immunizations, rates have been high and stable for the past several decades, namely, at or above the 80% to 90% range for nearly all ACIP recommended childhood vaccinations. Similarly, recent reports suggest that a majority of parents have favorable beliefs or perceptions with regard to recommended childhood vaccines. A 2009 Health Styles survey of parents of children 6 years old and younger, for instance, found 79% were "confident" or "very confident" in the safety of routine childhood vaccines.[13,53] A 2010 Health Styles survey found 72% of parents were confident in the safety of vaccines, with slightly more parents expressing confidence in the effectiveness of vaccines (78%) and the benefits of vaccines (77%).[13,53] Further analyses of these data showed that 2 factors—confidence in vaccine safety and confidence in vaccine effectiveness—were a major source of influence on parents' self-reported vaccination behavior.[9] Overall, however, these studies also suggested that about 1 in 5 parents were not fully confident in the safety or importance of recommended vaccinations.

The Cultural Cognition Project at the Yale Law School has collected data involving or related to confidence.[54] They also found that about 27% of adults strongly to slightly disagreed with the statement, "I am confident in the judgment of public health officials who are responsible for identifying generally recommended childhood vaccinations." About 62% had moderately or extremely high confidence in "the judgment of the American Academy of Pediatrics that vaccines are a safe and effective way to prevent serious disease," but about 20% had relatively low confidence.[13,54]

HEALTH CARE PROVIDER CONFIDENCE

It is clear from published studies that health care providers—the frontline people who interact with parents and who administer vaccines—are critically important when it comes to vaccine confidence.[13,51] Studies consistently find that the vast majority of parents (80% or more) look to their child's health care provider for information and advice on vaccine-preventable diseases, vaccines, and the recommended immunization schedule.[55] When providers are able to communicate effectively with parents about vaccine benefits and risks, the value and need for vaccinations, and vaccine safety, parents are more confident in their decision to adhere to the recommended schedule. In a study involving both parents and health care providers, Mergler and colleagues[56] found a strong association between parental and provider vaccine-related attitudes and beliefs. For example, parents had a 45 times higher odds of agreeing that the community benefits from having children fully vaccinated if their provider agree, compared with parents whose provider did not agree. They also noted that some parents likely chose providers who are similar vaccine beliefs as their own—and, as such, providers with doubts about recommended vaccinations can foster or support hesitancy.[57] Finally, it has also been found that reliance on vaccine information sources other than providers is associated with exemptions from school entry requirements. Rosenstock,[13,58] for instance, found that parents who sought vaccine information on the Internet were more likely to have lower perceptions of vaccine safety, vaccine effectiveness, and disease susceptibility and were more likely to have a child with a nonmedical exemption. From the perspective of vaccine confidence, it is thus important to recognize that health care providers are key players when it comes to establishing, maintaining, and building parent confidence in vaccines. Thus, health care providers need to demonstrate vaccine confidence by becoming fully vaccinated.[13,57,58]

In many instances, however, health care providers have not met their responsibility to be fully immunized against vaccine-preventable disease.[3,4,9,13] They continue to put themselves and the public at risk. For influenza, vaccination coverage among physicians and dentists (84.2%) was similar to coverage among nurse practitioners and physician assistants (82.6%), and was significantly higher than for those working in all other occupational groups. Coverage also was significantly higher among health care providers aged 60 years or greater (74.2%), compared with those aged 18 to 29 years (56.4%) and those 30 to 44 years (57.8%).[13] An in-depth literature review describing universal influenza vaccination attitudes in hospital-based health care provider identified a number of reasons commonly cited for not receiving the vaccine. In 21 studies in 9 countries, the authors reported that the 5 most frequently reported categories for vaccine refusal included:

1. Fear of adverse reactions;
2. Lack of concern (ie, perception that influenza does not pose a serious public health risk);
3. Inconvenient delivery;
4. Lack of perception of own risk; and
5. Doubts regarding vaccine efficacy.

These studies also found that health care providers are more likely to be vaccinated to protect themselves against influenza than to be vaccinated for the protection of patients. Similarly, a recent CDC report found that the prevalence of beliefs regarding influenza and influenza vaccination differ between vaccinated and unvaccinated health care provider. This study found that 92.7% of vaccinated health care provider believed getting vaccinated could protect them from influenza infection, whereas only 54.2% of those who were unvaccinated shared that belief. Notably, the CDC study also indicated that 55.4% of unvaccinated health care provider do not believe that vaccination better protects those around them from influenza infection. The most important factor facilitating vaccine acceptance was a desire for self-protection, previous receipt of influenza vaccine, perceived effectiveness of vaccine, and older age. These studies highlight the importance of educating health care providers on the seriousness of influenza and vaccine-preventable disease as a public health threat.[13]

SUMMARY AND FUTURE DIRECTIONS

Vaccination and immunization to prevent the transmission of infectious diseases remain a major dynamic force for all health care specialists and their patients around the globe and, as such, all health care workers should be candidates for immunizations to prevent the spread of disease within the communities they serve. The evidence presented in this article represents a need for greater awareness toward immunizations by and within the oral health care arena because numerous vaccine-preventable diseases are frequently transmitted in the dental care setting (**Fig. 1**). Future directions include a closer evaluation of vaccine effectiveness as a preventive strategy in the dental health care setting to develop an algorithm for an immunization program that the oral health care provider can specifically play a pivotal role. It is essential that every dental practitioner be immunized against the vaccine-preventable diseases described throughout their oral health care career. Continuing education that focuses on vaccine-preventable diseases will increase vaccine

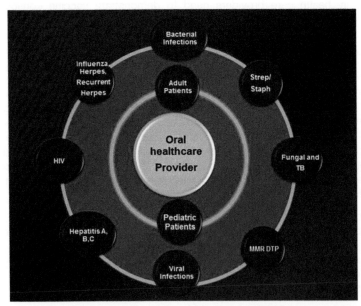

Fig. 1. Vaccine-preventable diseases in oral health care. HIV, human immunodeficiency virus; Strep/Staph, *Streptococcus*; *Staphylococcus*; TB, tuberculosis.

awareness and decrease the transmission of infectious diseases within the oral health practice setting.

REFERENCES

1. Coppola N, De Pascalis S, Onorato L, et al. Hepatitis B virus and hepatitis C virus infection in healthcare workers. World J Hepatol 2016;1893:273–81.
2. Elseviers MM, Arias Guillen M, Gorke A, et al. Sharps injuries amongst healthcare workers: review of incidence, transmissions and costs. J Ren Care 2014;40: 150–6.
3. Petti S, Messano GA, Polimeni A. Dentist's awareness toward vaccine preventable diseases. Vaccine 2011;29:8108–12.
4. Quaranta P. Immunization and oral health care providers. Dent Clin North Am 2003;47:641–64.
5. Ciesielski C, Marianos D, Ou CY, et al. Transmission of human immunodeficiency virus in a dental practice. Ann Intern Med 1992;116(10):798–805.
6. Dahlya P, Kamal R, Sharma V, et al. "Hepatitis" – prevention and management in dental practice. J Edu Health Promot 2015;4:1–6.
7. Bindra S, Reddy KVR, Chakrabarty A, et al. Awareness about needle stick injuries and sharps disposal: a study conducted at Army College of Dental Services. J Maxillofac Oral Surg 2014;113(4):419–24.
8. Cleveland JL, Cardo DM. Occupational exposure to human deficiency virus, hepatitis B virus and hepatitis c virus: risk, prevention, management. Dent Clin North Am 2003;47(4):681–96.
9. Cleveland JL, Gray SK, Harte JA, et al. Transmission of blood-borne pathogens in US dental health care settings. J Am Dent Assoc 2016;147(9):729–38.
10. Centers for Disease Control and Prevention (CDC). Healthcare-associated hepatitis B and C outbreaks reported to the Centers for disease Control and Prevention (CDC) 2008-2014. Available at: www.cdc.gov/hepatitis/outbreaks/ HealthcareHepOutbreakTable.htm. Accessed June 12, 2016.
11. Wolfe RM. Update on adult immunizations. J Am Board Fam Med 2012;25(4): 496–510.
12. Hillson CM, Barash JH, Buchanan EM. Adult vaccination. Prim Care 2011;38: 611–32.
13. National Vaccine Advisory Committee. Assessing the state of Vaccine confidence in the united states: recommendations from the National Vaccine Advisory Committee. Public Health Rep 2015;130:573–95.
14. Hadler SC, Hutchins SS, LeBaron CW, et al. General recommendations on immunization recommendations of the Advisory Committee on Immunization Practices (ACIP). MMWR Morb Mortal Wkly Rep 1994;43(RR01):1–38.
15. Baxter D. Active and passive immunity, vaccine types excipients and licensing. Occup Med 2007;57:552–6.
16. Nguyen GT, Altshuler M. Vaccine –preventable diseases and foreign –born populations. Prim Care 2011;38:633–42.
17. Atkinson W, Wolfe S, Hamborsky J, et al. Hepatitis A. Epidemiology and prevention of vaccine-preventable diseases. Washington, DC: Public Health Foundation; 2009. p. 85–96.
18. Klevens RM, Miller JT, Iqbal K, et al. The evolving epidemiology of Hepatitis A in the United States: incidence and molecular epidemiology from population-based surveillance 2005-2007. Arch Intern Med 2010;170(20):1811–8.

19. Mealy BL, Klokkevold PR, Corgel CO. Periodontal treatment of medically compromised patients. Carranza's Clinical Periodontology. 10th edition. Amsterdam (Netherlands): Elsevier Publication; 2010.
20. Center for Disease Control, Prevention. A comprehensive immunization strategy to eliminate transmission of Hepatitis B virus infection in the United States. Recommendations of the Advisory Committee on Immunization Practices (ACIP). Part II: vaccination in adults. MMWR Recomm Rep 2006;55(RR16):1–33.
21. Immunization safety review: hepatitis B vaccine and demyelinating neurological disorders overview of the Institute of Medicine (IOM) report. CDC web site. 2002. Available at: http://www.cdc.gov/nip/news/iom-hepb-5-2002/iom.htm. Accessed June 2, 2010.
22. Guss P, Havlichek D, Rosenman K, et al. Age-related Hepatitis B seroconversion rates in healthcare workers. Am J Infect Control 1997;25(5):418–20.
23. Abeulhassan W. Hepatitis C virus infection in 2012 and beyond. South Afr J Epidemiol Infec 2012;27:93–7.
24. WHO guidelines Approved By the Guidelines Review Committee. Guidelines for the screening, care and treatment of persons with hepatitis C infection. Geneva (Switzerland): World Health Organization; 2014. Available at: http://apps.who.int/medicinedocs/documents/s22180en/s22180en.pdf.
25. Mass S, Berg T, Rosktroth J, et al. Hepatology. 6th edition. Flying Publishers; 2015.
26. Centers for Disease Control. Prevention. In: Atkinson W, Wolfe S, Hamborsky J, editors. Mumps. Epidemiology and prevention of vaccine-preventable diseases. 12th edition. Washington, DC: Public Health Foundation; 2011. p. 205–14.
27. Rubella Vaccines: WHO position paper. Wkly Epidemiol Rec 2011;86(29):301–16.
28. Centers for Disease Control. Notice to readers: revised ACIP recommendation for avoiding pregnancy after receiving a rubella-containing vaccine. MMWR Morb Mortal Wkly Rep 2001;50(49):1117.
29. Tseng H, Harpaz R, Bialek S. Herpes zoster vaccine in older adults and the risk of subsequent herpes zoster disease. JAMA 2011;302(2):160–6.
30. Atkinson W, Wolfe S, Hamborsky J, et al, editors. Varicella. Epidemiology and prevention of vaccine preventable diseases. Washington, DC: Public Health Foundation; 2009. p. 283–304.
31. Atkinson W, Wolfe S, Hamborsky J, et al, editors. Influenza. Epidemiology and prevention of vaccine preventable diseases. Washington, DC: Public Health Foundation; 2009. p. 135–56.
32. Centers for Disease Control. Prevention. Prevention and control of Influenza with Vaccines. Recommendations of the Advisory Committee on Immunization Practices (ACIP). MMWR Recomm Rep 2010;59:1–63.
33. Muszkat M, Greenbaum E, Ben-Yehudah A, et al. Local and systemic immune response in nursing-home elderly following intranasal or intramuscular immunization with inactivated influenza vaccine. Vaccine 2003;21(11–12):1180–6.
34. Healthy People 2020, US Department of Health and Human Services. Available at: http://www.healthypeople.gov/2020/default/aspx. Accessed June 26, 2013.
35. Talbot TR, Herbert TV, Mitchel E, et al. Asthma as a risk factor for invasive pneumococcal disease. N Engl J Med 2005;352(20):2082–90.
36. Centers for Disease Control, Prevention. Updated recommendations for prevention of invasive pneumococcal disease among adults using the 23-valent pneumococcal polysaccharide vaccine (PPSV23). MMWR Morb Mortal Wkly Rep 2010;59:1102–6.

37. Pickering LK, Baker CJ, Freed GL, et al. Immunization programs for infants, children, adolescents, and adults: clinical practice guidelines by the Infectious Diseases Society of America. Clin Infect Dis 2009;49:817–40.
38. Centers for Disease Control and Prevention (CDC). Updated recommendations for use of tetanus toxoid, reduced diphtheria toxoid and acellular pertussis vaccine (Tdap) in pregnant women and persons who have or anticipate having close contact with an infant aged <12 months-Advisory Committee on Immunization Practices (ACIP), 2011. MMWR Morb Mortal Wkly Rep 2011;60:1424–6.
39. Parkin DM, Breay F. Chapter 2: The burden of HPV-related cancers. Vaccine 2006;24(Suppl 3):S11–25.
40. Weinstein LC, Buchanan EM, Hillson C, et al. Screening and prevention: cervical cancer. Prim Care 2009;36(3):559–74.
41. Markowitz LE, Dunne EF, Saraiya M, et al. Quadrivalent human papillomavirus vaccine: recommendations of the Advisory Committee on Immunization Practices (ACIP). MMWR Recomm Rep 2007;56(RR-2):1–24.
42. Center for Disease Control and Prevention. FDA licensure of bivalent human papillomavirus (HPV2, Cervarix) for use in females and updated HPVC vaccination recommendations from the Advisory Committee on immunization Practices (ACIP). MMWR Morb Mortal Wkly Rep 2010;59:626–9.
43. International tuberculosis incidence rates. Internet web page. 2011. World Health Organization. Available at: http://www.who.int/immunization_monitoring/diseases/en/. Accessed July 9, 2016.
44. Lalvani A. Diagnosing tuberculosis infection in the 21st century: new tools to tackle an old enemy. Chest 2007;131(6):1898–906.
45. CDC. Development of new vaccines for tuberculosis: recommendations of the Advisory Council for the elimination of Tuberculosis (ACET). MMWR Recomm Rep 1998;47(RR13):1–6.
46. Shepherd SM, Shoff WH. Immunization in travel medicine. Prim Care 2011;38: 643–79.
47. Emmett GA, Schneider M. Office immunization. Prim Care 2011;38:729–45.
48. Eibl MM, Wolf HM. Vaccination in patients with primary immune deficiency, secondary immune deficiency and autoimmunity with immune regulatory abnormalities. Immunotherapy 2015;7(12):1273–92.
49. Omer SB, Enger KS, Moulton LH, et al. Geographic clustering of nonmedical exceptions in school immunization requirements and associations with geographic clustering of pertussis. Am J Epidemiol 2008;168:1389–96.
50. Lieu TA, Ray GT, Klein NP, et al. Geographic clusters in under immunization and vaccine refusal. Pediatrics 2015;135:280–9.
51. Centers for Disease Control and Prevention (CDC) (US). National Immunization Survey. Available at: http://www.cdc.gov/nchs/nis.htm. Accessed July 28, 2015.
52. World Health Organization. Report of the SAGE working group on Vaccine Hesitancy: 2014. Available at: http://www.who.int/immunization/sage/meetings/2014/october/1_report_working_group_vaccine_hesitence_final.pdf. Accessed August 1, 2016.
53. Nowak GJ, LaVail K, Kennedy A, et al. Insights from public health; a framework for understanding and fostering vaccine acceptance. In: Chattergee A, editor. Vaccinophobia and vaccine controversies of the 21st century. New York: Springer; 2013. p. 459–79.
54. Kahan DM. Vaccine risk perceptions and ad hoc risk communication: an empirical assessment. 2014. Available at: http://papers.ssrn.com/so13/papers.cfm?abstract_id=2386034. Accessed August 10, 2016.

55. Kennedy A, LaVail K, Nowak G, et al. Confidence about vaccines in the United States; understanding parents' perceptions. Health Aff (Millwood) 2011;30: 1151–9.
56. Mergler MJ, Omer SB, Pan WK, et al. Association of vaccine-related attitudes and beliefs between parents and healthcare providers. Vaccine 2013;31:4591–5.
57. Gargano LM, Weiss P, Underwood NL, et al. School-located vaccination clinics for adolescents: correlates of acceptance among parents. J Community Health 2015;40:660–9.
58. Rosenstock I. Historical origins of the Health Belief Model. Health Educ Behav 1974;2:328–35.

Role of Oral Microbial Infections in Oral Cancer

Brett L. Ferguson, DDS[a,b,*], Scott Barber, DDS[c], Imani H. Asher, DDS[c], Chalmers R. Wood, DDS[c]

KEYWORDS

- Viral • Microbial • Carcinogenesis

KEY POINTS

- The role of bacterial and viral carcinogenesis in the oral cavity is becoming increasingly a subject of interest, as a means to provide more methods of cancer prevention.
- There have been suggestions of relationships between bacteria and multiple strains of viruses in the progression of malignancy in some studies.
- Cancer cause is closely related to the type of carcinogen, as well as the synergistic or additive actions of combined risk factors, the susceptibility of the host, and the duration of interaction between host and exposure to risk factors.
- Different bacterial species are reviewed in detail, as well as the main viruses identified as contributive factors in carcinogenesis, including human immunodeficiency virus, human papilloma virus, Epstein-Barr virus, and human herpesvirus.
- Because most of the current studies maintain a contributive relationship and very few legitimize a definitive causal relationship, much research is being done to further define the role that these microbial and bacterial agents play in the progression of malignancy.

INTRODUCTION

Head and neck cancer refers to a group of biologically similar cancers that start in the lip, oral cavity, nasal cavity, paranasal sinuses, nasopharynx, and larynx. About 40% of head and neck cancers occur in the oral cavity, 15% in the pharynx, 25% in the larynx, and the remaining 20% are in the salivary glands and thyroid. Overall, they account for more than 500,000 cases annually worldwide. They account for 3% of all

Disclosure: The authors have nothing to disclose.
[a] University of Missouri-Kansas City, Kansas City, MO, USA; [b] Oral and Maxillofacial Surgery, Head and Neck Clinic, University Health, Truman Medical Center, American Association of Oral and Maxillofacial Surgery, 2101 Charlotte Street, Suite 310, Kansas City, MO 64108, USA; [c] Department of Oral and Maxillofacial Surgery, University Health Oral and Maxillofacial Surgery Clinic, 2101 Charlotte Street, Suite 310, Kansas City, MO 64108, USA
* Corresponding author. Oral and Maxillofacial Surgery, Head and Neck Clinic, University Health, Truman Medical Center, American Association of Oral and Maxillofacial Surgery, 2101 Charlotte Street, Suite 310, Kansas City, MO 64108.
E-mail address: brett.ferguson@tmcmed.org

Dent Clin N Am 61 (2017) 425–434
http://dx.doi.org/10.1016/j.cden.2016.12.009
0011-8532/17/© 2016 Elsevier Inc. All rights reserved.

cancers in the United States. In 2015, it was estimated to affect 61,760 people (45,330 men and 16,430 women). Men are affected significantly more often, ranging from 2:1 to 4:1. It is estimated that more than 13,000 people will die from head and neck cancer. Most of these cancers are squamous cell carcinoma (**Fig. 1**).

Risk factors for head and neck cancer include smoking, alcohol consumption, ultraviolet light, viral infections, and possibly even bacterial infections. Human papillomavirus (HPV) and Epstein-Barr virus (EBV), herpes simplex virus, and human immunodeficiency virus (HIV) have been identified as significant risk factors. Cancer cause is closely related to the type of carcinogen, as well as the synergistic or additive actions of combined risk factors, the susceptibility of the host, and the duration of interaction between host and exposure to the risk factor.[1] The possible involvement of oncogenic viruses and bacteria in oral and oropharyngeal cancers has become a field of increasing interest.

The oral cavity contains a delicate balance of microbial flora. Studies have shown that the human oral carcinoma surface biofilms harbor significantly increased levels of both aerobes and anaerobes. They have also shown that the tumor microenvironment is suitable for bacteria to thrive. Strains such as *Escherichia coli* and facultative oral streptococci are among those that have been noted to highly colonize sites of oral squamous cell cancer (OSCC).

The role of bacterial carcinogenesis in the oral cavity is becoming increasingly a subject of interest, as a means to provide more methods of cancer prevention. There have been some suggestions of a relationship between bacteria and progression of malignancy in certain studies. Some of the bacterial causes include streptococci, *Helicobacter pylori*, and *Salmonella typhi*. However, the relationship between some of these, namely *H pylori* and *S typhi*, is complex. Some species are carcinogenic, whereas the presence of others is required to prevent carcinogenesis, depending on location. For example, research has shown that *H pylori* can cause gastric cancer or mucosa-associated lymphoid tumors in some individuals. In contrast, exposure to *H pylori* seems to reduce risk of esophageal cancer in other individuals. It is now recognized that bacteria bind to and colonize the mucosal surfaces in a highly selective manner via a lock-and-key mechanism. Bacterial infections have been linked to malignancies because of their ability to induce chronic inflammation. They can also produce cell toxins that disturb cell cycles and lead to altered cell growth. Another mechanism that has been of interest in recent research studies is the ability to facilitate tumorigenesis by converting ethanol into its carcinogenic derivative, acetaldehyde, to levels capable of inducing DNA damage, mutagenesis, and secondary hyperproliferation of the epithelium. This ability is especially evident in the streptococci species in

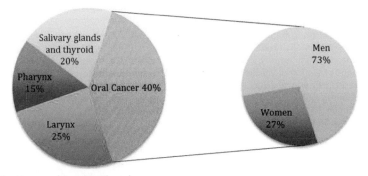

Fig. 1. Incidence of head and neck cancer.

the clinical setting of heavy ethyl alcohol and tobacco abusers. Gram-positive bacteria and yeasts are associated with high acetaldehyde production, which could explain the synergistic carcinogenic action of alcohol and smoking on upper gastrointestinal (GI) tract cancers.[2]

Viral Carcinogenesis

Human papilloma virus

More than 90% of HPV-related head and neck squamous cell cancers (HNSCCs) are associated with the HPV-16 strand. The HPV virus is strictly tissue-specific and associated with malignancies of skin, head and neck, and anogenital region, which is thought to be because these tissues have a squamocolumnar transition zone. This transition zone allows easy access to the basal epithelial cells for viral entry. For advanced and persistent infections with HPV, the demonstration of over-expressed cellular p16 protein (because of E7-binding retinoblastoma protein) in infected tissues supports this diagnosis. HPV-16 DNA is present in high copy numbers in HPV-positive HNSCC cells and its genomic DNA is frequently integrated into HPV-positive HNSCC with active transcription of major viral oncoproteins E6 and E7. The virus' affinity for lymphoepithelium is why it is so heavily documented in high incidences of oropharyngeal cancers. Other theories for its prevalence in oropharyngeal sites include that there are deep invaginations of the tonsillar crypts that function as a reservoir for HPV, that the reticulated epithelium has a discontinuous basement membrane allowing easy viral entry, and that the deep crypts within the lymphoid tissue represent immune-privileged sites that favor persistent HPV infection and allow tumors to evade immune surveillance.[3–6] A systematic review of studies used polymerase chain reaction to detect HPV DNA in 26% of HNSCCs.[7] Reports show that approximately 36% to 73% of oropharyngeal cancers are caused by HPV infection, and that HPV DNA has been detected in 25% and up to 31% of oral cavity and laryngeal cancers respectively. Oral HPV infections have classically been associated with concomitant smoking, older age, HIV, and larger numbers of sexual partners.

More recently, the study of the relationship between HPV and head and neck cancers has become increasingly relevant, because there has been a documented increased in incidence and mortality of HPV-related oropharyngeal cancers in younger generations (**Table 1**). The dramatic increase, particularly in developed nations, has raised concerns for an emerging cancer epidemic.[3] In recent studies, it has also been noted that patients with HPV-HNSCC are more likely to have a primary oropharyngeal tumor, be diagnosed at a later stage, and be less likely to have an extensive history of alcohol and tobacco use. The incidence is higher by 3-fold in men than in women.[7] HPV-positive tumors are more likely to occur in young white men who are of a higher socioeconomic status. Because of the consistent evidence supporting that HNSCC with HPV is largely found in the oropharyngeal region, it is thought to be caused by the affinity that HPV has for the lymphoepithelial tissue. As previously mentioned, there is a confirmed causal relationship that is increasingly being

Table 1	
Relationship between human papilloma virus and oropharyngeal cancers	
Risk Type	**HPV Type**
Low	6, 11, 42, 43, 44
Intermediate	31, 33, 35, 39, 45, 51, 52, 58
High	16, 18

investigated. Differences in molecular genetic profile support that HPV-related HNSCC is biologically distinct from HNSCC related to tobacco and alcohol use.

It is not as clear whether there is a causal relationship between HPV and nonoropharyngeal head and neck sites. Several viruses, particularly HPV-16, HPV-18, and HPV-32, are present in 25% to 30% of oral squamous cell carcinomas and 70% of cases diagnosed as proliferative verrucous leukoplakia.[1] HPV has been identified as the causative agent of several benign and malignant tumors, but the relationship and exact association are difficult to study and trend. Most HPV infections are cleared rapidly and do not cause malignancy, so the persistence of the infection is a central risk factor for carcinogenesis. In one study of patients with newly diagnosed base-of-tongue cancers, it was suggested that periodontal pockets were associated with an increased risk of HPV-positive tumor status. This finding is likely caused by the chronic presence of inflammatory markers in the periodontal pocket epithelium that serve as receptors for HPV, as well as the pocket serving as a reservoir for latent HPV. Based on mechanisms previously discussed, the junctional epithelium in the periodontal pocket also provides easy access for viral entry. The study revealed that every additional millimeter of alveolar bone loss was associated with a 4-fold increased risk of HPV-positive tumor status[8] (**Table 2**).

The problem with studies of HPV carcinogenesis is that it has not been established whether biomarkers of carcinogenesis are required to be present and detected at the sites of HNSCC. More studies are therefore required to establish a difference between passenger versus carcinogenic HPV infection. Despite these limitations, systematic reviews and meta-analysis of studies estimate that the HPV-attributable fraction is approximately 40% for oropharyngeal squamous cell carcinoma, and 7% to 16% for oral cavity squamous cell carcinoma worldwide (0%–9% in developed regions; ie, North America and Europe).[3] Although no causal relationship can be confirmed for the oral cavity, the results encourage larger studies to be done to determine the relationship between chronic inflammation in the oral cavity and HPV infections. It is of equal interest to delve deeper into the influence of HPV infection/carcinogenesis and the presence of other critical factors such as tobacco, alcohol, and other concomitant bacterial coinfections.

Human immunodeficiency virus

HIV/acquired immunodeficiency syndrome (AIDS) currently ranks as the seventh-leading cause of death worldwide. HIV has multiple oral manifestations, including Kaposi sarcoma. It is also found to exacerbate HPV infections, which also contribute to the carcinogenesis of head and neck cancers.[1] Patients with HIV tend to show a higher incidence of lip, oral cavity, and pharyngeal cancers.[3] The incidence of malignancy, such as squamous cell carcinoma, is especially noted in the populations of patients in later stages of immunocompromise. Head and neck lesions associated with HIV occur in approximately 80% of all patients with AIDS.[9] Epidemiologic data support the view that HIV infection increases the risk of HPV-associated OSCC. At the protein level, direct interaction has been found between HPV and HIV, because it was shown

Table 2	
Human papilloma virus types associated with oral lesions	
Oral Disease	**HPV Type**
Oral leukoplakia	16, 18
Verrucous carcinoma	6, 11, 16
Oral squamous cell carcinoma	16, 18, 32

to increase expression of E6 and E7 oncoproteins in HPV-16–positive oral keratino-cytes (discussed in detail elsewhere in this issue) as well as to enhance the prolifera-tive capacity of the oral keratinocytes.[10] Studies have shown that oral mucosal Langerhans cells are also the target of HIV infections. Cytopathic changes of the cells caused by HIV infection may contribute to the depletion of the cells and impair mucosal immunologic protection against colonization by microorganisms causing HIV-associated oral mucosal lesions.[11] Definitive pathogenesis of malignant transfor-mation remains unclear.

Human herpesvirus 8

Kaposi sarcoma is a vascular neoplasm associated with the Kaposi sarcoma herpes-virus/human herpesvirus (HHV) 8. It can involve the skin, mucosa, and viscera, and continues to be the most prevalent malignancy in patients with AIDS. Research has shown that HHV8 infection alone seems to be insufficient for development of Kaposi sarcoma, but that it also relies on some degree of host immunoinsufficiency. The sus-pected pathogenesis of Kaposi sarcoma begins with circulating blood mononuclear and endothelial progenitor cells that are reprogrammed by HHV8 infection. The host's blood endothelial cells are reprogrammed to resemble lymphatic endothelium, which upregulates several lymphatic receptors. Malignant transformation also requires a de-gree of host immune dysfunction and local inflammation. Studies have shown that detection of HHV8 DNA in mononuclear cells in individuals infected with HIV-1 and in transplant patients was associated with an increased risk of subsequent Kaposi sar-coma development. However, there are conflicting studies that deny a significant as-sociation between viral load and subsequent Kaposi sarcoma development or disease progression. These conflicting results were addressed in a retrospective study recently published in the *Journal of Clinical Virology* that showed that either the detec-tion or plasma level of HHV8 DNA is strongly associated with the presence of, and sub-sequent progression of, Kaposi sarcoma. The HHV8 DNA viral load was also an independent factor significantly associated with the AIDS–Kaposi sarcoma clinical status.[12]

Human herpesvirus 4

EBV has been identified as a major risk factor for malignancy. EBV is a group I double-stranded DNA virus that belongs to the family Herpesviridae with subfamily Gamma-herpesvirinae, genus Lymphocryptovirus, and species HHV4. The most common malignancies caused by this are Burkitt lymphoma and nasopharyngeal carcinoma. EBV-related epithelial cancers, such as nasopharyngeal carcinomas and EBV-positive gastric cancers, encompass approximately 80% of EBV-related malig-nancies. It has also been detected in other epithelial cancers, including carcinoma of the palatine tonsil, supraglottic laryngeal carcinoma, salivary gland cancer, and oral squamous cell carcinoma. EBV has the ability to affect the proliferation and sur-vival of its infected host cell that likely renders it oncogenic. Although there are con-flicting data that show strong association of EBV with head and neck cancer (HNC) and others showing weak or no association, there is compelling recent evidence iden-tifying specific micro-RNAs that contribute to epithelial tumorigenesis.

In humans, EBV is thought to initiate infection in the epithelial cells of the oropharynx, which is susceptible to viral replication. Lymphocytes are then infected. The B cells are thought to be the source of the continued viral spread. Following the latent EBV infection and immortalization of B cells, EBV induces RNA synthesis and cell division. Several oncogenic gene products that are capable of malignant tumor formation are induced by the latent EBV infection. Certain EBV nuclear antigens have been shown to be oncogenic on their own. There is strong evidence that certain micro-RNAs are induced by EBV, which cooperatively downregulates cell-specific epithelial metastatic suppressor proteins.[13] However, there is much more to be investigated in the genomics of the virus, as well as its mechanism of action to facilitate carcinogenesis in epithelial cells.

Bacterial Carcinogenesis

It has been reported that most head and neck cancer is related to tobacco use and heavy alcohol consumption; however, it is now thought that bacteria may play an equally important role in carcinogenesis in head and neck cancer. There is a delicate balance between the microbial flora and the immune system, which allows the microbial flora to live as a commensal organism. When disease occurs, the microbial flora become aggressive and gives rise to host diseases. Such is the case in certain species like *Porphyromonas gingivalis*, which disrupts this microbial equilibrium and results in dysbiotic host-microbiota interaction.[14,15] Some of these diseases are inflammatory, whereas others are degenerative, cancerous, or transitory.[16] Interest in the possible relationships between bacteria and the different stages of cancer development has increased since the classification of *H pylori* as a definite (class 1) carcinogen.[3] It has been shown that bacteria can cause chronic infections or produce toxins that disturb the cell cycle and lead to altered cell growth.[7,17–19] Chronic infections induce cell proliferation and DNA replication through activation of mitogen-activated kinase pathways and cyclin D1. This process increases the incidence of cell transformation and the tumor development rate.[8,20] Some infections cause intracellular accumulation of the pathogen, leading to suppression of apoptosis. This suppression protects the pathogen from destruction from the host immune system via apoptosis. The cells can then evade the self-destructive process and ultimately become tumorigenic. Some bacteria also have the ability to alter the cell's signaling pathways, which enhances the survival of the pathogen.[21] The metabolism of carcinogenic substances is an additional mechanism of pathogenesis that is being explored. It is thought that this process may take place in the oral cavity, where the preexisting local microflora may facilitate tumorigenesis by converting ethanol into acetaldehyde, a carcinogen. Sufficient acetaldehyde levels are capable of inducing DNA damage, mutagenesis, and secondary hyperproliferation of the epithelium. This mechanism may explain why heavy drinkers are more at risk for oral cancers (**Fig. 2**).[22]

Certain bacterial infections may evade the immune system or stimulate immune responses that contribute to carcinogenic changes through the stimulatory and mutagenic effects of the cytokines released by the inflammatory cells. These cytokines include reactive oxygen species, interleukin-8 (IL-8), cyclooxygenase-2, and nitric oxide. Chronic stimulation of the substances, along with environmental factors such as smoking or a susceptible host, may contribute significantly to carcinogenesis.[12]

Recent studies have shown that podoplannin, a transmembrane glycoprotein, is expressed in various normal tissues, as well as in neoplastic tissues. Butyric acid is

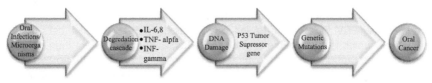

Fig. 2. Role of bacteria in causing oral cancer. IL, interleukin; INF, interferon; TNF, tumor necrosis factor.

an extracellular metabolite from periodontopathic bacteria that plays a significant role in the progression of periodontal disease. Butyric acid/sodium butyrate increases the podoplannin expression and cell migration in some lines of oral squamous cell carcinoma. This finding again suggests that bacteria associated with periodontal disease may prove to be an independent factor that promotes the progression of oral squamous cell carcinoma.[17] There is even increasing evidence that some pathogenic bacteria can contribute to specific stages of cancer development. Chronic infections triggered by bacteria can facilitate tumor initiation or tumor progression because the pathogen can alter the normal cell functions at various stages.

Porphyromonas gingivalis

This bacterium is known to have a major disruptive effect on local immune responses in the periodontal area, whereby the microbial balance is violated, giving way to inflammation and periodontal disease. The distinct link or role it plays in tumor development remains to be determined; however, there is strong evidence of its inherent ability to affect several aspects of epithelial cell signaling. P gingivalis is strongly antiapoptotic via multiple signaling pathways in epithelial cells. It also showed the ability to reduce the level of p53 tumor suppressor. These phenomena are being further researched in their relevance to carcinogenesis.

P gingivalis also has an impact on OSCC cells, in that the bacteria promote cellular invasion by inducing pro–matrix metalloproteinase expression and breakdown of the basement membrane. This process promotes carcinoma cell invasion and metastasis. This contributive mechanism is being explored in the dissemination and metastatic growth of OSCC at remote sites. Because this proMMP-p (ProMatrix metalloproteinases) induction occurs via multiple metabolic signaling pathways, and the presence of other proteins or factors may be required for progression into tumorigenesis, these mechanisms are being studied in more detail on the molecular level.[20]

Helicobacter pylori

H pylori is a gram-negative bacillus that colonizes the GI tract in more than 50% of the population and is one of the most common bacterial infections. The pathogen is closely associated with gastritis and peptic ulcers, and has been linked to the development of multiple malignancies associated with the GI tract, such as gastric mucosa– associated lymphoid lymphoma and gastric cancer. The mechanism of action by which H pylori leads to carcinogenesis in the GI tract is well known. Colonization of H pylori in the stomach results in a release of chemoattractants, such as neutrophil-activating protein-1 (NAP-1/IL-8), which recruits neutrophils into the gastric mucosa. This process in turn leads to gastritis or inflammation of the gastric lining. In addition, the H pylori virulence factor (cytotoxin-associated gene A) protein is injected into gastric epithelial cells and, via metabolic pathways, causes cellular changes that increase the risk of carcinogenesis.

There have also been studies investigating the association between H pylori infection and esophageal squamous cell carcinoma. The relationship between H pylori infection and atypical hyperplasia of esophageal epithelium is less understood and has been the subject of recent study. A study that was published in the International Journal of Cancer suggests that H pylori does lead to esophageal carcinogenesis. The results of the study showed a strong correlation between H pylori invasion and atypical hyperplasia of esophageal epithelial cells/esophageal carcinogenesis. It also confirmed that the severity of H pylori infection directly affected the severity of cellular change; severely dysplastic tissue showed a significantly higher infection rate. There was evidence that, as previously seen in gastric cancers, the CagA virulence factor protein has a significant influence in *H pylori* infection of the esophageal tissue. The mechanism of carcinogenesis was also proposed to be a function of the ability of *H pylori* infection to:

1. Induce modifications in mitochondrial DNA
2. Increase endogenous DNA damage
3. Generate a transient mutation that induces a nuclear DNA mutation[23,24]

Numerous studies have shown an increased presence of *H pylori* in the oral cavity of subjects with leukoplakia and oral lichen planus (well-documented lesions with potential for malignancy). Although studies indicate a need for further research, thus far it is relevant to acknowledge a possible relationship between the presence of *H pylori* and lesions of the oral mucosa. Research has identified *H pylori* in subgingival and supragingival dental plaques, as well as in saliva. When a study compared the detection of *H pylori* in patients with oral lesions (leukoplakia/lichen planus) with normal patients, the presence of the pathogen was significantly higher in patients with oral disease. However, there were no statistical differences in the presence of *H pylori* between the patients who had leukoplakic lesions and hose with oral lichen planus.[22] There remain questions about how significant a role *H pylori* plays in the progression of oral disease, because it is not always detected in cases of oral disease and it is not usually present in great quantity. It would be easy to apply its known molecular properties that encourage carcinogenesis in esophageal and gastric epithelium, but more studies need to be done to identify *H pylori* infection as an independent factor that promotes carcinogenesis in the oral cavity.

Future research

The population of microbial cells inhabiting the human body is 10-fold greater then all somatic and germ cells combined. This collective is termed the microbiome and is well documented to affect cancer susceptibility and progression both positively and negatively. Just as alterations of the microbial community are identified in saliva in oral squamous cell carcinoma, studies of patients with pancreatic and colorectal cancer have also shown changes in the microbiome compared with control groups. Animal models use gnotobiotic, or germ-free mice in which the microbiota can be manipulated to potentially elucidate a cause-and-effect relationship and these represent future directions for study. Current data using these animal models show that microbiota can increase, or even decrease, cancer susceptibility. Postulated mechanisms include the role of the microbiome in inflammation, influencing the genomic stability of cells, and altering cell metabolites that affect host gene expression, as discussed in detail earlier.

Individuals belonging to the microbiome have been identified as the possible causes of a disease process. Known examples are *H pylori* being implicated in gastric cancer and HPV being associated with cervical cancer. Other studies have linked the alteration of the microbiome in colorectal tumors specifically to a single organism in the microbiota. *Fusobacterium nucleatum*, an anaerobe found in periodontitis and appendicitis, was found to be profoundly over-represented in colorectal tumors compared with normal, adjacent colonic tissue in the same patient.[16] However, this raises questions regarding the potential causative nature of the microbiota, and whether it represents a consequence of the tumor state. The overwhelming opinion is that further clinical study and animal models may be necessary to answer that question.

Another malignancy of interest, glioblastoma multiforme, is the most common primary brain tumor and has been linked to cytomegalovirus (CMV) after 80% of newly diagnosed tumors had detectable CMV. Additional data suggested in cases of newly diagnosed glioblastoma multiforme that CMV infection in early childhood may have been protective, but infection in later childhood or adulthood may be a risk factor for malignancy.

By identifying a specific organism or manipulating a host microbiome, therapeutic modalities are being developed and serve as the underlying methodology for some chemotherapeutic agents or cancer virotherapy. In particular, the oncolytic poliovirus is being used to treat recurrent glioblastoma and is currently showing positive results in clinical trials. Even in recurrent head and neck squamous cell carcinoma, the oncolytic measles virus has been added to the existing standard regimen of chemotherapy with 5-fluorouracil and cetuximab and represents an emerging method of treatment referred to as chemovirotherapy. This budding field of therapy has led to the development of an oncolytic measles virus vaccine and has been shown to also have properties against other malignancies, such as mantle cell lymphoma.

The population and composition of a microbiome is affected by the specific environment it inhabits. This relationship raises questions about the role that even diet plays in affecting the microbiological community of the digestive tract: the oral cavity, the esophagus, the gastric epithelium, down to the colorectal epithelium. Continuing to study all potential factors may provide valuable contributions to establishing cause-and-effect relationships, including the mechanism of carcinogenesis and potential innovative avenues for therapeutic intervention.

Summary

The role of bacterial and viral carcinogenesis in the oral cavity is becoming increasingly a subject of interest, as a means to provide more methods of cancer prevention. There have been some suggestions of relationships between bacteria and multiple strains of viruses in the progression of malignancy in certain studies. Cancer cause is closely related to the type of carcinogen, as well as the synergistic or additive actions of combined risk factors, the susceptibility of the host, and the duration of interaction between host and exposure to risk factor. Different bacterial species are reviewed in detail, as well as the main viruses identified as contributive factors in carcinogenesis, including HIV, HPV, EBV, and HHV. Because most of the current studies maintain a contributive relationship and very few legitimize a definitive causal relationship, much research is being done to further define the role that these microbial and bacterial agents are playing in the progression of malignancy.

REFERENCES

1. Marx, Robert E, Diane Stern. Oral and Maxillofacial Pathology: A Rationale for Diagnosis and Treatment. Chicago: Quintessence Pub. Co; 2003.
2. Khajuria N, Metgud R. Role of bacteria in oral carcinogenesis. Indian J Dent 2015;6(1):37–43.
3. Chi AC, Day TA, Neville BW. Oral cavity and oropharyngeal squamous cell carcinoma - an update. CA Cancer J Clin 2015;65(5):401–21.
4. Ernster JA, Sciotto CG, O'Brien MM. Rising incidence of oropharyngeal cancer and the role of oncogenic human papilloma virus. Laryngoscope 2007;117: 2115–27.
5. Schwartz J, Pavlova S, Kolokythas A, et al. Streptococci-human papilloma virus interaction with ethanol exposure leads to keratinocyte damage. J Oral Maxillofac Surg 2012;70:1867–79.
6. Radu O, Pantanowitz L. Kaposi Sarcoma. Arch Pathol Lab Med 2013;137:289–94.

7. Joseph AW, D'Souza G. Epidemiology of human papillomavirus-related head and neck cancer. Otolaryngol Clin North Am 2012;45:739–64.
8. Tezal M, Nasca MS, Stoler DL, et al. Chronic periodontitis - human papillomavirus synergy in base of tongue cancers. Arch Otolaryngol Head Neck Surg 2009; 135(4):391–5.
9. Shanti RM, Aziz SR. HIV-associated salivary gland disease. Oral Maxillofac Surg Clin North Am 2009;21:339–43.
10. Syrjanen S. Human papillomavirus infection and its association with HIV. Adv Dent Res 2011;23(1):84–9.
11. Chou LL, Epstein J, Cassol SA, et al. Oral mucosal Langerhans' cells as target, effector and vector in HIV infection. J Oral Pathol Med 2000;29:394–402.
12. Broccolo F, Chiara TD, Vigano MG, et al. HHV-8 DNA replication correlates with the clinical status in aids-related Kaposi's sarcoma. J Clin Virol 2016;78:47–52.
13. Kanda T, Miyata M, Kondo S, et al. Clustered microRNAs of the Epstein-Barr virus cooperatively downregulate an epithelial cell-specific metastasis suppressor. J Virol 2015;85:2684–97.
14. Whitmore SE, Lamont RJ. Oral bacteria and cancer. PLoS Pathog 2014;10(3):1–3.
15. Campo-Trapero J, Cano-Sanchez J, Palacios-Sanchez B, et al. Update on molecular pathology in oral cancer and precancer. Anticancer Res 2008;28:1197–206.
16. Kostic AD, Gevers D, Pedamallu CS, et al. Genomic analysis identifies Association of *Fusobacterium* with colorectal carcinoma. Genome Res 2012;22(2):292–8.
17. Schwabe RF, Jobin C. The microbiome and cancer. Nat Rev Cancer 2013;13: 800–12.
18. Sewell DA, Zhen KP, Paterson Y. Listeria-based HPV-16 E7 vaccines limit autochthonous tumor growth in a transgenic mouse model for HPV-16 transformed tumors. Vaccine 2008;26:5315–20.
19. Eslick GD. Infectious causes of esophageal cancer. Infect Dis Clin North Am 2010;24:845–52.
20. Inaba H, Sugita H, Kuboniwa M, et al. Porphyromonas gingivalis promotes invasion of oral squamous cell carcinoma through induction of ProMMP9 and its activation. Cell Microbiol 2014;16(1):131–45.
21. Grimm M, Munz A, Exarchou A, et al. Immunohistochemical detection of *Helicobacter pylori* without association of TLR5 expression in oral squamous cell carcinoma. J Oral Pathol Med 2014;43:35–44.
22. Kazanowska-Dygdala M, Dus I, Radwan-Oczko M. The presence of *Helicobacter pylori* in oral cavities of patients with leukoplakia and oral lichen planus. J Appl Oral Sci 2016;24(1):18–23.
23. Li W-S, Tian DP, Guan XY, et al. Esophageal intraepithelial invasion of *Helicobacter pylori* correlates with atypical hyperplasia. Int J Cancer 2014;134: 2626–32.
24. Schmidt BL, Kuczynski J, Bhattaharya A, et al. Changes in abundance of oral microbiota associated with oral cancer. PLoS One 2014;9(6):1–12.

Infection Control in the Dental Office

Francesco R. Sebastiani, DMD[a,*], Harry Dym, DDS[b], Tarun Kirpalani, DDS[a]

KEYWORDS

- Hand hygiene • Blood-borne pathogens • Personal protective equipment
- Sterilization and disinfection • Environmental infection control

KEY POINTS

- The Centers for Disease Control and Prevention (CDC) has developed infection control guidelines intended to improve the effectiveness and impact of public health interventions and inform clinicians, public health practitioners, and the public.
- This article highlights current scientific rationale and technique for performing proper infection control practices in the dental office.
- Although the principles of infection control remain unchanged, new technologies, materials, equipment, and data require continuous evaluation of current infection control practices.

WHY IS INFECTION CONTROL IMPORTANT IN THE DENTAL OFFICE?

During dental treatment, both patients and dental health care personnel (DHCP) can be exposed to pathogens through contact with blood, oral and respiratory secretions, and contaminated equipment. Following recommended infection control protocols described in the 2003 CDC guidelines and 2016 CDC summary can prevent transmission of infectious organisms among both patients and DHCP.[1] Dental patients and DHCP may be exposed to a variety of disease-causing microorganisms that are present within the oral cavity and respiratory tract. These pathogens include cytomegalovirus, hepatitis B virus (HBV), hepatitis C virus (HCV), herpes simplex virus types 1 and 2, HIV, tuberculosis (TB), staphylococci including methicillin-resistant *Staphylococcus aureus*, and streptococci, among others. The modes of infection of these organisms in dental settings are through multiple routes:

1. Direct contact of blood, saliva, teeth, or other potentially infectious patient materials with intact or nonintact skin

---

[a] Department of Oral and Maxillofacial Surgery, The Brooklyn Hospital Center, 121 Dekalb Avenue, Brooklyn, NY 11201, USA; [b] Department of Dentistry and Oral Maxillofacial Surgery, The Brooklyn Hospital Center, 121 Dekalb Avenue, Box 187, Brooklyn, NY 11201, USA
* Corresponding author.
E-mail address: fsebastiani@tbh.org

Dent Clin N Am 61 (2017) 435–457
http://dx.doi.org/10.1016/j.cden.2016.12.008
0011-8532/17/© 2016 Elsevier Inc. All rights reserved.

2. Indirect contact with a contaminated object, such as instruments, operatory equipment, or environmental surfaces
3. Direct contact of conjunctival, nasal, or oral mucosa with droplets containing microorganisms
4. Inhalation of airborne microorganisms that can remain suspended in the air for long periods of time

Infection through any of these routes requires that all of the following conditions be present:

- An adequate number of pathogens, or disease-causing organisms, to cause disease
- A reservoir or source, such as blood, that allows the pathogen to survive and multiply
- A mode of transmission from the source to the host
- An entrance through which the pathogen may enter the host
- A susceptible host, one who is not immune

The occurrence of all these events is the chain of infection (**Fig. 1**). Effective infection control strategies prevent disease transmission by interrupting 1 or more links in the chain of infection.

The CDC is widely recognized as the leading national public health institute of the United States. Previous CDC recommendations on infection control for dentistry in 1986 and 1993 described the use of universal precautions to prevent transmission of blood-borne pathogens. Universal precautions were based on the concept that all blood and certain body fluids should be treated as infectious because it is impossible to know who may be carrying a blood-borne virus. Thus, universal precautions should apply to all patients.

The relevance of universal precautions applied to other potentially infectious materials was recognized, and in 1996, the CDC replaced universal precautions with standard precautions.[1] Standard precautions integrate and expand universal precautions to include organisms spread by

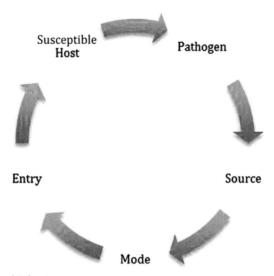

Fig. 1. The chain of infection.

- Blood
- All body fluids, secretions, and excretions except sweat, regardless of whether they contain blood
- Nonintact skin
- Mucous membranes

Standard precautions include respiratory hygiene with cough etiquette, sharp safety, safe injection practices, sterile instruments and devices, clean and disinfected environmental surfaces, and the use of personal protective equipment (PPE). Saliva has always been considered a potentially infectious material in dental infection control; thus, no operational difference exists in clinical dental practice between universal precautions and standard precautions.

When standard precautions alone cannot prevent transmission, they are supplemented with transmission-based precautions. This second tier of infection prevention is used when patients have diseases that can spread through contact, droplet or airborne routes in addition to standard precautions. Despite that most dental practices are not designed to carry out all transmission-based precautions, DHCP should carry out systems for early detection and management of potentially infectious patients at initial points of entry into the dental setting.

Standard precautions include

- Hand washing
- The use of PPE, such as gloves, masks, eye protection, and gowns, intended to prevent the exposure of skin and mucous membranes to blood and other potentially infectious materials
- Proper cleaning and decontamination of patient care equipment
- Cleaning and disinfection of environmental surfaces
- Injury prevention through engineering controls or safer work practices

The Occupational Safety and Health Administration (OSHA) retains the use of the term, *universal precautions*, because they are concerned primarily with transmission of blood-borne pathogens.

IS HAND HYGIENE THE SINGLE MOST IMPORTANT FACTOR IN PREVENTING THE SPREAD OF PATHOGENS IN HEALTH CARE SETTINGS?

The CDC estimates that each year approximately 2 million patients in the United States acquire infections in hospitals, and approximately 90,000 of these infections result in patient mortalities.[1] The hands are the most common mode of pathogen transmission. Hand hygiene is a general term that applies to routine hand washing, antiseptic hand wash, antiseptic hand rub, and surgical hand antisepsis.

- Hand washing refers to washing hands with plain soap and water.
- Antiseptic hand wash refers to washing hands with water and soap or other detergents containing an antiseptic agent, such as triclosan or chlorhexidine.
- Using a waterless agent containing 60% to 95% ethanol or isopropanol alcohol-containing preparation is referred to as an alcohol hand rub.[2] These agents are a new addition to the dental guidelines and have become more frequently used in the United States to improve compliance with hand washing in hospitals. In dental practices, however, sinks are readily available and the need for alcohol preparations is not as great.
- Surgical antisepsis refers to an antiseptic hand wash or alcohol-based hand rub (if using an alcohol-based hand rub, the hands should first be washed with soap

and water) performed preoperatively by surgical personnel to eliminate microorganisms on hands. Antiseptic preparations for surgical hand hygiene should have persistent (long-lasting) antimicrobial activity.[2]

Hand washing can reduce the spread of antibiotic resistance in health care settings and the likelihood of health care–associated infections (**Table 1**).

Table 1
Methods of hand hygiene

Method	Agent	Purpose	Area	Duration (Minimum)
Routine hand wash	Water and nonantimicrobial soap[a] (plain soap)	Remove soil and transient microorganisms	All surfaces of the hands and fingers	15 s[b]
Antiseptic hand wash	Water and antimicrobial soap (chlorhexidine, iodine and iodophors, chloroxylenol [PCMX], triclosan)	Remove or destroy transient microorganisms and reduce resident flora (persistent activity)	Remove or destroy transient microorganisms and reduce resident flora (persistent activity)	15 s[b]
Antiseptic hand rub	Alcohol-based hand rub	Remove or destroy transient microorganisms and reduce resident flora (persistent activity)	All surfaces of the hands and fingers[c]	Until the hands are dry
Surgical antisepsis	Water and antimicrobial soap (chlorhexidine, iodine and iodophors, chloroxylenol [PCMX], triclosan)	Remove or destroy transient microorganisms and reduce resident flora (persistent activity)	Hands and forearms	2–6 min
	Water and nonantimicrobial soap (plain soap) followed by an alcohol-based surgical hand scrub product with persistent activity	—	—	Follow manufacturer instructions for surgical hand scrub product with persistent activity

[a] Use of liquid soap with hands-free dispenser is preferred. Pathogenic organisms have been found on/or around bar soap during and after use.
[b] Reported effective time in removing most transient bacteria flora from skin. A vigorous rubbing together of all surfaces of premoistened lathered hands and fingers for ≥15 seconds, followed by rinsing under a stream of cool water is recommended. Dry hands thoroughly before donning gloves.
[c] Alcohol-based hand rubs should contain 60% to 95% ethanol or isopropanol and should not be used with visible soil or organic material.
Adapted from Centers for Disease Control and Prevention (CDC). Guidelines for infection control in dental health-care settings — 2003. MMWR Morb Mortal Wkly Rep 2003;52:161.

WHAT ARE INDICATIONS FOR HAND HYGIENE?

Hand hygiene substantially reduces potential pathogens on the hands and is considered a primary measure for reducing the risk of transmitting organisms to patients and health care personnel (HCP). Hospital-based studies have shown that noncompliance with hand hygiene practices is associated with health care–associated infections and the spread of multiresistant organisms and has been a major contributor to outbreaks.[1] Studies also have shown that the prevalence of health care–associated infections decreased as hand hygiene measures improved.[2]

Specific indications for hand hygiene include

- Before and after treating each patient (before glove placement and after glove removal)
- After bare hand touching of inanimate objects likely contaminated by blood, saliva, or respiratory secretions
- Before leaving the dental operatory
- When hands are visibly soiled; before regloving, after removing gloves that are torn, cut, or punctured
- For oral surgical procedures, perform surgical hand antisepsis before donning sterile surgical gloves.

Alcohol-based hand sanitizers are the most effective products for reducing the number of germs on the hands of health care providers.[2] Antiseptic soaps and detergents are the next most effective and nonantimicrobial soaps are the least effective. When hands are not visibly dirty, alcohol-based hand sanitizers are the preferred method of cleaning a provider's hands in the health care setting. Soap and water are recommended for cleaning visibly dirty hands (**Table 2**).

POTENTIAL INFECTIOUS DISEASES IN THE DENTAL OFFICE

Blood-borne viruses, such as HBV, HCV, and HIV, are of particular concern to DHCP. These viruses

- Can be transmitted to patients and HCP in health care settings
- Can produce chronic infection
- Are often carried by persons unaware of their infection

Table 2 Centers for Disease Control and Prevention recommendations during routine dental care	
Wash with Soap and Water	**Use an Alcohol-Based Hand Sanitizer**
• When hands are visibly dirty • After known or suspected exposure to *Clostridium difficile* if facility is experiencing an outbreak or higher endemic rates • After known or suspected exposure to patients with infectious diarrhea during norovirus outbreaks • If exposure to *Bacillus anthracis* is suspected or proved • Before eating • After using a restroom	• For everything else

From Centers for Disease Control and Prevention (CDC). Hand hygiene in healthcare settings. Available at: http://www.cdc.gov/handhygiene/providers/index.html. Accessed April 2, 2016.

The risk of infection with a blood-borne virus is largely determined by

- Its prevalence, or frequency, in the patient population
- The risk of transmission after an exposure to blood (risk varies by type of virus)
- The type and frequency of blood contacts. If HCP are frequently exposed to blood, especially if they are working with sharp objects, such as needles, their risk of exposure to a blood-borne virus would be higher than if they rarely come into contact with blood.

OSHA requires that all dental practitioners receive training in standard precaution practices at the time of employment and annually thereafter.[3]

Table 3 highlights the average risk of transmission after a single needlestick from an infected patient by type of blood-borne virus. As displayed, risk varies greatly by the type of virus.

The risk of HBV transmission after a needlestick to HBV-infected blood varies from 1% to 62%, depending on the hepatitis B e antigen (HBeAg) status of a source patient. If a source patient's blood is positive for HBeAg, a marker of increased infectivity, the risk of transmission can be as high as 62%.[1] If the patient's blood is hepatitis B surface antigen (HBsAg) positive but HBeAg negative, the risk varies from 1% to 37%.

The average risk of HCV transmission after a percutaneous exposure to HCV-infected blood is 1.8%. The average risk of HIV infection after a percutaneous exposure to HIV-infected blood is 0.3%.[1] Thus, 1 in 3 needlesticks from an HBeAg-positive source patient results in infection compared with only 1 in 300 needlesticks from an HIV-infected patient.

The critical 2011 recommendations from the CDC regarding HBV vaccination and influenza control for infection control in dental health care settings are discussed. Each recommendation is categorized on the basis of existing scientific data, theoretic rationale, and applicability. Rankings are based on the system used by the CDC and the Healthcare Infection Control Practices Advisory Committee to categorize recommendations (**Boxes 1–3**).

CONTROL OF 2009 H1N1 INFLUENZA

A hierarchy of control measures should be applied to prevent transmission of 2009 H1N1 influenza in all health care settings. To apply the hierarchy of control measures,

Table 3	
Percutaneous exposure risk in dental practice	
Source	**Risk**
HBV	
HBsAg⁺ and HBeAg⁺	22.0%–31.0% clinical hepatitis; 37%–62% serologic evidence of HBV infection
HBsAg⁺ and HBeAg⁻	1.0%–6.0% clinical hepatitis; 23%–37% serologic evidence of HBV infection
HCV	1.8% (0%–7% range)
HIV	0.3% (0.2%–0.5% range)

Data from Centers for Disease Control and Prevention (CDC). Division of Oral Health. Infection prevention & control in dental settings. Questions & Answers: Occupational Exposure to Blood. Available at: http://www.cdc.gov/oralhealth/infectioncontrol/questions/occupational-exposure.html. Accessed April 2, 2016.

Box 1
Categories for recommendations on infection control in dental health care settings

- Category IA—strongly recommended for implementation and strongly supported by well-designed experimental, clinical, or epidemiologic studies

- Category IB—strongly recommended for implementation and supported by experimental, clinical, or epidemiologic studies and a strong theoretic rationale

- Category IC—required for implementation as mandated by federal or state regulations or standards. When category IC is used, a second rating can be included to provide the basis of existing scientific data, theoretic rationale, and applicability. Because of state differences, readers should not assume that the absence of a IC recommendation implies the absence of any state regulations.

- Category II—suggested for implementation and supported by suggestive clinical or epidemiologic studies or a theoretic rationale

Adapted from Centers for Disease Control and Prevention (CDC). Guidelines for infection control in dental health-care settings — 2003. MMWR Morb Mortal Wkly Rep 2003;52:1–61.

---

facilities should take the following steps, ranked according to their likely effectiveness:

1. Elimination of potential exposures (deferral of treatment of ill patients and source control by masking persons who are coughing)
2. Engineering controls that reduce or eliminate exposure at the source without placing primary responsibility of implementation on individual employees
3. Administrative controls, including sick leave policies and vaccination, that depend on consistent implementation by management and employees
4. PPE for exposures that cannot otherwise be eliminated or controlled (PPE includes gloves, surgical face masks, respirators, protective eyewear, and protective clothing, such as gowns.)

Box 2
Hepatitis B virus vaccination

Offer the HBV vaccination series to all DHCP with potential occupational exposure to blood or other potentially infectious material (category IA or IC).

Always follow US Public Health Service/CDC recommendations for hepatitis B vaccination, serologic testing, follow-up, and booster dosing (category IA or IC).

Test DHCP for anti-HBs 1 to 2 months after completion of the 3-dose vaccination series (category IA or IC).

DHCP should complete a second 3-dose vaccine series or be evaluated to determine if HBsAg positive if no antibody response occurs to the primary vaccine series (category IA or IC).

Retest for anti-HBs at completion of the second vaccine series. If no response to the second 3-dose series, nonresponders should be tested for HBsAg (category IC).

Counsel nonresponders to vaccination who are HBsAg negative regarding their susceptibility to HBV infection and precautions to take (category IA or IC).

Provide employees appropriate education regarding the risks of HBV transmission and availability of the vaccine. Employees who decline the vaccination should sign a declination form to be kept on file with the employer (category IC).

Adapted from Centers for Disease Control and Prevention (CDC). Guidelines for infection control in dental health-care settings — 2003. MMWR Morb Mortal Wkly Rep 2003;52:1–61.

Box 3
Preventing exposures to blood and other potentially infectious material

General recommendations

Use standard precautions (OSHA blood-borne pathogen standard retains the term universal precautions) for all patient encounters (category IA or IC).

Consider sharp items (eg, needles, scalers, burs, laboratory knives, and wires) that are contaminated with patient blood and saliva as potentially infective, and establish engineering controls and work practices to prevent injuries (category IB or IC).

Implement a written, comprehensive program designed to minimize and manage DHCP exposures to blood and body fluids (category IB or IC).

Engineering and work practice controls

Identify, evaluate, and consider devices with engineered safety features at least annually and as they become available on the market (eg, safer anesthetic syringes, blunt suture needle, retractable scalpel, or needleless intravenous systems) (category IC).

Place used disposable syringes and needles, scalpel blades, and other sharp items in appropriate puncture-resistant containers located as close as feasible to the area in which the items are used (category IA or IC).

Do not recap used needles by using both hands or any other technique that involves directing the point of a needle toward any part of the body. Do not bend, break, or remove needles before disposal (category IA or IC).

Use a 1-handed scoop technique or a mechanical device designed for holding the needle cap when recapping needles (eg, between multiple injections, before removing from a nondisposable aspirating syringe) (category IA or IC).

Postexposure management and prophylaxis

Follow current CDC recommendations after percutaneous, mucous membrane, or nonintact skin exposure to blood or other potentially infectious material.

Handling of biopsy specimens

During transport, place biopsy specimens in a sturdy, leak-proof container labeled with the biohazard symbol (category IC).

If a biopsy specimen container is visibly contaminated, clean and disinfect the outside of a container, or place it in an impervious bag labeled with the biohazard symbol (category IC).

Handling of extracted teeth

Dispose of extracted teeth as regulated medical waste unless returned to the patient (category IC).

Do not dispose of extracted teeth containing amalgam in regulated medical waste intended for incineration (category II).

Clean and place extracted teeth in a leakproof container, labeled with a biohazard symbol, and maintain hydration, for transport to educational institutions or a dental laboratory category (IB or IC).

Heat-sterilize teeth that do not contain amalgam, before they are used for educational purposes (category IB).

Adapted from Centers for Disease Control and Prevention (CDC). Guidelines for infection control in dental health-care settings—2003. MMWR Morb Mortal Wkly Rep 2003;52:1–61.

Vaccination

Vaccination, an administrative control, is one of the most important interventions for preventing transmission of influenza to HCP. More information on this hierarchy of controls is available in the CDC *Interim Guidance on Infection Control Measures for 2009 H1N1 Influenza in Healthcare Settings, Including Protection of Healthcare Personnel* (CDC: H1N1 Flue Clinical and Public Health Guidance, http://www.cdc.gov/h1n1flu/guidance/).

Specific Recommendations for Dental Health Care

- Encourage all DHCP to receive seasonal influenza and 2009 H1N1 influenza vaccinations.
- Use patient reminder calls to identify patients reporting influenza-like illness, and reschedule nonurgent visits until 24 hours after patients are free of fever without the use of fever-reducing medicine.
- Identify patients with influenza-like illness at check-in; offer a face mask or tissues to symptomatic patients; follow respiratory hygiene/cough etiquette and reschedule nonurgent care. Separate ill patients from others whenever possible if evaluating for urgent care.
- Urgent dental treatment can be performed without the use of an airborne infection isolation room, because transmission of 2009 H1N1 influenza is thought not to occur over longer distances through the air, such as from one patient room to another.
- Use a treatment room with a closed door, if available. If not, use one that is farthest from other patients and personnel.
- Wear recommended PPE before entering the treatment room.
- DHCP should wear a National Institute for Occupational Safety and Health fit-tested, disposable N95 respirator when entering the patient room and when performing dental procedures on patients with suspected or confirmed 2009 H1N1 influenza.
- As customary, minimize spray and spatter (eg, use a dental dam and high-volume evacuator).

Dental Health Care Personnel

- DHCP should self-assess daily for symptoms of febrile respiratory illness (fever plus 1 or more of the following: nasal congestion or runny nose, sore throat, or cough).
- Personnel who develop fever and respiratory symptoms should promptly notify their supervisor and should not report to work.
- Personnel should remain at home until at least 24 hours after they are free of fever (100°F/37.8°C), or signs of a fever, without the use of fever-reducing medications.
- Personnel with a family member who is diagnosed with 2009 H1N1 influenza can still go to work but should self-monitor for symptoms so that any illness is recognized promptly.

TRANSMISSION RISK OF MYCOBACTERIUM TUBERCULOSIS IN DENTISTRY

Mycobacterium TB is spread from person to person through the air. When a person with pulmonary or laryngeal TB coughs or sneezes, tiny particles, known as droplet nuclei, are expelled into the air. The particles are an estimated 1 μm to 5 μm in size, and normal air currents can keep them airborne for prolonged periods of time and spread them throughout a room or building.[4] Infection may occur when a person inhales droplet nuclei containing TB organisms.

During the first few weeks after infection, organisms can spread from the initial location in the lungs to the lymph nodes in the center of the chest and then to other parts of the body by way of the bloodstream. Within 2 to 12 weeks, the body's immune system usually prevents further multiplication and spread, although they can remain alive in the lungs for years.[3] This condition is referred to as latent TB infection. Overall, the risk for transmission of TB in most dental settings is low.

Table 4 lists the CDC recommendations on work restrictions for HCP infected with or exposed to major infectious diseases at work in the absence of state and local regulations.

PERCUTANEOUS INJURIES AMONG DENTAL HEALTH CARE PROVIDERS

Current literature substantiates that percutaneous injuries among dentists have declined from an average rate of 11 injuries per year in 1987 to fewer than 3 injuries per year in 1993.[1] Most injuries among general dentists were found to be caused by burs, followed by syringe needles and other sharp instruments. Injuries are found to occur while a dentist's hands are outside a patient's mouth. The frequency of percutaneous injuries among oral surgeons is similar to that reported among US dentists. Injuries among oral surgeons may occur more frequently during procedures using surgical wire, such as during fracture reductions.

Primary methods used to prevent occupational exposures to blood in health care settings include standard precautions, engineering controls, work practice controls, and administrative controls.[2]

EXPOSURE PREVENTION STRATEGIES
Engineering Controls

Engineering controls are the primary method to reduce exposures to blood, such as sharps containers and self-sheathing needles. Safe practices include handling, using, or processing sharp devices.[2] OSHA code mandates that employees be given the opportunity to review and help select needlestick prevention devices. In addition, employers are responsible for maintaining a log of needlestick exposures to help in the annual review so that the workplace protocol may be modified to reduce the number of exposures.[5]

Work Practice Controls

Work practice controls are behavior based and are intended to reduce the risk of blood exposure by changing the manner in which a task is done. These include using instruments instead of fingers to retract or palpate tissue during suturing and anesthesia administration, 1-handed needle recapping, and not passing an unsheathed needle to another dental health care provider.[2]

Administrative Controls

Administrative controls include policies, procedures, and enforcement measures to prevent exposure to disease-causing organisms. The placement in the hierarchy varies by the problem addressed, such as early identification and referral of a patient suspected of having TB.[2]

Personal Protective Equipment

PPE, or barrier precautions, is a major component of standard precautions. It is essential to protect the skin and mucous membranes of personnel from exposure to

Table 4
Work restrictions for health care personnel exposed to infectious diseases

Disease/Problem	Work Restriction	Duration
Conjunctivitis	Restrict from patient contact and contact with patient's environment.	Until discharge ceases
Cytomegalovirus infection	No restriction	
Diarrheal disease		
Acute-stage (diarrhea with other symptoms)	Restrict from patient contact and contact with patient's environment.	Until symptoms resolve
Convalescent stage, *Salmonella* species	Restrict from care of patients at high risk.	Until symptoms resolve; consult with local and state health authorities regarding need for negative stool cultures.
Enteroviral infection	Restrict from care of infants, neonates, and immunocompromised patients and their environment.	Until symptoms resolve
Hepatitis A virus	Restrict from patient contact and contact with patient's environment.	Until 7 d after onset of jaundice
HBV		
Personnel with acute or chronic hepatitis B surface antigenemia who do not perform exposure-prone procedures	No restriction[a]; refer to state regulations. Standard precautions should always be followed.	
Personnel with acute or chronic hepatitis B e antigenemia who perform exposure-prone procedures	Do not perform exposure-prone invasive procedures until counsel from a review panel has been sought; panel should review and recommend procedures that personnel can perform, taking into account specific procedures as well as skill and technique. Standard precautions should always be observed. Refer to state and local regulations or recommendations.	Until HBeAg is negative
HCV	No restrictions on professional activity.[a] HCV-positive HCP should follow aseptic technique and standard precautions.	

(continued on next page)

Table 4
(continued)

Disease/Problem	Work Restriction	Duration
Herpes simplex virus		
Genital	No restriction	
Hands (herpetic whitlow)	Restrict from patient contact and contact with patient's environment.	Until lesions heal
Orofacial	Evaluate need to restrict from care of patients at high risk.	
HIV; personnel who perform exposure-prone procedures	Do not perform exposure-prone invasive procedures until counsel from an expert review panel has been sought; panel should review and recommend procedures that personnel can perform, taking into account specific procedures as well as skill and technique. Standard precautions should always be observed. Refer to state and local regulations or recommendations.	
Measles		
Active	Exclude from duty	Until 7 d after the rash appears
Postexposure (susceptible personnel)	Exclude from duty	From 5th day after first exposure through 21st day after last exposure, or 4 d after rash appears
Meningococcal infection	Exclude from duty	Until 24 h after start of effective therapy
Mumps		
Active	Exclude from duty	Until 9 d after onset of parotitis
Pediculosis	Restrict from patient contact	Until treated and observed to be free of adult and immature lice
Pertussis		
Active	Exclude from duty	From beginning of catarrhal stage through 3rd week after onset of paroxysms, or until 5 d after start of effective antibiotic therapy
Postexposure (asymptomatic personnel)	No restriction; prophylaxis recommended	
Postexposure (symptomatic personnel)	Exclude from duty	Until 5 d after start of effective antibiotic therapy

(continued on next page)

Table 4
(continued)

Disease/Problem	Work Restriction	Duration
Rubella		
Active	Exclude from duty	Until 5 d after rash appears
Postexposure (susceptible personnel)	Exclude from duty	From 7th day after first exposure through 21st day after last exposure
Staphylococcus aureus infection		
Active, draining skin lesions	Restrict from contact with patients and patients' environment or food handling.	Until lesions have resolved
Carrier state	No restriction unless personnel are epidemiologically linked to transmission of organism.	
Streptococcal infection, group A	Restrict from patient care, contact with parent's environment, and food handling.	Until 24 h after adequate treatment started
Tuberculosis		
Active disease	Exclude from duty	Until proved noninfectious
Purified protein derivative (PPD) converter	No restriction	
Varicella (chicken pox)		
Active	Exclude from duty	Until all lesions dry and crust
Postexposure (susceptible personnel)	Exclude from duty	From 10th day after first exposure through 21st day (28th day if varicella-zoster immune globulin administered) after last exposure
Zoster (shingles)		
Localized; in healthy person	Cover lesions; restrict from care of patients[b] at high risk.	Until all lesions are dry and crust
Generalized or localized in immunosuppressed person	Restrict from patient contact	Until all lesions are dry and crust
Postexposure (susceptible personnel)	Exclude from duty	From 10th day after first exposure through 21st day (28th day if varicella-zoster immune globulin administered) after last exposure or, if varicella occurs, when lesions crust and dry

(continued on next page)

Table 4 (continued)		
Disease/Problem	**Work Restriction**	**Duration**
Viral respiratory infection, acute febrile	Consider excluding from the care of patients at high risk[c] or contact with such patients' environments during community outbreak of respiratory syncytial virus and influenza.	Until acute symptoms resolve

[a] Unless epidemiologically linked to transmission of infection.
[b] Those susceptible to varicella and who are at increased risk of complications of varicella (eg, neonates and immunocompromised persons of any age).
[c] Patients at high risk as defined by ACIP for complications of influenza.
Adapted from Weissfeld AS. Infection control in the dental office. Clin Microbiol Newsl 2014;36(11):81, 82; with permission.

infectious or potentially infectious materials in spray or spatter and the should be removed when leaving treatment areas. The various barriers available include[5]

1. Gloves – these include powder-free latex gloves, vinyl gloves, and nitrile gloves. These minimize the risk of HCP acquiring infections from patients or of transmission from HCP to patients. Wearing gloves does not eliminate nor replace the need for hand washing. Gloves that are torn, cut, or punctured should obviously be removed. Gloves should also not be washed, disinfected, or sterilized for reuse. Maintaining short fingernails and not wearing jewelry can minimize the risk of puncture.[3] Lastly, wearing sterile gloves or double gloving has not been mandated. After wearing gloves for a period of time, glove juice collects that is laden with skin flora. It is important to prevent glove juice from contacting instruments, for instance, when changing gloves during a long procedure. It is recommended that clinicians remove gloves slowly and deliberately, with their hands as far away from the instrument setup as possible.[6]
2. Masks – these include surgical masks that are fluid-resistant and isolation masks that cover the nose and mouth. Layers include an outer layer, a microfiber middle layer, and a soft inner layer that absorbs moisture.
3. Protective eyewear for dentist and patient – with side shields, this protects from aerosols and spatter that transmit infection, from debris projected from the mouth, and from injuries caused by sharp instruments. Face shields can be considered for procedures that involve a great potential for splatter or aerosol generation.[6]
4. Surgical head caps
5. Protective clothing – this include cotton gowns, if contamination of clothing is anticipated, and fluid-resistant isolation gowns, if contamination by significant volumes of blood or body fluids is anticipated. It should completely cover personal clothing and any skin likely to come in contact with blood-borne pathogens.[6]

Respiratory Hygiene/Cough Etiquette

Respiratory hygiene/cough etiquette infection prevention measures are designed to limit the transmission of respiratory pathogens spread by droplets or airborne routes. These were added to standard precautions in 2007. They include implementing measures to contain respiratory secretions in patients with signs and symptoms of a respiratory infection (eg, signs with instructions to cover their mouth/noses when coughing or sneezing), providing tissues and no touch receptacles for disposal of tissues, providing resources for performing hand hygiene in or near waiting areas, offering masks to coughing patients, and encouraging persons with symptoms of respiratory infections to sit as far from others as possible. Lastly, DHCP should be educated on the importance of infection prevention measures to contain respiratory secretions.[7]

POSTEXPOSURE MANAGEMENT

Despite best efforts, blood exposures will likely continue to occur. Postexposure management remains an important component of a complete program to prevent infection following exposure to blood. Elements of an effective postexposure management program include

- Policies and procedures that clearly state how to manage exposures
- Education of DHCP in prevention strategies (including evaluation of safety devices), principles of postexposure management, the importance of prompt reporting, and postexposure prophylaxis efficacy and toxicity
- Resources for rapid access to clinical care, postexposure prophylaxis, and testing of both source patients and exposed HCP (preferably with a rapid HIV test)

Except for institutional settings, coordination with off-site infection control or occupational health services likely is necessary. A health care professional who is qualified to manage, counsel, and provide medical follow-up should be selected before staff are placed at risk. Ensure that this person is familiar with the dental application of risk assessment and management. The key elements of postexposure management include wound management and exposure reporting. After a puncture wound, such as a needlestick, the area should immediately be thoroughly washed with soap and water. If blood or saliva contacts mucous membranes, immediate flushing with water is necessary.[3] The evaluating health care professional should assess the risk of infection by examining the type and severity of exposure, the blood-borne status of the source person, and the susceptibility (immune status) of the exposed person. All these factors should be considered in assessing the risk of infection and the need for further follow-up.

DISINFECTION VERSUS STERILIZATION

Disinfection and sterilization are both decontamination processes. Although disinfection is the process of eliminating most harmful microorganisms from inanimate objects and surfaces, sterilization is the process of killing all microorganisms, including a substantial number of resistant bacterial spores (**Table 5**).

Disinfection

Disinfection is a 2-step process — the initial step involves vigorous scrubbing of the surfaces to be disinfected and wiping them clean; the second step involves wetting the surface with a disinfectant and leaving it wet for the time prescribed by the manufacturer. The spray-wipe-spray technique enhances decontamination through mechanical cleansing with a paper towel followed by the chemical action of the disinfectant solution. The same process occurs when using the disinfectant wipes in the wipe-discard-wipe technique; the first wipe removes microbes and the second wipe provides disinfection.[8] The ideal disinfectant has a broad spectrum of activity; acts rapidly; is noncorrosive, environmentally friendly, free of volatile organic compounds, and nontoxic; and does not stain.[9]

Table 5
Categories of patient care items

Category	Definition	Dental Instrument	Management
Critical	• Penetrates soft tissue • Contacts bone • Enters bloodstream	Surgical instruments, periodontal scalers, scalpel blades, burs	• Heat sterilize between use.
Semicritical	• Contacts mucous membranes or nonintact skin • Do not penetrate soft tissue	Mouth mirror, amalgam condenser, impression trays, hand pieces	• For heat tolerant — heat sterilize. • For heat sensitive[10] — replace with a heat tolerant or disposable alternative. If not, then high-level disinfection (glutaraldehyde, peracetic acid, hydrogen peroxide).
Noncritical	• Contacts intact skin	Radiograph head and cone, pressure cuff, facebow, pulse oximeter	• Clean and disinfect using a low- to intermediate-level disinfectant. If low-level disinfection, OSHA requires a label claim for killing HIV and HBV. If bloody, an intermediate level disinfectant should be used. Protecting these surfaces with disposable barriers is an alternative.

Modified from Centers for Disease Control and Prevention (CDC). Guidelines for infection control in dental health-care settings — 2003. MMWR Morb Mortal Wkly Rep 2003;52:1–61.

Sterilization

Sterilization stages include presoaking, cleaning, corrosion control and lubrication, packaging, sterilization, handling sterile instruments, storage, and distribution. The physical agents used in sterilization can include sunlight, drying, dry heat, moist heat, filtration, radiation, ultrasonic and sonic vibrations. The chemical agents used can be alcohols, aldehydes, dyes, halogens, phenols, surface-active agents, metallic salts, and gases.[10]

DECONTAMINATION AND DISINFECTION METHODS

Cleaning is the first step in the decontamination process, which involves the physical removal of debris and reducing the number of microorganisms on the instrument. If visible debris or organic matter is not removed, it may interfere with the disinfection or sterilization process. This may be achieved by manual cleaning, or automated cleaning, and the Environmental Protection Agency (EPA) Web site lists registered approved cleansers.[5]

Manual Cleaning

The instruments should be soaked in a rigid container filled with disinfectant. This prevents drying of patient material and makes cleaning easier and less time consuming.

The disinfectant to hold the instruments should not be high level, such as glutaraldehyde. To avoid injury, it is recommended that personnel wear puncture-resistant, heavy-duty gloves.[2]

Automated Cleaning

a. Ultrasonic cleaner: involves the use of sound waves to form oscillating bubbles, a process referred to as cavitation. Instruments are kept in a perforated cassette where the bubbles act on remaining debris to remove it from the instruments. They are then rinsed and then carefully inspected for debris. Instruments likely to rust are dipped in a rust inhibitor solution and are then dried using an absorbent towel.[10]
b. Instrument washer: uses high-velocity hot water and a detergent; there is a cleaning and drying cycle in this process. Thermal disinfectors may also be used, which are similar to instrument washers except that it is the high temperatures of the water and chemical additives that are used to disinfect the instruments.[10]

STERILIZATION METHODS

In dentistry, the 4 accepted methods of sterilization include steam pressure sterilization (autoclave), unsaturated chemical vapor pressure sterilization (chemiclave), dry heat sterilization (dryclave), and ethylene oxide sterilization.

Autoclaving

Autoclaving usually involves a temperature of 121°C at 15 lb of pressure for 20 minutes.[6] It is the most rapid and effective method for sterilizing cloth surgical packs and towel packs, is dependable and economic, and the sterilization is verifiable. Items sensitive to elevated temperatures cannot be autoclaved, however, this process tends to rust carbon steel instruments and burs, and the instruments must be air dried at cycle completion. Types of autoclaves include downward displacement, positive pressure displacement, negative pressure displacement, a triple vacuum, and prevacuum.[10] In the commonly used gravity displacement sterilizers, steam enters the chamber and unsaturated air is forced out through a vent. Prevacuum sterilizers are fitted with a vacuum pump to create a vacuum in the chamber before the chamber is pressurized with steam to improve the speed and efficiency of the process.

Chemiclave

Chemiclave involves the use of an unsaturated chemical vapor system of alcohol and formaldehyde. This process is quick, the load comes out dry, the sterilization is verifiable, and corrosion-sensitive instruments do not rust. Items sensitive to elevated temperatures are damaged, however, must be dried before processing; aeration is needed due to offensive vapors; and heavy cloth wrappings of surgical instruments may not be penetrated.[10]

Dry Heat Sterilization

Dry heat sterilization involves the use of conventional dry heat ovens with a short cycle and high temperatures for items that cannot be subject to moist heat; either static air or forced air is used. Advantages include no corrosion (if instruments are dried well prior to the cycle), rapid cycles, low cost, and verifiable sterilization and it can be performed at a larger capacity with industrial hot air ovens. Disadvantages include that sterilization cycles are prolonged at lower temperatures, ovens must be calibrated, and the high temperatures may damage heat-sensitive items, including rubbers and plastics.[10]

Ethylene Oxide Sterilization

Ethylene oxide sterilization involves the use of a fumigator. It operates effectively at low temperatures, the gas is penetrative and can be used for sensitive equipment such as hand pieces, and the sterilization is verifiable. On the other hand, this method can be mutagenic and carcinogenic, requires an aeration chamber, and is usually only available at hospitals.[11]

Newer methods of sterilization under research and development include peroxide vapor sterilization, ultraviolet light, and ozone sterilization. Peroxide vapor sterilization involves an aqueous hydrogen peroxide solution boiled in a heat vaporizer and flowed as a vapor into a sterilization chamber containing instruments at low temperature and pressure. Ultraviolet light exposes the contaminants with a lethal dose of energy in the form of light at 240 nm to 280 nm, which results in the destruction of nucleic acid through the induction of thymine dimers (not effective against RNA viruses). Ozone sterilization is the newest low-temperature sterilization method suitable for many heat sensitive, moisture sensitive, and stainless steel devices. The sterilizer creates its sterilant internally from United States Pharmacopoeia–grade oxygen, steam-quality water, and electricity; the sterilant is converted back to oxygen and water vapor at the end of the cycle by a passing through a catalyst before being exhausted into the sterilization room. The ozone cycle parameters are approximately 4 hours and 15 minutes at 30°C to 35°C.[12]

Flash sterilization was originally defined as sterilization of an unwrapped object at 132°C for 3 minutes at 28 lb of pressure in a gravity displacement sterilizer for immediate use. It is acceptable for processing cleaned patient care items that cannot be packaged, sterilized, or stored before use. It is also used when there is insufficient time to sterilize an item by the preferred package method. This type of sterilization cycle should only be used after instruments have been thoroughly cleaned.[10]

INSTRUMENT PROCESSING

To prevent cross-contamination, the instrument processing area should be physically and spatially divided into areas for[2]

1. Cleaning – reusable contaminated instruments are received, cleaned, decontaminated, and sorted.
2. Packaging – for inspecting, assembling, and packaging clean instruments in preparation for sterilization. Critical and semicritical items should be wrapped or placed in containers before sterilization, and hinged instruments should be opened and unlocked so that all surfaces are exposed. Lastly, a chemical indicator should be placed inside each wrapped package.
3. Sterilization – contains sterilizers and incubators for analyzing spore tests.
4. Storage – should be dust proof, dry, well ventilated, and easily accessible for routine dental use. Sterile instruments must be at least 8 inches from the floor, 18 inches from the ceiling, and 2 inches from the walls. Items should be positioned so that packaged items are not crushed, bent, compressed, or punctured. Ultraviolet and formalin chambers can be used for storage.[9]

SPORE TESTING AND DUAL-MONITORING STRIPS IN STERILIZATION BAGS

The 3 methods for monitoring sterilization include mechanical techniques, chemical indicators (internal/external), and biological indicators. The mechanical and chemical techniques do not guarantee sterilization but help detect procedural errors and equipment malfunction.

Mechanical techniques

Mechanical techniques involve assessment of cycle time, temperature, and pressure by observing gauges on the sterilizer. Because these parameters can be observed during the sterilization cycle, this might be the first indication of a problem.

Chemical Techniques

Chemical techniques use sensitive chemicals that change color when a given parameter is reached, usually a heat-sensitive external tape or an internal chemical indicator strip. A chemical indicator should be used in every package to verify that the sterilization agent penetrated the package and reached the instruments inside. If the internal chemical indicator is not visible from the outside of the package, an external indicator should be used. These indicators can also help differentiate between processed and unprocessed items, eliminating the possibility of using instruments that have not been sterilized. It is recommended to use multiparameter internal chemical indicators that react to time, temperature, and presence of steam.[7]

Biological Techniques

Biological techniques, or a biological spore test, is the most valid process because it assesses the process directly by using the most heat-resistant microorganism, which is contingent on the sterilization method. A control biological indicator from the same lot, which has not been sterilized, should be incubated along with the test indicator. The control should show a positive result and the test should yield a negative result **(Box 4)**.[3]

PROPER DISINFECTION OF HAND PIECES, IMPRESSIONS, AND ENVIRONMENTAL SURFACES

Operatory asepsis is important because environmental surfaces can be contaminated during patient care. These surfaces include light handles, unit switches, counter tops, bracket trays, dental chairs, door handles, and drawer knobs that can serve as reservoirs of microbial contamination. The transfer of microorganisms from contaminated

---

Box 4
Protocol for positive spore text

- Recall and resterilize affected instruments.

- Remove autoclave from service.

- Review process to identify possible operator error (eg, packaging, loading, or monitoring).

- Retest unit with biological indicator and control.

- If unit fails a second test, affected instruments should be resterilized with an alternate autoclave.

- If second test is negative and chemical/mechanical indicators are satisfactory, place unit back in service.

- Incident should be documented in sterilization log.

Modified from Thomas MV, Jarboe G, Frazer RQ. Infection control in the dental office. Dent Clin N Am 2008;52(3):624; with permission.

environmental surfaces to patients occurs primarily through personal hand contact. These do not require as stringent decontamination procedures, and surface barriers can be used and changed between patients. If surface barriers cannot be used, clean and disinfect the surface with an EPA-registered hospital disinfectant effective against HIV and HBV.

Housekeeping surfaces, such as walls, floors, and sinks, must be cleaned with water and soap or a registered hospital detergent on a regular basis. They must be cleaned if visibly soiled. Treatment rooms should be free of extraneous materials to facilitate cleaning and disinfection. Loose items should be placed in draws or storage.[6]

Strategies for decontaminating spills of blood and other body fluids differ by setting and volume of the spill. The person assigned to clean the spill should wear PPE as needed. Visible organic material should be removed with absorbent material, such as disposable paper towels, and the manufacturer's instructions for proper use of intermediate level disinfectants with a tuberculocidal claim should be followed. If such products are unavailable, a 1:100 dilution of sodium hypochlorite could be used.[9] Because of their toxic nature, however, high-level disinfectants on environmental surfaces are not recommended.

Hand pieces are considered semicritical devices, but they must be heat sterilized between patients because studies have shown that their internal surfaces can become contaminated with patient materials during use.[7] Hand piece surface decontamination includes running it under the sink, scrubbing it thoroughly, cleaning the fiberoptic ends with alcohol, placing it in a clear view sterilization pouch, and then sterilizing the hand piece.[10] Because it is difficult for chemical germicides to reach the internal parts of the hand pieces, they should be heat sterilized with a steam autoclave or chemical vapor sterilizer.[2] This includes the associated attachments, including low-speed motors and reusable prophylaxis angles. Surface disinfection, liquid germicides, and ethylene oxide are not acceptable.

For ultrasonic scalers, inserts must be soaked in a container with 70% isopropyl alcohol to remove organic debris. The inserts must then be rinsed in warm water to remove all chemicals and can then run the scaler hand piece with the insert to flush out any remaining chemicals. The inserts are then dried thoroughly and packaged with spore tests and chemical indicators. Ethylene oxide is the preferred method of choice, with dry heat and chemical vapor considered ineffective with risk of damage to materials.[13]

Dental prosthesis and orthodontic appliances are also potential sources of contamination and should be handled in a manner that protects patients and DHCP from exposure to microorganisms. They should be disinfected with an intermediate-level disinfectant before sent to a laboratory or before delivery to a patient. Heat-tolerant items used in the mouth should be heat sterilized and appropriate PPE worn until disinfection has been completed.[2] According to a study by Omidkohda and colleagues,[14] autoclave and glutaraldehyde solution were the best methods for disinfection of orthodontic marking pencils but could also be disinfected with Deconex solution if the 2 aforementioned methods were not available. Laboratory equipment, such as pumice and buff wheels, should also be disinfected between patients. If ultrasonic cleaners are used to clean prostheses or other items that are going to be inserted into a patient's mouth, the prosthesis must first be placed in a sealed, impervious receptacle containing cleaner.[6]

Dental impression handguns are also easily contaminated during clinical use. A study by Westergard and colleagues[8] concluded that to minimize the cross-contamination with these items, the use of steam sterilization combined with plastic impression gun covers and disinfection was recommended.

Digital radiography sensors are also considered semicritical and should be protected with a Food and Drug Administration–cleared barrier to reduce contamination during use, followed by cleaning and heat sterilization or high-level disinfection between patients. These items vary by manufacturer and their ability to be sterilized or high-level disinfected also vary. The manufacturer's instructions for reprocessing should be referred to.[7]

MEDICAL WASTE MANAGEMENT

A majority of waste generated in a dental office is considered noninfectious and can be discarded in regular trash. This includes gloves, masks, and lightly bloodied gauze. Regulated medical waste, however, including needles, extracted teeth, and gauze soaked in blood, may pose a potential risk of infection. A leak-resistant biohazard bag is adequate to contain nonsharp regulated medical waste. Puncture-resistant containers with a biohazard label, such as sharps containers, are used as containment for scalpel blades, needles, syringes, and unused sterile sharps. Medical wastes are stored and disposed of in accordance with state and local EPA regulations. For regulated waste, this may involve autoclaving and incineration.[2]

To protect those handling and transporting biopsy specimens, the specimens should be placed in a leak-proof container with a secure lid to prevent leakage during transport. Contaminating the outside of the container should be avoided by placing it in a leak-proof bag. The container must also be labeled with a biohazard symbol.

Extracted teeth are considered regulated medical waste. Those containing amalgam should not be incinerated. Those to be used for shade comparison or given back to the patient on request should be cleaned and disinfected. Teeth to be used for educational settings and preclinical training should be cleaned, autoclaved, and hydrated in tap water or saline. Those containing amalgam should not be autoclaved because harmful mercury favors are released; they should be soaked in formalin instead.

The American Dental Association has published recommendations and guidelines for amalgam management in dental offices. In 2006, the American National Standards Institute and American Dental Association developed specifications describing the procedures for storing and preparing amalgam waste for delivery to recyclers. Containers for amalgam waste must have a silver or gray label and must be marked, "Amalgam Waste for Recycling." Containers must have a sealable closure and meet requirements set by the Department of Transportation and the International Safe Transportation Association. Some states require dental practices to install amalgam separators.[5]

DENTAL UNIT WATERLINES

Dental unit water systems are classified as open or closed based on the water source; open units are connected to a municipal water supply whereas closed units use a refillable reservoir attached to the unit. Studies have shown that biofilms can form inside the tubing that transport water within the dental unit to hand pieces and air/water syringes. A few pathogenic bacteria, such as *Legionella* species, *Pseudomonas aeruginosa,* and nontuberculous mycobacterium have been isolated from water systems, but a majority of them are heterotrophic bacteria with limited pathogenic potential. Regardless, untreated dental units cannot reliably produce water that meets drinking water standards of less than 500 colony-forming units/mL of heterotrophic water bacteria. Hence, removal of dental waterline biofilms is required to meet CDC standards. Using independent reservoirs, chemical treatment, microfilters, or sterile water delivery systems can do this. Monitoring of dental water quality may be performed by using commercial self-contained test kits. In-office water-testing systems are available that work at room temperature to culture medium to reveal bacteria colonies. Dentists should, however, follow recommendations provided by the manufacturer of the dental unit or waterline treatment protocol to monitor the water quality and disinfecting the waterlines.[2] For open water systems, it has been recommended that these units be flushed for varying periods. If no guidance is provided, then flush all dental unit waterlines for 5 minutes before patient care.[6]

For components of devices permanently attached to the air and water lines, waterproof barriers must be used and changed between uses. Examples include attachments of saliva ejectors, high-speed air evacuators, and air/water syringes. If an item becomes visibly soiled, an intermediate-level disinfectant with tuberculocidal claim must be used. With saliva ejectors, patients should be instructed to not close their lips tightly around the tips because this can cause reverse flow, potentially causing material from the mouth of the previous patient to be aspirated into the mouth of the next patient. Saliva ejectors and high-volume evacuation valves should be removed and sterilized, especially if the unit is used for surgical procedures. If this is not feasible, the valves should be cleaned thoroughly with an intermediate level disinfectant.[6]

INFECTION CONTROL PROGRAM PLAN AND GOALS

Each dental office should have a written plan for an infection control program that includes elements to protect personnel. These elements include

- Education programs for staff members
- Immunization plan for vaccine preventable diseases
- Exposure prevention and postexposure management, with follow-up of staff exposed to infectious organisms or potentially harmful materials
- Medical condition management and work-related illnesses and restrictions
- Maintenance of health records in accordance with all applicable state and federal laws

REFERENCES

1. Centers for Disease Control and Prevention. Division of Oral Health, Infection Control in Dental Settings. Available at: https://www.cdc.gov/oralhealth/infectioncontrol/index.html. Accessed April 2, 2016.

2. Centers for Disease Control and Prevention. Guidelines for infection control in dental health-care settings—2003. MMWR Morb Mortal Wkly Rep 2003;52: 1–61. Available at: http://www.cdc.gov/Mmwr/preview/mmwrhtml/rr5217a1.htm.

3. Weissfeld AS. Infection control in the dental office. Clin Microbiol Newsl 2014; 36(11):79–84.

4. Little JW, Falace DA, Miller CS, et al. Guidelines for infection control in dental health care settings. Little and Falace's dental management of the medically compromised patient. 8th edition. St Louis (MO): Mosby; 2013. p. 587–601. Appendix B.

5. Boyce R, Mull J. Complying with the Occupational Safety and Health Administration: guidelines for the dental office. Dent Clin North Am 2008;52:653–68.

6. Thomas MV, Jarboe G, Frazer RQ, et al. Infection control in the dental practice. Dent Clin North Am 2008;52:609–28.

7. Centers for Disease Control and Prevention. Summary of infection prevention practices in dental settings: basic expectations for safe care. Atlanta (GA): US Department of Health and Human Services, Centers for Disease Control and Prevention, National Center for Chronic Disease Prevention and Health Promotion, Division of Oral Health; 2016.

8. Westergard EJ, Romito LM, Kowolik MJ, et al. Controlling bacterial contamination of dental impression guns. J Am Dent Assoc 2011;142(11):1269–74.

9. Mante F. "Infection control," lecture. Philadelphia: University of Pennsylvania School of Dental Medicine; 2012.

10. Shanker S. "Sterilization in dentistry & infection control," lecture. Telangana (India): Mamata Dental College; 2013.

11. Gardner JF, Peel MM. Introduction to sterilization, disinfection and infection control. 2nd edition. Melbourne: Churchill Livingstone; 1991.

12. Rutala WA, Weber DJ, the Healthcare Infection Control Practices Advisory Committee (HICPAC). Guidelines for disinfection and sterilization in healthcare facilities. Atlanta (GA): Center for Disease Control and Prevention; 2008.

13. Parkes RB, Kolstad RA. Effects of sterilization on periodontal instruments. J Periodontol 1982;53(7):434–8.

14. Omidkhoda M, Rashed R, Bagheri Z, et al. Comparison of three different sterilization and disinfection methods on orthodontic markers. J Orthod Sci 2016; 5(1):14–7.

Index

Note: Page numbers of article titles are in **boldface** type.

A

Actinobacteria, 307–308
Actinomycetes, 307–308
Actinomycosis, in oral cavity, 288–290
Aggregatibacter, 308–309
Amoxicillin, in odontogenic infections, 248–249
    in osteomyelitis, 279
Amphotericin B, in candidiasis, 332–333
Anidulafungin, 336
Antibiotics, in acute and chronic osteomyelitis, **271–282**
    resistance to, in oral infections, epidemiology of, 221–227
    systemic, in periodontitis, 264, 265
Antimicrobials, locally delivered, in periodontitis, 265–266
Aspergillosis, 340–343
Azithromycin, in odontogenic infections, 249
Azoles, in candidiasis, 330, 333–336

B

Bacterial infections, human oral microbiome and, 305
    in oral cavity, 286–292, 306–307
    normal flora of oval cavity and, 305
    oral, 305–318
    sexually transmitted, of oral cavity, 292–296
Bacterial lesions, specimen collection and transportation of, 297
Bacteroides, 313
Bacteroidetes, 313–315
Bifidobacteria, 308
Blastomycosis, 340
Blood, exposures to, prevention of, 442
Buccal mucosa, aand dorsum of tongue, 203–204

C

Calculus, classification of, 210–211
    composition of, 210–211
    formation of, 210
Cancer, human papillomavirus-associated oropharyngeal, 228
    microbial, of oral cavity, epidemiology of, 227–228, 229
    oral, oral microbial infections in, **425–434**
Candidiasis, 320–336
    chronic mucocutaneous, 329

Dent Clin N Am 61 (2017) 459–466
http://dx.doi.org/10.1016/S0011-8532(17)30012-5
0011-8532/17

Moving?

Make sure your subscription moves with you!

To notify us of your new address, find your **Clinics Account Number** (located on your mailing label above your name), and contact customer service at:

Email: journalscustomerservice-usa@elsevier.com

800-654-2452 (subscribers in the U.S. & Canada)
314-447-8871 (subscribers outside of the U.S. & Canada)

Fax number: 314-447-8029

Elsevier Health Sciences Division
Subscription Customer Service
3251 Riverport Lane
Maryland Heights, MO 63043

*To ensure uninterrupted delivery of your subscription, please notify us at least 4 weeks in advance of move.

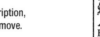